PRAISE FOR TH

"Alaine Duncan and Kathy Kain use contemporary neuroscience to bridge the classic Five Element model of Acupuncture and Asian Medicine (AAM) with Somatic Experiencing. Through this integration a new understanding of traumatic experiences emerges that leads to more effective treatment."

—STEPHEN W. PORGES, PhD, professor, Department of Psychiatry, University of North Carolina; distinguished university scientist, Kinsey Institute, Indiana University Bloomington, Indiana; developer, Polyvagal Theory

"We are a part of this natural world, and it is nature that heals our body, opens our mind, and awakens our spirit. In this pioneering book, Alaine Duncan and Kathy Kain draw on the wisdom of nature, and chart a rich and trustworthy pathway for working with trauma."

—TARA BRACH, PhD, psychologist, author of *Radical Acceptance* and *True Refuge*

"When trying to help people with complex and difficult symptoms and conditions, I have often found that the greatest insights and healing came when I looked at these problems through an entirely different lens or system than the biomedical model in which I was trained. *The Tao of Trauma* teaches us all to do just that. This important work will directly impact all clinicians who work with people living with traumatic stress, and the clients and patients they serve."

—TRACY W. GAUDET, MD, executive director, Office of Patient Centered Care and Cultural Transformation, Veterans Health Administration

"East meets West! *The Tao of Trauma* is a unique book and Alaine Duncan's compassion, sensitivity and skill as a practitioner shines through from every page."

—ANGELA HICKS, LAc, cofounder, College of Integrated Chinese Medicine, Reading, UK

"This pioneering method of combining Eastern and Western schools of thought creates a new model for healing trauma. This book is clear and highly readable, and will be educational not only for those affected by trauma but also for professionals who devote their practices to resolving it."

—STEPHEN J. TERRELL, PsyD, SEP, author (with Kathy Kain), *Nurturing Resilience: Helping Clients Move Forward from Developmental Trauma—An Integrative Somatic Approach*

"Duncan and Kain artfully describe the restoration of our natural healthy functioning via the balancing of *yin* and *yang*, and the return of regulated functioning of the autonomic nervous system. While our experience of trauma may be complex, understanding that our life force/*qi* is always available to support healing is simple and essential guidance for practitioners wanting a comprehensive resource for a somatic approach to trauma healing."

—BERNS GALLOWAY, somatic psychotherapist, senior faculty member, Somatic Experiencing® Trauma Institute

"*The Tao of Trauma* offers providers a new lens to understand the impact of trauma on human beings, and how and why integrative approaches are so critical. I highly recommend this book to all providers."

—ROBIN CARNES, MBA, certified yoga therapist, cofounder of Warriors at Ease

"Alaine Duncan has opened new doors of discourse for clinicians and new promise for those suffering from trauma. *The Tao of Trauma* is a must-read for integrative-minded clinicians."

—JANE GRISSMER, LAc, MAc (UK), director, Crossings Healing and Wellness, former dean of faculty and chair of AOM Theory Division, Maryland University of Integrative Health

"Duncan and Kain reveal themselves as healers and teachers with sensitivity, experience, skill, and scholarship."

—NANCY TAKAHASHI, LAc, MAc

"*The Tao of Trauma* fills a critical gap in the literature on trauma and healing. I recommend it as essential reading for all practitioners."

—DIANA FRIED, founder and president, Acupuncturists Without Borders

"I came to know Alaine Duncan's patience, clarity, and knowledge as a student in her workshops. Her teachings, now presented in *The Tao of Trauma*, should be required reading for everyone working in the field of healing minds, bodies, and souls."

—THE REVEREND CHERYL A. JONES, board certified institutional chaplain. Washington, DC

"*The Tao of Trauma* is a gem, filled with wisdom and profoundly beautiful ways to walk side by side, supporting another human being on their path toward profound healing following trauma."

—JANET DURFEE, RN/MSN/ANP-c, Navy Nurse Corps Veteran

The TAO *of* TRAUMA

A PRACTITIONER'S GUIDE FOR INTEGRATING FIVE ELEMENT THEORY AND TRAUMA TREATMENT

ALAINE D. DUNCAN

with KATHY L. KAIN

North Atlantic Books
Berkeley, California

Published by North Atlantic Books
Huichin, unceded Ohlone land
aka Berkeley, California

Cover design by Daniel Tesser
Book design by Happenstance Type-O-Rama
Printed in the United States of America

The Tao of Trauma: A Practitioner's Guide for Integrating Five Element Theory and Trauma Treatment is sponsored and published by North Atlantic Books, an educational nonprofit based in the unceded Ohlone land Huichin (*aka* Berkeley, CA) that collaborates with partners to develop cross-cultural perspectives; nurture holistic views of art, science, the humanities, and healing; and seed personal and global transformation by publishing work on the relationship of body, spirit, and nature.

MEDICAL DISCLAIMER: The following information is intended for general information purposes only. Individuals should always see their health care provider before administering any suggestions made in this book. Any application of the material set forth in the following pages is at the reader's discretion and is their sole responsibility.

North Atlantic Books's publications are distributed to the US trade and internationally by Penguin Random House Publisher Services. For further information, visit our website at www.northatlanticbooks.com.

Library of Congress Cataloging-in-Publication Data
Names: Duncan, Alaine (Alaine D.), author. | Kain, Kathy L., 1957- author.
Title: The tao of trauma : a practitioners guide for integrating five element theory and trauma treatment / Alaine D. Duncan with Kathy L. Kain.
Description: Berkeley, California : North Atlantic Books, [2018] | Includes bibliographical references and index.
Identifiers: LCCN 2018029979 (print) | LCCN 2018051931 (ebook) | ISBN 9781623172237 (e-book) | ISBN 9781623172220 | ISBN 9781623172220 q(paperback)
Subjects: LCSH: Psychic trauma—Alternative treatment. | Medicine, Chinese. | Touch—Therapeutic use.
Classification: LCC RC552.T7 (ebook) | LCC RC552.T7 D86 2018 (print) | DDC 616.85/21—dc23
LC record available at https://lccn.loc.gov/2018029979

3 4 5 6 7 8 9 KPC 26 25 24 23

North Atlantic Books is committed to the protection of our environment. We print on recycled paper whenever possible and partner with printers who strive to use environmentally responsible practices.

"Holding Up the Sky"—A Chinese Folktale

One day an elephant saw a hummingbird lying flat on its back on the ground. The bird's tiny feet were raised up into the air.

"What on earth are you doing, hummingbird?" asked the elephant.

The hummingbird replied.

"I have heard that the sky might fall today.

If that should happen,

I am ready to do my bit in holding it up."

The elephant laughed and mocked the tiny bird.

"Do you think THOSE *tiny little feet could hold up the* SKY*?"*

"Not alone," admitted the hummingbird.

"But each must do what he can.

And this is what I can do."[1]

We dedicate this book to all the hummingbirds in our families, communities, and workplaces; in the halls of government and commerce; on the land, sea, and air. Wherever you are, we thank you for your service.

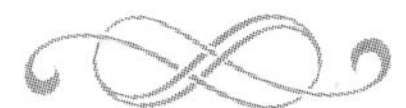

CONTENTS

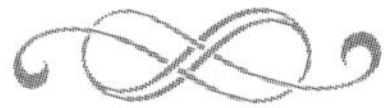

LIST OF ILLUSTRATIONS

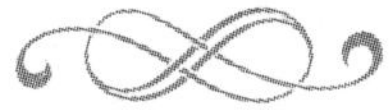

FOREWORD

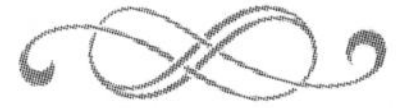

THE TAO OF TRAUMA is an important book for a number of reasons. First, the interface between the Five Element model of Acupuncture and Asian Medicine (AAM) and five steps or ways that trauma survivors engage in a self-protective response is fully described for the first time that I know of. Second, this lays the foundation for the model of healing trauma in which East meets West that Alaine Duncan has developed. And third, the book is about parallel journeys of patients and healers with the cycles of nature. I so resonate with the journey to find such an integrative model and healing path. As Alaine says in her preface, "experiences create vibrations."

About thirty-seven years ago, as a college graduate slightly soured on my lifelong dream of becoming a doctor, I set off with my friend Jeff to find my path, to discover a way—or *the* way—to become a healer and not just a technician. Since my independent study in college was on biofeedback and personal volition, our first stop was in Topeka, Kansas, at the Menninger Foundation. Arriving unannounced, in my youthful and hopeful way, I knocked on the door. It opened.

"Dr. Elmer Green?" I queried.

"Yes," he replied.

"Hi ... uh ... I just thought I might find you here and talk with you."

Quizzically gracious, he was willing to hear about a young man's dilemma of wanting to be a doctor but being horrified by his perceptions of Western medicine's reductionistic view. I shared my problem for a few minutes, during which he occasionally interjected into my somewhat coherent story things like, "they need to study energy," "they need to know about self-healing," "they need to know about," and so on.

Finally, he said, "You are on the right track, and some of your ideas will sound a bit ... um, well ... kooky to conventional folks. If you are on the outside, you will be dismissed, so you will need to get on the inside to be effective."

"Healing" and "integration" were not easily found in medical training in those days, in part because they are not easily learned or taught. Fast forward to 1998: Nityamo, an acupuncturist, was a research assistant in our group, and one day she suggested we apply for a grant to apply acupuncture to study post-traumatic stress disorder (PTSD). I honor her and other colleagues who respected the vibrations felt and gently pulled me into opening doors. In 2006 and 2007 we published our work about developing and testing an acupuncture intervention for PTSD. Which is how I came to meet Alaine Duncan.

We were on a panel together at the U.S. Army's annual Force Health Protection Conference in Albuquerque, New Mexico, in 2008, along with Colonel Charles Engel, USA, (Ret), MD, Nityamo Sinclair-Lian, and Richard Neimtzow, MD. Dr. Engel was completing the first study of acupuncture for PTSD in active-duty military personnel (for which Alaine was the assessing acupuncturist), which showed similar effects to our own study of acupuncture for PTSD in civilians completed a few years prior. I watched and marveled as Alaine presented in a way that almost seemed to be a beautiful dance, though with complete respect (and I mean that!) to Engel, Neimtzow, and me—we three had spoken in the usual linear way, propped up by the power points and data points typical of the medical sciences. I later attended a workshop by Alaine and colleagues about using acupuncture with Somatic Experiencing® and touch work to heal trauma survivors. Affixed with a sort of hazy upwelling of feeling-emotion, my whole body/mind was revisiting my journey years ago and my discussion with Elmer Green. What I was sensing was something I had partially lost—forgot—during my medical training: trauma and harm are freezes, interruptions, and a recoil to self for protection, while healing is motion, flow, and opening self to connections in a context of trust. Alaine was magically taking me back to a time and space when I had more of an innate sense of what healing was about but a fear to pursue my dreams because I was afraid of being gobbled up by "the reductionistic view." I now know my fear was one of doubt that I could become the healer, that I could integrate medical training with other healing practices. Now I am grateful for the amazing training and experience I have had in medicine and in acupuncture and Asian medicine, for the mentors I have been blessed to be in the presence of, and for the healers I have come across and learned from.

Alaine and I had some time to talk in Albuquerque about healing, about the neurobiology and physiology of trauma and repair, and about her developing work as a Somatic Experiencing (SE) practitioner and her views of how SE and acupuncture work together. She told me about her journey into AAM from both a personal and professional viewpoint. I learned about her work as an acupuncturist since 1990, in the private sector, and her work in the Veterans Administration's Integrative Health and Wellness Program in Washington, DC, where she worked for ten years bringing her much needed craft and presence to our nation's warriors. And, as we have kept connected over the years, I know about her exceptional work as the founder of two nonprofit organizations, again bringing her self and skill to trauma survivors, most of whom are veterans or refugees of war, or their family members. We also worked together a few years after our meeting in Albuquerque on a study to co-design two forms of acupuncture for treating headaches in combat veterans with mild to moderate traumatic brain injury.

The Tao of Trauma is first a journey. It is a journey of healers understanding the trajectory of their patients' trauma in the context of the cycles of the earth, of life, and of death and rebirth. Human life and all its experiences are inexorably part of the rest of nature and exist and are experienced through the lens of how the body has evolutionarily developed, informed by the cycles of the earth. Individual persons, too, are born, develop, and experience life (and trauma) entwined in the earth's cycles. The Five Element theory of Chinese medicine posits that all living things are made up of five primary elements—Metal, Water, Wood, Fire, and Earth—each of which corresponds in a functional way to one of the agricultural seasons and to certain organ systems. Just as winter precedes and gives rise to spring, Water nourishes Wood, and the Kidney and Bladder system nurtures the Liver and Gallbladder system. Just as a harsh winter begets a spring that is different from one that follows a mild winter, so too the balance between internal organ systems varies dependent on the timing and nature of one's birth and the conditions that occur during one's development. In Part One, Alaine beautifully dances the integration of Western and Eastern thought about developmental and biological influences relevant to the trauma spectrum response. She informs us about the balance in biological systems that make sense in both Western and Eastern terms, using Porges's exquisite polyvagal theory for illustration of its relationship using AAM terms. This foundation allows the reader to move into the principles for the remainder of the book, traveling through the effects of trauma for each of five survivor types and stages relating to the Five Elements, and learning how healing can occur using AAM principles by a practitioner keen to the parallel process he or she brings by knowing the individual and his or her type and stage of traumatic injury.

Parallel to taking us through the trauma spectrum response, the defensive protective response, and the path of healing, Alaine continues to give voice to a truth often lost in all healing arts, that trauma affects the body in its primal core. When we are born, we know and experience our world only through bodily sensation. Emotion is patterned and learned years after sensation first emerges—and cognition later yet—a sort of epiphenomenal process to the more primal body-feeling state. Emotions describe a central response to body sensation, and thoughts are organized ways to describe emotion and sensation. As we use cognition to learn and describe our world, we can largely forget about the primacy of sensation, about the wisdom of body and biology. In the *Tao of Trauma,* Alaine has spoken clearly about how traumatic stress is held in the body, about how symptoms from trauma conform to the natural world in which a body lives, and how healing best occurs by recognizing this fact and utilizing methods that restore balance and regulation in the body's tissues. And because betrayal and disconnection are central to trauma, Part Two is wisely dedicated to the principles of caring, connecting, and practice that are the core to any healing art, with specific reference to mindful ways to engage in sessions and use touch as a part of restoring coherence. Part Three then details the damages of trauma in each of the Five Element spaces and the concurrent healing that can and must occur for the survivor to move forward with fewer symptoms and with the ability to embrace the world again.

The Tao of Trauma is about what healing is about. In this case, with poignant descriptions and stories of specifically healing trauma with AAM and touch work—Alaine-style! And yet the book also calls to anyone who knows there is a healer inside, who longs to be connected with the healing power the vibrations of our earth provides. Listen to it. Feel it. It is the alpha and the omega. It is everyone's journey.

MICHAEL HOLLIFIELD, MD

President and CEO, War Survivors Institute, Long Beach, California

HS Associate Clinical Professor, Department of Psychiatry and Human Behavior, University of California at Irvine, Irvine, California

Angel Fire, New Mexico

PREFACE

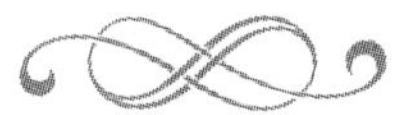

OUR LIVES ARE shaped by experiences that create vibrations that change the direction of our lives.

In 1977, working as a kidney dialysis technician, I was stuck by a needle from a patient infected with hepatitis C. I spent the next twenty-five years suffering extended and recurrent periods of debilitating weakness, fatigue, weight loss, and digestive upset.

At the time, Western medicine could neither diagnose nor treat hepatitis C. Unable to find any markers in their many tests, doctors found no basis for my symptoms. This experience of chronic, undiagnosable, and mysterious illness nearly consumed me.

I began my now lifelong experience with acupuncture in 1985. Western medicine had nothing it could offer me, and I was desperate for help. Acupuncture treatment helped me cope with these acute episodes and essentially kept me alive and functioning—and waiting. I was enthralled by both its power and its wisdom. In 1988, my experience at the business end of this very different kind of needle brought me to acupuncture school. I felt called to give what I had received to others.

I finally eliminated the virus in 2003, with the benefit of advances in Western medical treatment. While six months of interferon and ribavirin left me emaciated, debilitated, and nearly bald, I was now free of the disease that had crippled me for so long. I am now much healthier as an older adult than I ever was as a young adult.

Hepatitis C gave me my career, a tenderness toward those experiencing chronic illness, and a way of living that calls me to listen deeply and attend to the subtle messages of body, mind, and spirit—mine and others. I honor hepatitis C as my life's most commanding, demanding, compelling, exacting, and thoroughgoing teacher.

Not long after completing my treatment, I heard Kevin and Joyce Lucey interviewed on my car radio. They were telling the world about their son, Marine Lance Corporal Jeffrey Lucey, who returned home from Iraq in 2003. Unable to cope with what he had witnessed and what he had been asked to do, Jeffrey had committed suicide in his parents' basement. As I listened to his parents speak, it was clear to me that this young man could not have asked for more active, engaged, or loving parents. How could it be true that even that was not enough?

While I had no specialized training in working with trauma at the time, I had been in practice nearly fifteen years and knew in my heart, as well as my mind, that acupuncture could have made a difference for this young man and for his family. *What a shame his VA wasn't set up to offer acupuncture to him, to his fellow soldiers—and to their families* was my first thought. I was filled with a feeling, a knowing, that it didn't have to be this way for Jeff and far too many others.

Quakers call such a pull "a leading,"[1] a sense of being called to take a certain course of action. After hearing that interview, I was carried into the most meaningful work of my life. Young people—the age of my own children—were coming home from war so troubled they could no longer tolerate living. I needed to be part of a tangible response to Kevin and Joyce's longing for the world to see that their son's life, as well as his death, had meaning and purpose. I felt called to serve, within my own domain as an acupuncturist, to bring peace to those most personally impacted by war.

I knew that my newfound passion and even my compassion were not enough. I needed to know more about military culture and how to work with trauma survivors. Thankfully, the Somatic Experiencing Trauma Institute trains acupuncturists and body workers, as well as mental health providers, and I began my study of the neurophysiology of traumatic stress there.[2]

To my good fortune, I met Kathy Kain in 2007. She taught the final year of my Somatic Experiencing (SE) training, and I continued to study with her in her post-SE-certification workshops.[3] In those learning experiences, the intimate relationship between modern Western medicine's study of neurophysiology and the constructs of Acupuncture and Asian Medicine came alive in my hands. I saw principles of acupuncture emerge out of my patient's bodies as I integrated what I was learning. I had found a fellow seeker in Kathy's clear and accessible, grounded, humble, and powerful exploration of how to touch trauma, recognize embodied regulation, and understand developmental disruptions. I had found a home for my intellectual curiosity, as well as my passion for helping individuals and communities transform and heal from abuse, violence, and misunderstanding. *The Tao of Trauma* is, in large part, Kathy's work retold through the lens of Acupuncture and Asian Medicine.

Jeffrey Lucey's death, and his parents' love, set off a vibration in me that has carried me to places I never could have imagined. I find myself at home in military and veterans' hospitals. I have used my needles, my hands, and my heart to bring peace to the bodies and minds of survivors of war—and to their caregivers, families, and communities.

At first, the division between the military and civilian worlds felt more like a wall than a gate—and it existed as much inside me as it did around Walter Reed Army Medical Center. The more I let go of my sense of being different and separate, of the idea of an *us* and a *them*—the more welcoming the gates of my heart became. Coming to "be with" these service members, veterans, and their families and caregivers has been a journey of listening, learning, expanding, and softening—truly a wisdom journey.

Asian medicine taught me that the front of the hand cannot exist without the back of the hand. I would not have the compassion and commitment to bring acupuncture to people with chronic, complex, and mysterious illness without my experience with hepatitis C. I would not have the sense of purpose and courage to carry my tenacious and persistent spirit into the world of military medicine without the love and inspiration of Kevin and Joyce Lucey. I am profoundly grateful for all of it—except, of course, the tragic and unnecessary loss of Jeff.

With the publication of *The Tao of Trauma,* my domain as an acupuncturist and trauma healer expands to that of a writer, teacher, and philosopher on the impact of abuse, violence, and misunderstanding in our world. It is my hope that it also serves to expand your world—that through reading it, you will find yourself ever more curious about people who are different from yourself, in dynamic wonder at the profound power of our body's inherent healing wisdom, able to see a sense of possibility and hope for the challenges we face as a world community, more compassionate than ever for those who suffer, and more able to nurture the faces of trauma that manifest in your domain—and that beckon you to serve the transformation and healing of our troubled and beautiful world.

ACKNOWLEDGMENTS

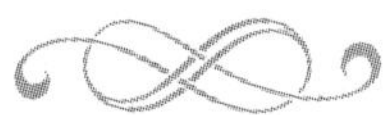

IT IS HUMBLING to think about all the individuals, the collective wisdom, and the many steps in the East-meets-West journey that has brought *The Tao of Trauma* into being.

We begin with honoring our teachers, the giants of intellect and compassion upon whose work and wisdom we stand:

- Dr. J. R. Worlsey, who brought Five Element acupuncture to the West
- Dr. Peter Levine, who articulated the five steps of the self-protective response and developed the Somatic Experiencing model of trauma resolution
- Dr. Stephen Porges, whose research led to the development of the polyvagal theory, providing a scientific basis for safety and relationship as the foundation for all healing

Each represents a powerful lineage. Each of their voices, in its own way, affirms what we all know implicitly—nature is our greatest healer and teacher—and experiences of safety, love, and understanding are the foundation for all healing. As in every dimension of life, our rope is stronger when it is made of diverse strands coming together as one.

The touch material we present has its foundation in Kathy's Touch Skills Training. Our hope is that the cross-pollination of that material with AAM and trauma recovery will provide a rich interdisciplinary exploration of a new way to approach the healing of trauma. We (Kathy and Alaine) have learned so much from each other as we have journeyed together.

We met through the Somatic Experiencing training program and have shared our curiosity for over ten years, exploring experiences with patients;

ideas about the interface of AAM, trauma resolution, and touch; and, ultimately, our thoughts about curriculum development, as our desire to present these intertwined lineages as a cohesive whole grew.

Our process became a series of workshops for clinical staff at the Washington DC Veterans Administration Medical Center and then a postgraduate series for acupuncturists. The curious and compassionate healers who participated in these workshops helped hone and sharpen the substance of *The Tao of Trauma.* Our gratitude to you is woven into its fabric.

We also acknowledge our clients, who have been our greatest teachers and mentors. You have inspired us to reflect, have been the fuel for our engines, the hope for our world, and are the heart of this book. We are profoundly grateful for your thumbprint on our lives and this work.

The name, *The Tao of Trauma,* came to Alaine while meditating with a group of veterans in an acupuncture group at the Integrative Health and Wellness Program at the Washington DC Veterans Administration Medical Center. A very special thank you goes to these amazing veterans, whose tender hearts helped me find a way to live with how very small I am in the face of how very big the vibration of war is. I will be forever grateful for the lessons learned, the people met, and the experiences had while working there.

While it is impossible to thank all the individuals who held space in their hearts and minds for what has become this book, we do wish to acknowledge the support of colleagues and friends in these institutions who generously gave their encouragement and support at every step: Adelphi Friends Meeting, Crossings Healing and Wellness, Maryland University of Integrative Health, and the Somatic Experiencing and Somatic Practice communities.

We particularly acknowledge the following individuals who read and reflected on the manuscript: Susan Berman, Heather Dorst, Ann Dunne, Jane Grissmer, Karen McCune, Jim Pastore, and Leah Turner. Particular thanks go to Leslie Eliel for her assistance in crafting our ideas into a coherent proposal to North Atlantic Books, Cecily Sailer for her thoughtful and reflective editing of the manuscript, and our North Atlantic Books editors, Alison Knowles, Louis Swaim, and Jennifer Eastman, for their consistently patient, kind, clear, and helpful guidance offered at each and every step.

From Alaine: Special and heartfelt acknowledgment goes to Rob, my sweet husband, who has tended the ventral vagal system of my heart for decades, and to our children, Will and Alison—together, you have been my most profound teachers of the compelling power of love.

From Kathy: As always, my family has given of themselves in so many ways to support me in my work and creative endeavors. To Gordon, Benjamin, and Dorothy—a special thank you for all the years of sharing so much love and laughter with you.

INTRODUCTION

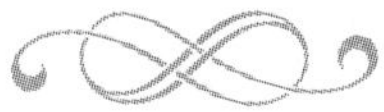

THE INFORMATION IN this book is rooted in an East-meets-West approach to restoring balance and regulation in survivors of traumatic stress. It marries theoretical and clinical concepts from Western neuroscience with Acupuncture and Asian Medicine (AAM) to elucidate body-informed clinical skills for somatic psychotherapists, acupuncturists, and physical care and medical providers.

Traumatic stress knows no geographic, chronological, or personal boundaries. Service members don't check their wartime experiences at the door when they leave a combat zone. People who have survived a violent sexual assault don't leave that experience behind when they leave the hospital. For years after the actual event, the tendrils of such experiences remain alive in cognitive memory and oftentimes more vividly in body memory. To the survivor, the event may feel very much in the here and now, instead of the "there and then." The survivor may live as if still under attack. Trauma's impact is far-reaching and vibrational in nature, not only for the individual survivor, but also for whole families and communities, who can also be affected by trauma's impact on any one of their members.

Many survivors come to care providers with elusive, intangible, and difficult-to-pin-down symptoms, such as insomnia; chronic pain; metabolic and digestive disturbance; obesity; problems with memory, cognition, or mood; interpersonal challenges; autoimmune illness; or endocrine disorders. The roots of many of these symptoms lie in autonomic nervous system dysregulation caused by traumatic stress—known or unknown, spoken or unspoken.

Advances over the past ten to twenty years in the study of the neurophysiology of traumatic stress have revolutionized mental health treatment of trauma spectrum disorders and are influencing program development in education, social work, public health, and criminal justice. A growing appreciation for the influence of traumatic stress on both mental *and* physical health calls *all* providers to look beyond their particular specialization, cultivate an understanding of the energetic imprint of traumatic stress, and include it in their assessment and interpretation of signs and symptoms, their management and pacing of clinical interactions, and, for acupuncturists, how and when needles are offered.

Integrating the approaches of Acupuncture and Asian Medicine into the treatment of traumatic stress invites the practitioner to focus on whole-body balance and regulation and dynamic coherence between systems. Rather than treating only the symptoms of trauma disruption, a broadened and combined perspective allows practitioners to utilize therapies that access deeper parts of the body, psyche, and spirit—the places where trauma has left its deepest and most profound imprint. *The Tao of Trauma* interprets the principles of AAM, takes them beyond needles and herbs, and applies them in a framework accessible to somatic psychotherapists and physical care and medical providers, as well as acupuncturists.

Our approach is primarily bottom-up, starting in the body and moving up to the mind. The problem with the "talking cure" for trauma survivors is that the trauma itself gets in the way of survivors reflecting on their experience. No matter how much cognitive insight or understanding survivors develop in their frontal cortex, their emotional limbic midbrain and most primal brain stem are unable to embrace a different reality.[1] Our clinical experience affirms that the body holds trauma's impact even after the analytical mind has considered and evaluated its narrative. Traumatic stress does not arise from the story of the event per se, but rather from the *lived experience* of that event, uniquely manifesting in an individual's body, mind, and spirit. It lives in what we call the "tissue memory" or "body memory" of survivors. Our goal is to help providers understand, identify, and work with the inherent order that lies within a survivor's disorder. We seek to help providers develop coherent clinical approaches that can access and resolve the traumatic stress responses that reside in survivors' physiology.

We bring together two lexicons—the technical, scientific language of neurophysiology and the poetic, vibrational, and nature-based language of Five Element theory. Integrating these two apparently disparate perspectives on science and healing will, we believe, provide a wide range of clinicians with new and nuanced ways to access the rich depth of knowledge contained in both lexicons.

This integrative approach will help providers:

- listen in a new way to body-based metaphors (e.g., I have been asked to digest too much; I feel it in my bones; my heart stood still; my stomach sank; or it made my blood boil);
- access the client's experience of his or her most resilient and coherent inner reality as a resource to anchor treatment and minimize overwhelm;
- bring embodied awareness and attention to support the completion of threat responses stored in body memory;
- know which tissue or body part will be most helpful to work with, how to use attention and intention to inform touch, and how to titrate interventions for the "just right" effect, neither overwhelming the client nor working so cautiously that treatments are ineffective; and
- create nuanced and individualized approaches that deepen the client's sense of relationship, safety, and attachment.

Note that using touch in the context of reregulating the autonomic nervous system is not about repairing physical injury. The training of physical care providers to conduct repair work after injury or surgery is distinctly different than what we are recommending.

Fundamental to our approach is an acknowledgment of the resilience and malleability of the human brain and body, mind and soul. The information and methods presented here seek to help clients experience embodied sensations that transform, in a somatically mindful way, the helplessness, rage, or collapse that often arises from incomplete responses to life threat.[2]

At its core, the material in this book makes use of these guiding principles:

- Trauma is held in the body and in the unique experience of survivors, not exclusively in their stories—and certainly not in *our* experience of *their* stories.
- Expressions of the body, mind, emotions, and spirit exist as a coherent whole; restoring balance and regulation in any one of these dimensions informs all dimensions.

- Trauma survivors' symptoms arise out of their incomplete self-protective response, together with their genetic predisposition to certain strengths and weaknesses.
- Just as humans are hardwired to respond to threats in specific ways, we are also evolutionarily equipped to transform and heal traumatic experiences.
- Supporting balance and regulation in trauma survivors builds a platform for our "inner physician,"[3] first described by Hippocrates, to create the healing that is inherently available to us all.

Our approach builds on the work of psychologist and ethnobiologist Peter Levine, who developed the Somatic Experiencing model of trauma treatment.[4] His exploration of predator-prey relationships in the animal kingdom gave rise to his recognition that humans share similar responses to threat. His study illuminated a cycle of five somewhat distinct phases that both four-legged and two-legged animals go through when threatened. He named them: *arrest/startle, defensive orienting, specific self-protective response* (fight, flight, or freeze), *completion,* and *integration.*

One of the building blocks of Levine's Somatic Experiencing model of trauma recovery is its focus on the completion of interrupted self-protection efforts. Levine observed that successful completion of each step in this cycle of response tended to limit traumatic stress responses afterward. He came to see that thwarted or interrupted self-protective efforts tended to "stick" in the physiology and to contribute to further disruptions in a survivor's capacity for self-protection and in his or her overall physiology. These disruptions, in turn, could lead to some of the classic symptoms associated with traumatic stress—anxiety, sleep disturbance, memory issues, and uncontrolled emotional responses like anger or fear, as well as pain patterns, digestive upset, autoimmune illness, and vulnerability to addiction.

Many of the maladies associated with traumatic stress are well recognized throughout AAM, and there is a clear overlap between Levine's biophysiological model and the ancient AAM model of the Five Elements. In fact, the cyclical movement inherent in the Five Element model parallels these five steps. By making a connection between the disrupted phase in the stress-response cycle and its corresponding AAM Element, we identify five *survivor types,* giving providers a lens through which to see their patients more deeply and to hone their interventions more precisely.

The impact of a lightning bolt hitting a tree does not exclusively impact that tree. Every bug in its bark, every bird on its branches, every bush crushed by its fall, and the soil disturbed by its uprooting are all affected—and, in fact, if a fire arises from this single lightning strike, the ecosystem of the entire forest is impacted. Recovery of the forest will require quality minerals, water, new sprouts, warm sun, and good soil. All Five Elements of AAM—*Metal, Water, Wood, Fire,* and *Earth*—are required for its recovery.

Similarly, when any one of us is hit by a lightning bolt of trauma, we are also impacted in a comprehensive way. The impact of this event reverberates throughout our body, mind, emotions, and spirit. Its impact cannot be pinned to a certain organ system or function—nor can the transformation of its impact be reduced to universally applicable formulas or prescriptions. Each one of us, struck by the same "lightning bolt," will have different elemental needs for recovering the health and vitality of our individual tree and the relationships we have in our communal forest.

A challenge for all clinicians working with trauma survivors is to know where to start, what signs to look for, and how to proceed. Trauma survivors experience a wide variety and intensity of symptoms, including impaired cognitive capacity and emotional and spiritual distress, as well as compromised functioning of diverse organs and body systems. A survivor may present an odd array of symptoms, disorders, or difficulties that may appear to be the result of terrible luck or poor self-care, when, in fact, all are tied to traumatic experiences that were never detected by a practitioner, much less resolved or healed. Trauma survivors are clearly tough—they have survived, after all. But their survival effort may be held together by the most tenuous of strings, resulting in a sense of inner and often overwhelming fragility.

Understanding the Five Elements of AAM will help providers to use imagery from nature to help them choose which Element to focus on and determine the required "dosage" of that Element. Each survivor will have different needs. Do they seem to require more "quality minerals" in their life? Do they need to be watered or be given support to sprout, or do they need light to illuminate their experience or the proper nourishing soil in which to grow? Not only will your choices impact that missing Element's function, but they will also, through the AAM lens of relationship and movement, affect the functioning of all other Elements. When you offer the Element a survivor needs most, in the proper context and quantity, his or her health, vitality, balance, and regulation can be restored.

We encourage you to read all chapters of this book before practicing any of its methods. The nature of AAM is that there are many interconnected threads that influence each other. It is likely to take some time to become comfortable with this nonlinear approach to healing, but our hope is that the material in this book will provide helpful support in developing your understanding.

The Tao of Trauma is organized in three parts:

Part One, "East Meets West for Integrative Healing," provides an overview of the historical context of traumatic stress in the West, how the autonomic nervous system functions, and why the perception of safety and threat are critical to understanding the impact of traumatic stress. It also describes the axiomatic principles underlying AAM, the interface of Five Element theory with the five steps of the self-protective response, and the dynamic theoretical and groundbreaking framework of the polyvagal theory put forth by Stephen Porges.

Part Two, "Preparing for Caring," presents information on the energetic nature of body tissues, an orientation to the overarching clinical approaches useful to all survivor types, considerations for the use of touch in this population, an exploration of critical elements in framing a session, and important considerations relating to scope of practice. Readers with extensive experience with touch may choose to skim this section—and move on to Part Three where a tour of the Five Elements and remedies appropriate to each survivor type are presented.

Part Three, "Restoring Balance and Regulation via the Five Elements," introduces the five survivor types in detail, the common categories of symptoms affiliated with each type, and suggested somatic and touch-oriented interventions to restore their regulation and balance. The public health and social impact of working with each survivor type is also highlighted.

Although the Five Element model lends itself to rich complexities, the essence of our message is simple: completing the threat response cycle and restoring balance through a greater understanding of the wholeness of the body-mind-spirit can initiate meaningful and lasting change in individuals, their families, their communities, and society at large.

A NOTE ON TRANSLATION OF AAM TERMS

We have adhered to the convention of translating all AAM terms, with the exception of *qi, yin,* and *yang*—which are so unique to the history and culture of Asian Medicine as to be nearly impossible to translate into English. We have also distinguished terms that carry a distinctly different and much broader sphere of influence and meaning than their names in Western physiology would indicate, by presenting them with an initial capital letter. Thus, the Heart of AAM, known as the *Supreme Controller* who sits in the center of the kingdom, supports whole-body coherence with its steady rhythm, and houses the spirit—is distinguished from the heart in Western physiology, which maintains the rhythm and regularity of our blood pulse. While we have not capitalized "blood," we do want to acknowledge that the sphere of influence and function ascribed to blood in *The Tao of Trauma* may feel foreign to an unfamiliar reader. We invite you to allow your concept of the role and nature of the fluid in our veins to expand and soften as you immerse yourself in the energetic and relational framework inherent in the physiology of AAM. AAM's poetic vocabulary describes subtle and nuanced patterns that we trust will come alive in your experience of this text, as they have in ours.[5]

Please refer to Appendix Two for the functions of the remaining AAM Organ Systems.

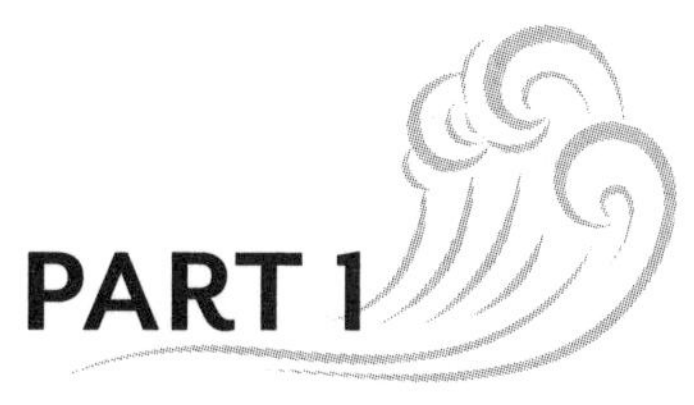

PART 1

EAST MEETS WEST FOR INTEGRATIVE HEALING

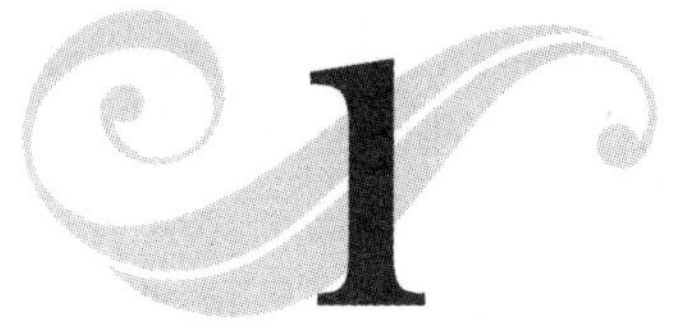

The Western Perspective on Traumatic Stress

HISTORY AND CONTEXT

THE IMPACT AND nature of traumatic life experiences has been a subject of interest for chaplains and shamans, poets and authors, historians and sociologists, as well as mental and physical health professionals since ancient Greece—characters suffering from traumatic experiences are portrayed in Homer's *Iliad* and *Odyssey,* as well as in some tragic plays, notably Sophocles's *Ajax.*[1]

"Hysteria," first described in the second millennium BCE in ancient Egyptian papyri, stands out as the first attempt to describe what we might today call PTSD. It is also the first mental health disorder ascribed exclusively to women. Hippocrates defined it in the fifth century BCE as arising from a "wandering uterus" within women's bodies, which was believed to be caused by a lack of sexual satisfaction and to cause both physical and psychological symptoms, including anxiety, shortness of breath, fainting, insomnia, irritability, and nervousness, as well as experiences of suffocation, tremors, and sometimes even convulsions and paralysis. Sigmund Freud, in the early 1900s, reversed this view on its etiology and named the cause for this wandering uterus and its complex symptomatology to be sexual trauma in childhood.[2] His exploration of the common experience of sexual exploitation in his patients, largely women who had been abused by their fathers, gave rise to modern psychoanalysis.

More than two thousand years after Hippocrates, American soldiers during the Civil War were said to suffer from *soldier's heart.* For troops during World War I, it was *shell shock,* and later in World War II, *combat stress reaction* (or *battle fatigue*), where the "two-thousand-yard stare" was named as a prominent indication. Treatment for these conditions most commonly included "three hots and a cot"—a few days of good food and rest before returning to the battlefield. It was not until 1980 that the American Psychological Association (APA) first formally described the features of the condition, which they named *post-traumatic stress disorder,* based on their research involving Vietnam War veterans, Holocaust survivors, and sexual assault victims.[3]

While the rate of PTSD among Vietnam War–era veterans can reach as high as 30 percent,[4] the good news is that the majority of those who have served in the military or have experienced sexual assault, street crime, or natural disasters do not go on to experience PTSD. In the United States, approximately 7 to 8 percent of people suffer from PTSD at some point during their lives, with approximately eight million adults experiencing PTSD in a given year. The lifetime prevalence of PTSD among men is 3.6 percent, and among women, it is 9.7 percent.

PTSD is defined in the fifth edition of the American Psychiatric Association's *Diagnostic and Statistical Manual of Mental Disorders (DSM-5)* as arising from "direct or indirect exposure to a known traumatic event involving actual or threatened death or injury, or a threat to the physical integrity of him/herself or others (such as sexual violence)."[5] The definition also stipulates that the affected person must have experienced some or all of the following symptoms for at least one month:

- intrusive thoughts, distressing dreams, or flashbacks of the traumatic event
- avoidance of certain people, places, activities, objects, and situations that bring on distressing memories

- negative cognitions or mood
- symptoms of arousal and reactivity, including having angry outbursts, behaving recklessly, being easily startled, or having problems concentrating or sleeping

The *DSM-5* definition provides the parameters used for diagnosis and related treatment in mental health settings and to determine veterans' benefits, insurance coverage, and the crafting of courtroom arguments.[6]

From our perspective, and that of many providers who work with survivors of traumatic stress, the fixed criteria in the *DSM-5*'s definition of PTSD does not reflect the full range of client presentations. Providers need a more accurate and complete representation of the depth, extent, and diversity of psychological, biological, and even spiritual effects that can arise from experiences of danger or a life-threatening situation.

For example, many survivors feel "wrong" or "odd" in a pervasive way—but will not be able to name a particular traumatic event. They may have experienced a life-threatening tragedy before they had language to name it, or the cumulative effect of repeated exposure to danger has overwhelmed their capacity to respond. They don't meet the criteria of "direct or indirect exposure to a known traumatic event," but their autonomic nervous system has surely been left disturbed or *dysregulated.*

In addition, the range of potential symptoms exhibited by patients is broader than those outlined in the *DSM-5,* and for some will include more physical or somatic expressions, rather than purely or exclusively psychological ones. The impact of traumatic stress goes well beyond the exclusive domain of mental health providers.

Survivors may suffer from many of the symptoms associated with dysregulation in the autonomic nervous system—things like irritable bowels, autoimmune disease, insomnia, chronic headaches, or other chronic pain patterns, as well as anxiety, mood disorders, or nightmares. But when survivors can't trace their symptoms to a specific cause, they may feel diminished, dismissed, or longing to understand why they are the way they are, especially if they do not feel understood and cared for by their providers or loved ones.

It is important to note that people exposed to the same or similar experiences of war, motor vehicle accidents, sexual assaults, street crimes, or natural disasters can come away with widely varying physical and emotional responses. Our assertion here is that the locus for defining an event as traumatic must rest in the experience of the individual, not in anyone else's interpretation of their experience. Constitution, genetic predisposition, history of previous stressful experiences, and availability of supportive relationships all influence a survivor's stress response and should be part of any plan of care.

In addition, a PTSD diagnosis isn't nuanced enough to be clinically useful. Traumatic stress manifests across a wide range of both hyper- and hypoarousal states—survivors may be agitated or lethargic, aggressive or passive, unable to sleep or consumed by fatigue. It has diverse physical and psychological symptoms, and can arise as assuredly from chronic emotional neglect in childhood as from the terror of witnessing a loss of life, the impact of a natural disaster, or an overwhelming experience in combat.

We believe strongly that what has come to be called PTSD is in fact a highly evolved, biologically dictated, and lifesaving response to an overwhelming situation. Our healing sometimes demands that we harness the power of the arousal that necessarily accompanied our effort to survive. It may also require that we make use of the collapse and immobility that may have been our most effective survival strategy "back then." These functions of arousal and collapse are not indications of pathology, but signs of incomplete or thwarted survival efforts—they are responses embedded in our physiology to help us survive life threat. PTSD is not a disorder, and the *D* in the acronym misrepresents and unfairly maligns the physiology of this experience.[7]

Perhaps most importantly, PTSD is not a permanent or static diagnosis. It is not a life sentence, nor is it a reflection of an unalterably broken person. Our body, mind, emotions, and spirit are designed to return to balance after arousal.[8] Just as our bodies mobilize extraordinary strengths to preserve and protect life when we are threatened, we are also evolutionarily predisposed to return to equilibrium and balance once our body/mind realizes—in an embodied and sensate way—that the threat has passed. We are hardwired to transform and heal traumatic experiences just as we are naturally predisposed to feel overwhelmed by them when they occur. Survivors can be helped to function more like a rabbit, which comes face to face with death every time a fox makes chase or a hawk flies overhead and yet never experiences insomnia, autoimmune disease, anxiety, depression, or suicidal ideation.[9]

In the context of clinical practice, we have found an energetic, body-based paradigm to be more useful. Rather than post-traumatic stress disorder, we prefer the term trauma spectrum response. Using this term affirms our observation that trauma survivors experience a wide range of symptoms with highly variable intensity. These symptoms do not exclusively reside in the brain or mind, and surely include body and spirit. They often affect multiple physiological systems, including the cardiovascular, neurological, digestive, immune, musculoskeletal, and endocrine. Trauma survivors may suffer from psychological, emotional, and spiritual distress, as well as cognitive impairment. Many experience various states of somatic dysfunction, including disturbances of sleep, appetite, digestion, sexuality, chronic pain, drug or opioid desensitization, and addiction. These phenomena are diversely expressed and highly variable in their intensity in any one survivor, and certainly between them.[10]

Thus, the trauma spectrum response as an expression of an energetic system that has been stimulated beyond a particular individual's ability to cope—physiologically, psychologically, and/or spiritually. This now highly disorganized system simply awaits restoration of its natural balance and equilibrium.

POSITIVE, TOLERABLE, AND TOXIC STRESS

Stress is part of life, but not all stress is the same. Short-term *positive* stress, such as walking quickly to work when you've overslept, is normal and quickly resolves. The immediate experience of *tolerable* stress may have a significant impact on our brain and body, but with appropriate support, it doesn't consume or overwhelm us in the long term. Experiences such as illness, divorce, or death may be difficult to bear, but our suffering can, in time, be ameliorated by our own resilience and by supportive personal—and perhaps professional—relationships or systems, as well as by our ability to access and make use of them. Positive and tolerable stressors actually promote greater resilience over the course of our lifetime. They teach us coping skills and can expand our consciousness.[11]

Allostasis is a term that describes the dynamic process of achieving stability by distributing the impact of stress across various body systems. Our capacity for allostasis is what helps us survive, learn from, and return to equilibrium (or homeostasis) after a stressful experience.[12]

For example, when our immune system is alerted to a pathogen, it mounts a response that makes use of resources in our cardiovascular, metabolic, autonomic, and central nervous systems. If we recover, all these body systems retain a memory of this particular pathogen and are better prepared to anticipate a similar pathogen and to fight it off in the future. Similarly, when we experience a physical threat and engage a flight response, several body systems respond together to help us survive. We pour energy from stored glucose and fat into our muscles. Our heart rate, blood pressure, and respiration all increase to transport nutrients and oxygen more efficiently. As long as this demand to flee is not made too often, our brain learns how to anticipate similar threats, coordinate its effort across multiple body systems, and respond more efficiently to future threats.[13]

This engagement of multiple systems not only helps us survive individual threats but also increases our overall resiliency in future life challenges. When these adaptive systems are turned on and off efficiently, and not too frequently, we become more able to cope effectively with circumstances we might not otherwise survive. While various stressors can create what is termed *allostatic load*—the wear and tear on the body systems that accumulates from a series of stressful events—we typically recover without a permanent strain on our vitality when the load is short-lived and sufficient support is readily available. Health-promoting behaviors like meditation, good sleep hygiene, regular exercise, and proper nourishment all support our capacity for system-wide and vital allostatic responses, as well as the subsequent return to homeostasis (the stable equilibrium in our physiological responses). These healthy behaviors promote our overall resiliency.

Chronic, repetitive, or overwhelming acute stress is considered *toxic stress*. When this level of stress sets in, we have exceeded our allostatic capacity to manage stress by distributing its impact across multiple systems. There are long-term consequences to toxic stress, because it places us in a state of *allostatic overload,* which leaves not just one, but multiple body systems depleted of energy and struggling to return us to homeostasis. The multisystem impact of allostatic overload is one framework for understanding the complex, multi-symptom illnesses associated with traumatic stress.[14]

If we are already experiencing a high allostatic load, what might be a tolerable stress for someone else, like getting a small burn while cooking dinner, can cause our system to become hyperaroused. We then move into allostatic overload, which, in turn, results in responses like flare-ups of chronic pain patterns or autoimmune or digestive disorders. Sustained allostatic overload causes significant, system-wide changes in our physiology with considerable impact on both our morbidity and mortality.[15]

Our allostatic load can be thought of as the price we pay for carrying repeated chronic or overwhelmingly acute stress—and the cost can be considerable. Either we are unable to return to neutral after yet another stressful experience, or the responsive interplay between body systems is no longer operative, and we feel unable to meet the next life challenge.[16] Because challenges are always part of life, allostatic overload can leave an individual feeling unable to manage day-to-day tasks. It can place a devastating burden on individuals and dramatically impact their role and capacity to function in the communities in which they live and work.[17]

UNDERSTANDING TOXIC OR TRAUMATIC STRESS

As will be discussed more fully in the next chapter, there are particular physiological systems that support various aspects of our response to both our external and internal environments. The autonomic nervous system (ANS) is the overall neurophysiological system governing responses that require an increase or decrease in automatic functions—the things that are outside our conscious control, such as heart rate, breathing, digestion, circulation, and perspiration. For our purposes here, we will use a simplified version of the ANS to illustrate how the physiology of traumatic stress can influence our exposure to allostatic overload. A more detailed discussion of this system will follow in Chapter Two.

The ANS has two branches, each of which has a distinctive physiological function. The branch of the ANS that prepares us for an active response to a threat is called the sympathetic nervous system (SNS). Its other branch, the parasympathetic nervous system (PNS), prepares us for rest, relaxation, and quiet contemplation.

Below is a depiction of the dynamic tension between the SNS and PNS, showing its movement as a wave. In everyday life, we naturally flow between the sympathetic awake-and-alert state and the parasympathetic rest-and-digest state, responding to what the situation calls for from moment to moment. Ideally, the rise and fall of these physiological functions will be contained inside what Daniel Seigel first named the "Window of Tolerance."[18]

We will use our preferred term, the "zone of resiliency," because it supports our focus on creating more regulation and greater resiliency in trauma survivors. The boundaries of this zone are similar to those of a thermostat, allowing a measured, easy rise and fall to maintain a comfortable average temperature. The space between these boundaries is where we experience a natural and fluid state of regulation. We have greater access to more positive states of being. We feel more respected, safe, hopeful, loved, and cared for when we are inside this zone. From here, we can negotiate life with a sense of safety and competency, even when traveling into new or unfamiliar territory.

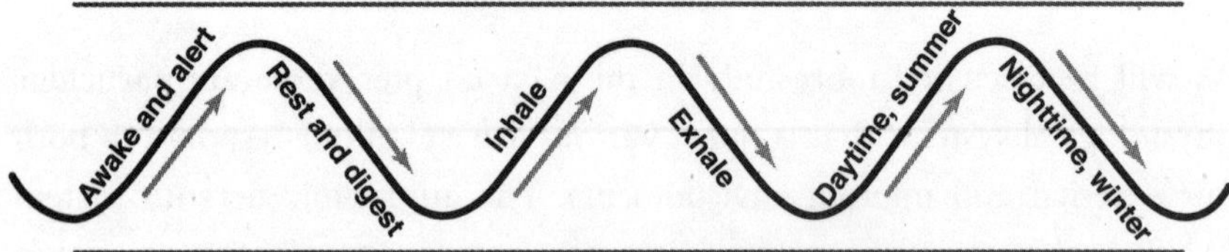

FIGURE 1.1. Zone of Resiliency

As will be discussed more fully in the next chapter, in order to avoid extreme dysregulation as adults, we need to have had an experience of loving and safe connection as infants. When our system expressed arousal by crying, it needed to be met with loving attention—food, touch, or a fresh diaper. This established an embodied and reliable experience of a balanced wave in which discomfort is met by comfort. This foundational experience helps wire our neurological systems for greater resilience and capacity for regulation of our physiology and behavior. Loving connection with those who cared for us early in our development helps us distinguish which people and circumstances are safe, and it enhances our capacity to make eye contact and maintain intimate emotional connections as adults. Healthy, engaged caregivers also leave us better equipped to notice and respond to our primal biological needs, like recognizing hunger or fatigue. Those who lacked this healthy connection as infants can experience pronounced dysregulation in their autonomic nervous system and are at greater risk for significant health problems as adults.[19]

When our zone of resiliency is wide, our capacity to manage life's challenges is greater. We return to regulated homeostasis more quickly and with less effort. But when our zone is narrow, we are at greater risk of overwhelming our allostatic capacity and developing allostatic overload, leaving us vulnerable to either sympathetic activation (a state of arousal in which we are actively mobilizing a response to danger or life threat—that is, fight or flight) or parasympathetic collapse (a physiologically compelled state of paralysis—that is, freeze)—even in response to small provocations.

The width of our zone of resiliency varies in relation to external circumstances and our internal vitality. When we feel safe and loved, we manage insults or threats with more equanimity. How resilient we feel may vary, depending on a number of circumstances: when we are older or younger, during different seasons of the year, or in the presence or absence of certain people or animals.

When a life-threatening event occurs, like the lightning bolt in Figure 1.2, fear or terror will send a signal to activate our sympathetic nervous system (SNS). We suddenly become stronger, faster, more focused, and more capable of responding successfully to danger or life threat. The high-energy survival state produced by the SNS will typically exceed the boundary of the easy rise and fall of everyday life found inside our zone.

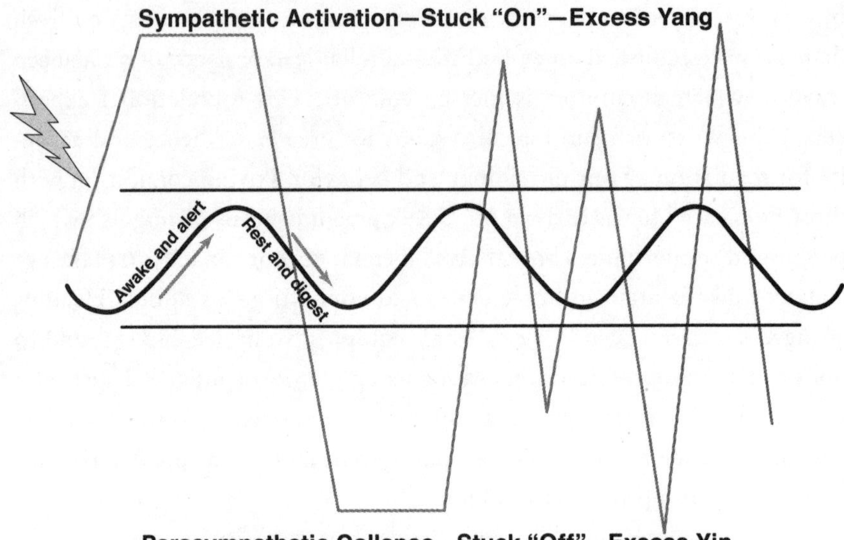

FIGURE 1.2. Zone of Resiliency with Overlay of Traumatic Stress

This hyperaroused state is designed to be short-lived. We survive, *experience* our successful survival effort, and our heart signals this success to the rest of the body in the form of a coherent, regulated, and calm heartbeat. We harvest new skills to help us manage similar threats in the future and then return to a state of open curiosity, with its normal rhythmic flow between our parasympathetic (PNS) and sympathetic (SNS) nervous systems. Our energy has returned to the range defined by our zone of resiliency.

Sometimes, however, we don't have the time, circumstances, or support we need for our energy to return to the area defined by this boundary—and thus restore our balance and regulation. Repeated lightning bolts strike again—or perhaps a single super-sized lightning bolt. Perhaps we are in combat, and a bomb explodes on our right—and before our system could recognize we were okay and could settle—another explodes on our left, and then another. Or, perhaps we survived the hurricane, but then the ensuing power outage and lack of clean water and adequate food became too much to bear.

Our allostatic load increases with each lightning bolt, along with our inner experience of disorganization, lack of regulation, and declining resilience. We experience a massive disruption in the organization, flow, function, and vitality of our energy. If this happens repeatedly, and if we don't find the means to recover, we can become stuck in the *on* position—in the mobilization of the fight-or-flight response—or what is called *sympathetic hyperarousal.* Here, our energy resides above the upper level of our zone of resiliency.

If we are unable to fight or flee, if our capacity to respond has been snuffed out by previous trauma, if we are too young or too small, if the threat is too big or too powerful, or if our efforts at self-protection are otherwise thwarted or inaccessible, we will fall into a physiologically compelled state of paralysis—what is called *parasympathetic collapse,* the *freeze* state, the *off* position. Here, our energy resides below the lower level of the same zone.

The fight, flight, and freeze responses are the primary survival responses articulated in the classical description of the physiological options available when we are faced with danger or life threat. We will discuss these categories as survival responses in more detail in Chapters Two and Three.

When we are very young, we lack the physical capacity to fight or flee, so our most likely response to threat is to "drop" physiologically into at least a mild version of the freeze state. Over time, this may become our habitual physiological response to high levels of stress. We may first experience the surge of the activation associated with our SNS turning on, but our early experiences of being overwhelmed have now predisposed us to plunge into the collapsed, numb state produced by our PNS. This can then become a chronic state, which limits our ability to access healthy arousal states, because each burst of arousal again plunges us into collapse.

Imagine an infant born with severe cardiac arrhythmia. She survived this life-threatening condition, but it likely required extended hospitalization and separation from her caregivers. Developmentally unable to self-soothe, she came to rely upon this freeze response to manage the arousal that was part of her experience of life threat. Because this response was deployed multiple times, there's a good chance this strategy has become her go-to physiological method for dampening sympathetic arousal.

The freeze state is meant to be a short-lived survival strategy; it is designed to plunge our physiology into an extreme conservation state. Under the influence of the freeze response, we slow our heart rate, limit oxygen consumption by restricting movement, digestion and other energy-consuming metabolic processes, and reduce the activity of our immune system. Extended and chronic exposure to this physiological state, and the suppression of the body processes it involves, creates a chronically and dangerously high allostatic load.[20]

Chronic exposure to either of these survival responses—either high sympathetic arousal or the collapsed and frozen state—creates a high allostatic load. When these survival states become habitual at an early age, they can have devastating consequences on development. For example, if a boy's caregiver is abusing him, and he is unable to run from or fight this threat because of his size, age, and dependency on that adult, this may produce a chronic state of hyperarousal, perhaps manifesting in constant anxiety or crying. Alternatively, he may make use of the numbing of his freeze response, which may give him relief from the constant activation and anxiety but compromises his ability to engage with the world. In either case, we would expect to see consequences that could extend throughout his adulthood.

One of the more damaging versions of dysregulation that can occur with unresolved survival responses is one of a coexisting high arousal and freeze response. The physiology moves erratically—oscillating between arousal and collapse—causing varied and complex symptoms in our physical, mental, emotional, and spiritual health and well-being. This is why we, as providers and educators, favor approaches that aim to restore overall regulation rather than parsing out discrete symptoms for our attention.

Our capacity to heal from the complex side effects of this chronic dysregulation is influenced by our ability to return to the regulated and balanced wave of energy within our zone of resiliency. A clinician's job is to help restore the natural, fluid, and measured rise and fall inside the client's zone. Restoring regulation to this intangible flow creates a foundation for healing the tangible symptoms common in trauma survivors.

It's important to understand that humans are biologically compelled to complete a successful defense to a life threat. For example, if we're hiking in the mountains and a falling rock pins us beneath it, our first impulse will be to try to push the rock off with as much force as we can muster. Our sympathetic nervous system will engage all the power in our musculoskeletal system. But if the rock is too heavy to move, our parasympathetic system will ultimately take over, and we will collapse and freeze beneath it. Our best chance of survival, in part, is to stop struggling—drastically reducing our need for oxygen and glucose—so that we will hopefully remain alive long enough for someone to come along and rescue us.

Imagine that a group of burly and kind people did hike by, lifted the rock, and brought medical help; we survived to hike another day. However, even though we're alive, the incomplete impulse to push the rock off—that hyperaroused state—may remain buried beneath the collapse we experienced in our autonomic nervous system. Without an embodied experience of successfully engaging our muscles to free ourselves from the rock, the initial state of unresolved hyperarousal may remain in our tissue memory. It can manifest in what we have come to call "strange, rare, and peculiar ways," like difficult-to-diagnose muscle weakness, unremitting pain, an elusive sense of powerlessness, or fear of hiking in rocky areas or of being alone in the mountains.

As we discuss in Chapter Three, our sense of powerlessness arises from having been challenged or interrupted in one or more of the five phases of the self-protective response. Where we experience this interruption—that is, which phase of the self-protective response we are at when the interruption occurs—will influence the nature of the physiological, psychological, spiritual, or energetic imprint this overwhelming sense of helplessness leaves behind.

The incomplete or thwarted survival response gives rise to highly disorganized energy that begins to dictate the physiological responses of the autonomic nervous system. This disorganization lives in our tissue memory. Depending on the history, circumstances, and constitution of the individual, this thwarted response can manifest in the various ways noted in this chart.

INCOMPLETE SURVIVAL RESPONSE

AUTONOMIC NERVOUS SYSTEM	COMMON SYMPTOMS
Hyperarousal or activation	*Anxiety, insomnia, anger, hypervigilance*
Hypoarousal or collapse	*Lethargy, fatigue, emotional vulnerability, forgetfulness*
Mixed hyperarousal and hypoarousal	*Complex, multi-symptom illness with symptoms of both activation and collapse*

Such taxing states of disorganized physiology and the resulting responses in the autonomic nervous system may occur after experiences of life threat, particularly if the traumatic event occurs very early in our life, such as a premature birth requiring an extended period of time in an incubator. They may also appear as the result of nonphysical experiences of life threat extended over time, like chronic emotional abuse in childhood. Or they may appear in the wake of overwhelming sympathetic activation as an adult, such as may occur with war trauma, natural disasters, automobile accidents, or street crime. In each of these scenarios, the dynamic balance and co-regulatory capacity of the parasympathetic and sympathetic nervous systems is at risk of being severely compromised.

Our inability to complete a successful "push" to lift the rock, fight off the mugger, run away from an aggressive dog, or escape the tsunami can give rise to unconscious and ineffective impulses toward self-defense, such as road rage, domestic violence, unrelenting anger, or consuming fear.[21] Most likely, we don't really want to kick our dog, beat our child, or run another car off the road—we are simply compelled by our unresolved survival impulse to take action. Our dog, child, or that other car becomes the target of these unfulfilled impulses. Those of us who struggle with an inability to control our responses and who are likely suffering from physical issues (such as autoimmune illness, chronic pain, metabolic disturbance, obesity, and substance abuse or addiction) need understanding and treatment, not shame or marginalization.

Trauma-informed care can help us access the permanent, regulated wave of resiliency that remains unbroken despite the overlay of dysregulation caused by overwhelming life experiences. Restoring access to this wave builds our inherent capacity for healing and helps return our bodies, minds, emotions, and spirits to resilient function. The more we experience this wave, the wider our zone of resiliency and the greater capacity we have for managing stressful experiences without moving into allostatic overload. We become better able to transform the imprint of past traumas and navigate future threats more successfully.

Healing is built on finding quiet for jangled nerves, restoring our ability to see clearly and navigate obstacles smoothly, cultivating compassion for self and others, breaking down and digesting the gristle remaining from difficult life experiences, discovering inspiration, and letting go. When we find these qualities, our inner physician—our innate capacity to heal—can do its job, and we can transform the underlying basis for the complex, multi-symptom illness we are suffering from. If the balance and rhythm between sympathetic (awake and alert) and parasympathetic (rest and digest) can be restored, if restful sleep returns, and if focus and clear thoughts arise again, then our inner physician can do the rest.

From the perspective of energy medicine, like Acupuncture and Asian Medicine (AAM), the essential and balanced rhythm inside our zone of resiliency is always available to us, even when the overlying, overwhelming, and powerful dysregulation in our autonomic nervous system makes it difficult to access without help from a compassionate, present, engaged, and mindful human being. It is a profound experience when we touch the sacred place inside each of us that can be neither broken nor destroyed and is the essence of our true nature.

It is worth noting that trauma today is experienced differently than in ancient times, when people were more likely to return home from war, natural disasters, or human tragedies to intact communities. These communities also lived a more agrarian lifestyle characterized by the regulating influences of the lunar and solar cycles, social and religious rituals, and strong cultural traditions—all of which support resiliency and homeostasis.

Many survivors in modern times do not have—or are not given—the opportunity to resolve their experiences through similar regulating influences. They do not necessarily belong to an intact and healthy community. Veterans return from war to a society that doesn't understand their experience or know how to acknowledge or welcome them. Many people today don't have or can't find opportunities for connection to the rhythms of nature in our highly urbanized and technology-driven culture.

Trauma-informed care is critical to helping survivors move incomplete mobilization responses out of their tissues, allowing them access to more life-giving and relationship-enhancing choices, and freeing them from the incomplete processing of trauma memories frozen in time.

In our view, it is essential that we cultivate integrative clinical practices that recognize the complexity of twenty-first-century traumatic stress and its related spectrum of chronic illness. We assert that the body holds the memory of the impact of trauma even after the analytical mind has considered and evaluated the story. We cannot restore our harmony, balance, and fundamental resiliency without including both the subtle and profound expression of the energy that influences our body, mind, emotions, and spirit after we experience life threat.

INTEGRATIVE HEALING CREATES MORE POSSIBILITIES

Clearly, traumatic stress manifests in diverse forms, affects survivors profoundly, and can influence the entire body, mind, emotions, and spirit. Integrative approaches that place a premium on relationship-centered care and that focus on whole-body regulation and whole-person healing offer survivors more compassionate, effective, and longer-lasting care.

Acupuncture is one such modality. In 2006, psychiatrist and physician acupuncturist Michael Hollifield, now Section Chief at the Program for Traumatic Stress at Tibor Rubin VA Medical Center, published the first research on the potential of acupuncture to treat PTSD.[22] Subsequent research by Hollifield and others has affirmed acupuncture as perhaps the most promising complementary and integrative medicine intervention for the trauma spectrum response.[23]

There is mounting evidence of the promise that AAM can offer for the "strange, rare, and peculiar" symptoms survivors of traumatic stress often experience.[24] The Five Elements and the resonant networks (or what AAM calls the *correspondences*) between each Element and various organs, emotions, tissues, psychological tasks, and spiritual gifts can help clinicians develop more tailored, more nuanced, and more meaningful care for survivors.[25]

The Tao of Trauma expands the AAM framework beyond needles and herbs to include touch and presence. Integrating the theoretical framework of AAM with Western neurophysiology, a variety of providers can incorporate these ideas into their existing knowledge of trauma and be supported to design approaches that make use of AAM's many gifts.

Leaders and policy makers—such as Dr. Tracy Gaudet, director of the Office of Patient Centered Care and Cultural Transformation of the

Veterans Health Administration,[26] Dr. Josephine Briggs, director of the NIH's National Center for Complementary and Integrative Health,[27] and researchers in the field of integrative medicine [28]—are paving the way in promoting relationship-centered, integrative health approaches, including acupuncture and mindfulness practices,[29] yoga,[30] and conscious touch by chiropractors[31] and massage therapists[32] in the U.S. health care system.

In addition to a growing understanding of trauma-informed care in public-health settings, grassroots, home, and community interventions can also be profoundly transformative. A loving and coherent community is critical.

THE IMPACT OF TRAUMA ON INDIVIDUALS, FAMILIES, AND COMMUNITIES

Traumatic stress affects both mental and physical health. It impacts educational success, criminal behavior, driving habits, work, family, and community life, as well as survivors' capacity for joy, pleasure, and intimacy in relationships of all kinds. It is not extreme to posit that new and creative treatment approaches to the impact of trauma is critical to our national and even our global well-being. It's quite possible that the impact of traumatic stress may be our most urgent public health issue.[33]

The clearest research on the pervasive role of traumatic stress in our society comes from the Centers for Disease Control's (CDC) work with the adverse childhood experiences (ACE) study.[34] The original researchers within the Kaiser Permanente Health Maintenance Organization (HMO) in California surveyed more than seventeen thousand of their members between 1995 and 1997, inquiring about adverse childhood experiences. Their survey[35] specifically asked about a parent's incarceration or drug addiction, as well as experiences of domestic abuse and sexual trauma, emotional and physical neglect, experiencing or witnessing violence, family mental illness, and the loss of a parent through divorce or death.

Of particular interest is the fact that the ACE study was carried out on working adults with middle-class lifestyles—indicating that low socioeconomic status is not the only source of life stress.[36] Further research focusing on low socioeconomic status has shown an even greater likelihood of stressors in these communities, including toxic chemical agents such as lead. Children impacted by toxic stress manifest with poor self-regulation, deficiency in language skills, depression, and early cardiovascular disease—with related physiological impact including smaller hippocampal volume,[37] reduction in prefrontal cortical gray matter,[38] and greater amygdala reactivity to angry or sad faces.[39]

The ACE study findings are striking and are considered so critical to public health that the CDC has taken over the monitoring of study participants' data. The greater the number of ACEs, the higher the risk for every major public health concern of our time—ischemic heart, chronic lung, liver, metabolic, and autoimmune diseases, as well as obesity, cancer, skeletal fractures, alcoholism, drug abuse, depression, and suicidality. The increase in these health risks is exponential—hundreds of percents higher than those who do not report multiple ACEs.

The ACE research is clear: experiences of safety in infancy and childhood support healthier decisions about the use of addictive substances,[40] sexual practices,[41] and the people we associate with as adults.[42] They also support better physical health and a greater capacity to recover from challenges, both physical and emotional. Every public health concern, from obesity[43] to drug addiction; cardiac,[44] pulmonary,[45] hepatic,[46] and autoimmune disease;[47] as well as sleep disturbance,[48] depression,[49] and suicidality,[50] can be influenced by—or perhaps even originate from—childhood trauma. The study's research also confirms a relationship between ACEs and criminal behavior,[51] domestic violence,[52] and success in the workplace.[53]

While we are focused primarily on the role of providers in this book, we would argue that the tremendous impact of trauma on every public health statistic also demands the attention of neighborhood leaders, social welfare advocates, public health specialists, educators, civil servants, and elected officials. Growing up in loving, intact families, and within communities governed by policies that support the safety and well-being of children, provides a foundation for the health of individuals and the communities in which we live and work.[54]

Taken together, the extraordinary burden that traumatic stress and interpersonal violence places on individuals and communities demands that we address trauma and its effects across all systems of care.[55] Expanding the capacity of health care systems to respond to this critical public health need in increasingly sophisticated and effective ways is crucial.

Communities need healers who can play an important role in nurturing a culture of safety, supporting relationships across differences, and taking effective action to protect vulnerable populations. Consider the results if practitioners offer more comprehensive, trauma-informed treatment to survivors:

- We can help bring peace to families and communities. Unresolved trauma is a principal cause of violent, impulsive acts. Traumatic reenactment is one way our unconscious minds attempt to bring closure to life-threatening experiences.
- We can help trauma survivors make thoughtful, flexible, and creative contributions to our social discourse, rather than ideologically rigid or divisive reactions rooted in fear or terror.
- We can create new possibilities for children. Children's futures are transformed when parents restore balance in their own inner worlds and overcome patterns likely formed over multiple generations, in the life experiences of known and unknown ancestors.

Dr. Vincent Felitti, who originated the ACE study within the Kaiser Permanente HMO, and Dr. Robert Anda, his colleague at the CDC, have laid a critically important and scientific foundation for what AAM also affirms—that we cannot separate the body from the mind and spirit. What we attribute to one aspect of our being is actually registered and recorded in all facets of our selves. Our body, mind, emotions, and spirit—and the health and vitality of our families, communities, and nation—are each highly textured strands in one essential fabric of personal and public health.[56]

Thankfully, the impact of healing is also far-reaching. The influence of devoted friends and family, time spent in cohesive group activities—such as playing an instrument in an orchestra or band, enjoying a team sport, engaging in social dance, participating in community theater, or spending time in nature—all help to restore coherence to every member of a system impacted by trauma. A healing vibration does indeed spread like honey on warm toast.

2

Polyvagal Theory Illuminates and Informs Acupuncture and Asian Medicine

THREE NEUROPHYSIOLOGICAL PLATFORMS

POLYVAGAL THEORY HIGHLIGHTS the special role that a sense of safety in relationships plays in mitigating the impact of stress in mammals, particularly in primates (including humans). Polyvagal theory was developed through decades of research and observation by psychologist Stephen Porges.[1] Textbooks of neuroscience traditionally taught that the autonomic nervous system was made up of two opposing functions: a sympathetic (activating) and a parasympathetic (inhibiting) branch. Porges came to understand that the mammalian autonomic nervous system differs from that of lower forms of animals, in that mammals have *three* branches in their ANS, each supporting distinct functions that inform and support a response to stress: one sympathetic branch and *two* parasympathetic branches.

By revealing the more complex functions of our stress neurophysiology, Porges's polyvagal theory helps us understand the highly variable responses to life threat—and the phenomena they engender—by describing these three branches as neurological "platforms." Each platform supports a different category or quality of behavior. The sympathetic branch supports excitation and alertness at the low end of its functional range (referred to as *tone* in the vocabulary of the nervous system), and at its high function, or tone, it empowers mobilization of fight or flight.

The two parasympathetic platforms are regulated by the dorsal and ventral branches of the tenth cranial, or vagus, nerve. They interact with the sympathetic system in different ways. The *ventral vagus* (VV) acts as a braking mechanism to inhibit the sympathetic system in a nuanced way, while the more primitive *dorsal vagus* (DV) supports deep rest and all silent metabolic functions at its low tone and, at its extreme high tone, supports the freeze response (death feigning). The *ventral vagus* (VV) supports our use of social engagement to mitigate arousal when we feel threatened.[2] Both emerge from the brain stem, with the dorsal branch arising toward the back and the ventral arising toward the front of the brain stem.

The dorsal vagus is considered an evolutionarily more primitive system. It remains unmyelinated throughout our lifetime. Myelination (the wrapping of a nerve cell in myelin, a fatty material that functions similarly to electrical insulation) aids nerve function. It supports a nerve to send more accurate and rapid messages. Lacking this sheath, the DV does not possess the quick, accurate function of its myelinated companion, the ventral vagus, which provides a faster, more responsive, and nuanced component to the parasympathetic braking mechanism. The myelination process of the ventral vagus nerve unfolds over time. It begins at about thirty weeks gestationally, with most myelination occurring in the first eighteen months after birth. The most rapid period of myelination is during the time between birth and six months.[3] This process continues through childhood and adolescence, giving us full access to its highly nuanced function in early adulthood.[4]

Porges's model postulates that we use each of these three different neurophysiological platforms in sequential order, opposite that of their development in evolution.

1. When threatened, we first attempt to mitigate that threat via our most recently developed neurological platform, the ventral vagus system. This more nuanced portion of our parasympathetic braking system supports mammalian social-engagement behaviors such as

bonding, attachment, and appeasement. It enables us to look softly into each other's eyes and express and understand subtle nuances of meaning in speech and facial expression.

2. If our social-engagement system is unable to mitigate this threat, we resort to our fight-or-flight response, which is supported by our sympathetic arousal system. The "vagal brake," regulated by our ventral vagus, is lifted, allowing us to mobilize active responses for self-protection. Our SNS increases our heart rate and blood pressure, shunts blood to our periphery to power our musculoskeletal system for active survival effort, and escalates our breathing.
3. If our fight-or-flight responses are unsuccessful or somehow thwarted, we will resort to the most evolutionarily primitive portion of our ANS: our dorsal vagus system, which mediates the freeze response. The DV is considered a residual physiological system—one that is present in diving mammals that land-based mammals have repurposed as an emergency braking mechanism. A partial freeze response, with muscle tone maintained, is a blended state—with a combination of the dorsal vagus and the sympathetic system together. However, the extreme plunge into the "death-feigning" response, with its affiliated loss of muscle tone and collapse, is associated with a pure surge of the dorsal vagus. This rapidly and precipitously slows our heart rate and respiration and lowers our blood pressure. It essentially helps us conserve energy. At its highest level of tone, the DV produces extreme conservation by mimicking what would happen if we were suddenly underwater: we collapse as this system shunts oxygenated blood away from our muscles and sends it to our more critically important brain and vital organs. Digestion and anything else we don't need to survive the next few minutes is shut down. In fact, immersing our face in icy water can trigger this dorsal vagal response, instigating what is referred to as the *dive reflex*.

While polyvagal theory indicates that these different neurophysiological platforms are used in the sequence noted above, Porges acknowledges that in actual practice, we typically use these systems in a blended way, with one or the other in dominance at any given time, but rarely in exclusive control of our physiology. As an example, imagine we are at a lively party (despite the term *fight-or-flight response,* these stress responses are functioning at all times, helping us navigate active engagement in all aspects of our lives). At this party, we are moving around and talking, then sitting more quietly, then we bump into old friends and again begin gesticulating and perhaps dancing. In this instance, we would likely move from a more SNS-dominant physiology to the ventral vagal system and then back to SNS as dominant, but with the VV still at least somewhat engaged and available to constrain the SNS. This is what helps us shift our mobilization response from defense to active play.

Of course, our own history—particularly if we have experienced trauma—will influence how and when we use each of these neural platforms. In the following sections, we will take each of these portions of the ANS in turn and provide more detail about their relationship to traumatic stress—one of the fields in which Porges has made unique and profound contributions.

We will begin our exploration with the SNS system, which supports arousal and activity. We will then explore the two branches of the PNS—the dorsal vagus and the ventral vagus. As noted previously, the primary source of the braking mechanism on the SNS is the VV, with the DV coming into play when the SNS can no longer viably recruit resources for fight or flight.

THE SYMPATHETIC NERVOUS SYSTEM AND SELF-PROTECTION

The SNS supports alertness (at its lower tone, or level, of function) and physiologically active states (at its higher tone). It will be dominant when we are exercising, dancing, or engaging in active play. It will also dominate when we feel nervous about an upcoming event or anxious, angry, or excited. At its high tone, it will support our most active states—including both the fight and flight responses to threats.

When we experience or anticipate a threat, our physiological system undergoes a massive mobilization process that supports our ability to protect both ourselves and others. Under the influence of the SNS, our heart will pound, our blood pressure will rise, our breathing escalates, and our muscle system will be infused with blood to facilitate action and physical activity.

Because we are mobilizing in response to a life threat, other parts of our physiology—such as digestion—are inhibited so as not to expend energy that might be needed for our immediate self-protection. We power up for the fight-or-flight response, which will be covered in more detail in the following chapter. For our purposes here, the important element to understand is that this activation of the arousal system is the equivalent of stepping on the gas.

While mobilizing a response to threats is critical for our survival, there is a limit to how much escalation of this physiological response we can tolerate—a pounding heart and high blood pressure can be detrimental if it goes on too long. For the sake of survival, we need a way to temper this alarmed state and reduce it to levels that do not harm our physiology, particularly our heart, when this arousal has little hope of success. For this, we have the parasympathetic system, with both of its branches using different methods to apply the brakes.

THE VENTRAL VAGUS/SOCIAL ENGAGEMENT SYSTEM

As noted above, the most significant rates of ventral vagus myelination occur during our early years. This myelination makes the nerve's expressions quick and accurate, and it provides the capacity for a delicate interplay between the VV and the arousal states of the SNS. We can delicately apply the brakes when we need to slow our arousal and then gently release the brake to allow our SNS to support more active interaction.

Because the VV supports this nuanced interplay between the excitation of the sympathetic system and the calming of the parasympathetic system, it reinforces the neural platform of social engagement particularly well. The VV protects our physical vitality as well as our relationships in our community. The critical importance of this platform is in its capacity to support our use of social engagement to mitigate threat. The VV allows us to disagree with others but remain in a relationship with them. It enables us to inhibit violent impulses when we are angry. This beautiful VV helps us join with others for protection, negotiate and apologize, have compassion for the suffering of others, and meet aggression with thoughtfulness and empathy. A healthy VV is critical for both individual and community life. Porges has provided us with a "science for love."[5]

We humans *require* community for our survival. Our capacity for social engagement, including our ability to collaborate with others in a joint response to a common threat—as well as to seek out kind people to help mitigate our individual arousal in more personal contexts, is a reflection of the vitality and health of the functions supported by our ventral vagus nerve. Our physiology supports our capacity to cultivate trusting relationships and live in community. We are meant to be tribal animals.[6]

Polyvagal theory applies the rigor of science to what we all know implicitly: when we feel safe, we connect with others more easily. The reverse is also true: when we feel connected to others, we feel safer. The functions of our frontal cortex are more available when we feel safe and connected—it is easier to engage with others, think clearly, and access our memories. We make more inclusive and thoughtful choices in our interpersonal relationships and social discourse. Safety, social engagement, and our frontal cortex together bridge our inner self with the outer world.

The VV's capacity for nuanced and gentle lifting of its braking mechanism allows the sympathetic system to subtly rise to support social interaction—speaking, gesturing, or connecting with others—without demanding the secretion of stress chemicals. The VV can be so accurate in lifting its vagal brake that the heart's own pacemaker, via the sinoatrial node, can increase our heart rate without the release of stress chemicals from the adrenal glands that would initiate a more intense physiological response. We can erupt in laughter, pat our friend on the back, and pass the potatoes without resorting to stress chemistry to support those actions. This capacity to increase our heart rate without relying on adrenalin or other stress chemicals is less physiologically depleting and more protective of our essential vitality.

The ventral vagus predominantly regulates the organs above the respiratory diaphragm, essentially the heart and lungs. It also influences the functions of the face, eyes, vocal cords, and ears via related nerves. It gives us the capacity to look at each other with soft eyes, to understand the subtleties of meaning in speech, and to communicate emotional nuance with facial expression and voice tone. When we are in a safe relationship with others, the VV also brings our heartbeat and breathing into co-regulation with our companion, which contributes to our experience of feeling "connected." Without these capacities, our ability to cultivate relationships and create community becomes compromised.

Dr. Porges essentially established a scientific justification for the importance of the feeling of safety and connection for the healthy development of multiple aspects of our physical health and capacity for social engagement. We experience greater intellectual success, engage in healthy and more prosocial behavior, and enjoy both physical and mental health when our ventral vagus system is uninhibited by fear or social isolation. In establishing this principle, Porges created a critical foundation for program development in sectors where trauma and its effects play out in communities—particularly in public health, social services, education, and law enforcement. Bringing Porges's work into these sectors puts high value on creating experiences of safety over punishment and relationship over isolation—and, perhaps most profoundly, it brings a depth of understanding and compassion instead of shame and blame for many of the symptoms that overwhelm our public health system, such as obesity and addiction.

As noted above, our ventral vagus nerve is only partially myelinated at birth—enough to facilitate coordination between sucking, swallowing, breathing, and calming. Preterm and high-risk infants have virtually no myelination and thus no resources from their ventral vagus to support them with these critical functions.[7] Myelination develops most rapidly in the first six months of life and continues into young adulthood. We are born without the physiological capacity to mitigate hyperarousal in our heart when we feel threatened, which means we cannot self-soothe. We are dependent on caregivers to provide that function for us. We need them to coo over us and respond to our needs for food, toileting, and bathing. We need them to hold and comfort us when we cry out, in order to protect our heart and its many functions, including regulating our vulnerable frontal cortex. Loving responses to experiences of threat or arousal in infancy are critical for building the function of our VV. Without them, our capacity for relationship with others and for regulation of our body's autonomic functions in adulthood will be compromised. Our physiology actually develops its capacity both to digest and assimilate nutrients and, of critical importance, *to feel safe* in both loving connection and rough and tumble play with thoughtful and caring adults.

It is something of a physiological irony that consistent access to safety prepares us for responding effectively to threats. In the process of healthy social development, we also develop better discrimination between threat and safety, a wider range of potential physiological responses to threats, and more resilience in our recovery after stressful events.

Our best survival strategy includes using this accurate and nuanced VV system as our go-to system. A healthy and vital ventral vagal system helps us look to our community to find support when we feel threatened. Rather than mounting an aggressive fight-or-flight response—or cascading into the primitive and rather blunt freeze response, we can maintain access to our more complex, refined social-engagement system. We stay in relationship with our social group, which helps us in our efforts toward survival. Our survival actually *requires* a capacity to connect with others to mount communal or tribal responses to threat. This connectedness, in turn, supports the healthy functioning of our frontal cortex and overall success in life—in work, family, and relationships.[8]

In addition to outlining the important role of social engagement for navigating normal stress and low-level danger, polyvagal theory provides an explanation for the physiology of life threat. In these instances, the braking mechanisms supported by the VV are not strong enough to limit the escalation of our arousal system, so we use an emergency braking mechanism instead: the dorsal vagus system.

THE DORSAL VAGUS SYSTEM

As noted previously, if the more evolutionary recent VV system of social engagement has not effectively mitigated the threat, we will resort to increasingly more primitive systems (a process referred to as *dissolution*) as part of our self-protective efforts. The SNS system will cause our level of arousal to escalate as we move toward active mobilization of a fight-or-flight response. If this physiological escalation continues unabated, eventually we can no longer viably recruit resources for self-protection—our own physiology becomes dangerous to us. In that instance, our most primitive neural platform, the DV, will intervene to shut down this escalation of arousal. This is the DV working at the "defensive," high-tone end of its function, where it decelerates cardiac hyperarousal by physiologically slamming on an emergency brake.

(Conversely, the involvement of the DV in its optimal, nonemergency range of function, is its resting-state interplay with the SNS to support homeostatic function.)

This portion of the vagus nerve is unmyelinated, and while it is neurologically slower than the ventral vagus, it has a powerful capacity to apply an inhibition system using something like blunt force. In this deep energy-conservation state, or freeze, we feel less pain and our memories of terror become blurred. We are meant to use this state exclusively in extreme danger.[9] High-tone DV is an effective management strategy in circumstances of abject life threat, but it is a dangerous option for mammals. Shutting down the heart too forcefully or for too long can be lethal, resulting in suppressed breathing or heart rate. Medical providers in emergency rooms are all too familiar with the risks that patients face when they are in a state of shock.

As noted above, the DV system is a conservation system; it helps us slow everything down to conserve oxygen and other metabolic resources. But even though the DV shunts blood away from our muscles and directs it toward our brain and vital organs, we still remain at risk from the impact of reduced oxygenation to our brain. Our large frontal cortex requires a steady flow of highly oxygenated blood in order to function well. Limiting our access to a robust supply of oxygen has significant negative consequences, so consistently relying on the DV system for slowing arousal will impair rather than support survival in the long term.

The high-tone DV response (freeze) should be used only when *not* using it poses a greater life threat than does activating a shutdown response. Unfortunately, as we will discuss in the next section and later chapters, trauma—especially trauma that occurs early in life—can predispose us to overuse of this powerful neurophysiological platform.

The physiology of the freeze response has dire implications for our overall health if it is used chronically. Physiologically, we have slammed into a metaphorical brick wall of immobility while at the center of a massive mobilization effort. Raging underneath this freeze state is the unresolved arousal that plummeted us into collapse. If we cannot find a way to resolve these two contrary survival responses, we are likely to end up in a chronic state of hyperarousal while trapped in this freeze, like putting one foot firmly on the gas and the other, equally firmly, on the brakes. We will cycle rapidly between hyperarousal and hypoarousal or experience being tugged in both directions at the same time. The gentle rise and fall within our zone of resiliency is now elusive.

Our autonomic nervous system is highly adaptive and flexible. It subscribes to the essential maxim of the animal kingdom: "Eat lunch, don't be lunch." There is no inherent preferential value in using one neurological platform over another in the context of life threat, and it is not about choice. A person's response during trauma is not influenced by their ethics, morals, or courage. There is nothing wrong with reacting more like a deer, a wolf, or a possum; each has a role and a place in creation. Our self-protective response is an instinctive, flexible negotiation for our essential existence. It is only about our survival, and it is hardwired in our genetics and our neurological development.

As we will discuss next, the high sympathetic tone coupled with equally high parasympathetic tone in complex trauma is mirrored in the language of Acupuncture and Asian Medicine (AAM). *Yin* is struggling to soothe, quiet, or cool *yang*, while at the same time, *yang* is struggling to activate, enliven, or warm *yin*. Traumatic stress overrides the essential regulation provided by *yin* and *yang*.

POLYVAGAL THEORY AND ACUPUNCTURE AND ASIAN MEDICINE

Dr. Porges refers to the impact of using each of these three neurological platforms—the ventral vagus, sympathethic, and dorsal vagus—as "the cost of doing business." He notes that each platform serves to save our life in certain circumstances but also comes with some metabolic or physiological cost. With his theory, Porges has given providers a framework for understanding the physiological impact of the different impulses available to humans to ensure our survival.

In the coming chapters, we will build on Porges's model, integrating his focus on the metabolic demands of these three neurological platforms with AAM's body-mind-emotions-spirit orientation to include the three platforms' psychological, emotional, and social costs as well. Extending his concept of "cost" to include these less tangible burdens will support our exploration of the impact of traumatic stress on children in our schools, newcomers in our communities, violence in our neighborhoods, and burdens on our public health system.

Ventral Vagus

When we operate from our ventral vagal platform, there is little metabolic demand and essentially no social cost. We feel safe. We feel connected to others in a heartfelt way. Our heart is providing a coherent rhythm that regulates every autonomic function of our body—we are functioning like a well-oiled machine.

High-Tone Sympathetic

The costs of a high-tone SNS state are significant. This neurological response uses a great deal of stored energy—all of which pours into our muscles and joints to support our fight-or-flight response. Digestion is necessarily and temporarily shut down. However, if we become habituated to high-tone SNS, this digestive shutdown will become dominant, and we won't assimilate nourishment well. This also compromises the gut's role in the production of neurotransmitters like serotonin and immune cells, and leaves us prone to both musculoskeletal and emotional constriction and rigidity.

While the physiological burden of high-tone SNS is enormous, it also places a burden on our interpersonal relationships and community engagement. Others may feel turned away by our rigid and reactive interpersonal bearing. We may struggle to find softness and warmth in interpersonal relationships, and our flexibility in thinking and planning may be compromised. We will explore approaches to softening the constriction and rigid bearing of survivors living in constant SNS arousal in Chapter Eight.

Low-Tone Dorsal Vagal

In contrast, in a low-tone DV state, our autonomic functions related to digestion, assimilation of nutrients, heart rate, breathing, and immune and endocrine functions are well supported. We can meditate, contemplate deep thoughts, and sleep well. There is little metabolic demand. In fact, this is a profoundly restorative inner state. However, there are social and interpersonal costs to this neurological state as well. This platform will not support active social engagement or mobilization in response to a threat. We need to wake up our SNS and cultivate a healthy ventral vagus to temper excess arousal the SNS can manifest in order to engage in life's pleasures and respond to life's challenges without social and interpersonal costs. We will explore approaches to restoring regulation in the SNS in Chapter Eight and ways to nourish interpersonal engagement and mitigate SNS arousal using the VV in Chapter Nine.

High-Tone Dorsal Vagal

If we are in high-tone DV, on the other hand, tone in other systems—especially digestion, circulation, and respiration—will necessarily be suppressed. This state places a tremendous burden on our whole physiology, because it shuts down these essential services. A high-tone DV state is designed to be short-lived—only lasting long enough to save our lives in an acute life threat. If we become habituated to this state, our capacity to assimilate nutrients and convert food into energy will be severely compromised, and we may also develop cardiac or pulmonary symptoms.

This habituation can happen if we experienced pervasive neglect or abuse as an infant or young child. Seeking the protection of a high-tone DV state was our best survival strategy at the time, but it takes a substantial physiological toll. This state will be carried in our viscera and affect its function. It also carries a significant but intangible emotional and psychological cost: our capacity to assimilate our experiences and convert them into life lessons and to integrate new skills for managing our lives will also be compromised, leaving us unprepared to manage similar challenges in the future. We may feel unable to cope and be consumed by fear. It may be hard to *not* feel like a victim, which can have profound effects on our interpersonal relationships and the role we play in our "tribe." We will explore approaches to restoring healthy, low-tone parasympathetic movement and transformation in both our bodies and our minds in Chapter Ten.

High-tone freeze in the DV also compromises all the functions of our frontal cortex. As a result, our decision making is less thoughtful and may not be relationship-based. High-tone DV has a profound impact on how we navigate unfamiliar people or situations and the choices we make in how we engage with others in our communities and workplaces. High-tone DV exacts a high tax on the health and welfare of the communities in which we live. The greater the capacity in our VV for connection with others, the less likely we are to go into either high-tone SNS supported violence or collapse into a DV freeze state. We will explore approaches to working with chronic fear and the freeze state in Chapter Seven, working with chronic anger and restoring regulation in the SNS in Chapter Eight, and with enhancing VV function in Chapter Nine.

While it may seem that survivors who find high-tone SNS their "home" are the most troubled, because of their habituation to emotional constriction and rigid bearing, those carrying the greatest burden to their health and welfare from their traumatic experience are those whose DV remains frozen in high tone.

This DV high tone arises from terror in the Kidney and adrenal system. It releases a powerful and overwhelming signal that life threat is imminent. It quickly spreads to every function, tissue, and organ throughout the body. Its pervasive impact is the basis for the complex and diverse symptoms that are too often found in trauma survivors.

As you can see, the Five Element model is a dynamic one. It mirrors the experience of many survivors who have diverse and complex symptoms that are intertwined, interconnected, and nearly impossible to tease apart as discrete phenomena.

Integrating Porges's findings with AAM's Five Element theory—with its system of correspondences and body-mind-emotions-spirit approach—offers clinicians additional information about how to engage the neurological platform most needing attention to restore balance and regulation in their clients.

Treating trauma survivors is a little like playing pick-up sticks. So much complexity—how and where do we focus an intervention and get the best results? Providers who specialize in a single body system or only one category of symptoms risk overlooking the dynamics between systems, as well as the underlying dysregulation that may be critical to understanding the client's whole-body, whole-person experience.

To continue the pick-up sticks image—providers need to choose the stick that relates most closely to this client's incomplete step in the five steps of the self-protection response (5-SPR). Choosing this stick will help our clients to complete their self-protective responses and bring greater coherency, rather than more turmoil, to their entire system. As will be explored in Part Three of this book, AAM can help providers to locate and work with the tissue, organ, or function where an incomplete step in the 5-SPR remains in body memory.

Thankfully, neuroscience affirms what AAM has long known: healing is always available to us. Our brains are plastic—they are malleable and can change and heal. A traumatic stress response is not a life sentence, and there is much we can do to change the impact that traumatic stress is having on our clients. In the coming chapters, we will provide orientation to how clinical interventions can become more effective and how we can make use of not only modern neuroscience but also the ancient wisdom of AAM.

3

Acupuncture and Asian Medicine's Perspective on Traumatic Stress

IN CHAPTER TWO, we discussed how polyvagal theory illuminated and deepened the understanding of trauma in the West and began our exploration of trauma in Acupuncture and Asian Medicine. Porges's framework describes the impact of traumatic stress in terms of Western anatomy and physiology—its impact on nerves, neurotransmitters, and hormones, as well as immune, endocrine, and digestive function. In this chapter, we turn our attention more fully to the contributions of AAM, and examine how this lens can expand our understanding of trauma with an appreciation of the underlying energy that influences our physiological responses to threat. Through this integration, we can see the impact of Porges's work even more deeply—and we can consider clinical applications to better serve our clients. We are fortunate to live in a time and place where the best of Western medicine and the wisdom of Eastern medicine can come together in service of healing.

AXIOMS OF ACUPUNCTURE AND ASIAN MEDICINE

The Tao

The Taoist school emerged in China during the Han Dynasty, more than two thousand years ago. The foundations of Taoist scholarship lie in affirming the intrinsic order of nature. Taoism accepts as an axiom (something that is self-evidently true) that all of creation arises from a single, essential, unnameable, and primal source called the Tao. While this is held as a fundamental axiom that explains the nature of the universe and life within it, Taoism also acknowledges the cosmic ineffability of the magnificence of creation. It is embraced as incomprehensible: "the Tao that can be understood is not the eternal, cosmic Tao, just as an idea that can be expressed in words is not the infinite idea, and yet this ineffable Tao is the source of all spirit and matter. Expressing itself, it is the mother of all created things."[1]

Everything emerges out of the oneness of the Tao, and so it follows that all of nature is interdependent and connected. The Tao is "the way," or the essential "principle" that underlies, organizes, unites, and informs all of nature's manifestations. This essential impulse is inherent in both great and small movements—from the fluid movement of a butterfly's wings in Brazil to the power of the tides in the Bay of Fundy. It is said to be inherent in endless "changes and transformations."[2] Humans are, of course, part of the Tao, neither separate from nor above the rest of nature. We exist as an integrated part of creation. The Taoists instruct us that our health is maintained by aligning with nature's laws.[3]

Taoism later became the foundation for acupuncture and Asian medicine, and its wisdom continues to teach us today:

> *What is good for nature is good for humanity, what is good for one is good for all, what is good for the mind is good for the body.... To harm a part is to harm the whole. What is bad for the heart is bad for the body, what damages one person damages all people, what injures the earth injures me. Conversely, to restore and preserve the good health of one body and mind is to foster the well-being of the whole, the earth, and all life upon it.*[4]

Yin and Yang

Nature was the Taoists' teacher, and observation and contemplation were their tools. These scholars observed the rising and setting of the sun, the waxing and waning of the moon, and the movement from summer to winter, noting how the Tao revealed itself in the dynamic movement between paired opposites. The Tao came to be understood as a container for dualities that unite and oppose each other, such as heaven and earth, male and female, day and night, life and death, inner and outer, and physical and metaphysical.

The primal distinction of the rising and setting of the sun gave rise to the associations of light, activity, and heat with *yang*, and darkness, rest, and coolness with *yin*. This exploration of dualities grew to include the nature of all things. *Yin* is seen as feminine and relates to interior, structure, and substance; *yang* is masculine, and relates to exterior, function, and energy. The day is the time for activity, while night is the time for rest. The law of *yin* and *yang* became an essential component of Taoism. This is a radically different paradigm from the common sensibilities of the Western world. While Aristotelian logic asserts that, "*A* cannot equal *B*," Taoism teaches that *A* is intimately connected to *B*, and, in fact, *A* requires *B* for its existence. The front of the hand cannot exist without the back of the hand, and neither can warmth be experienced without knowing coolness. *Yin* is both connected to *yang* and requires *yang* for its existence, as *yang* requires *yin*.

Like Einstein, who saw energy and matter as interchangeable, and who understood energy as both a wave and a particle, the Taoists saw the world around them similarly: *yin* and *yang* are fluid, not static states. Each state emerges out of its opposite. Day arises out of night, and night appears as day retires. Not only do day and night give rise to one another, their functions and attributes require the other. The rest of nighttime is essential to sustain the activity of daytime, which is again necessary to support deep rest at night. Similarly, traditional farmers leave productive fields unplanted from time to time, as lying fallow helps to restore their fertility. All things are born, decay, and die. Light and action are always paired with darkness and rest. *Yin* and *yang* emerge from one another and are fundamentally connected to each other.

The small white dot in the black half and the black dot in the white half of the *Taiji* symbol illuminate the axiom that nothing is exclusively *yin* or *yang*. Each pole also contains an aspect of its opposite—every woman *(yin)* has a masculine *(yang)* aspect and every man *(yang)* has a feminine *(yin)* aspect.

We can trust the regularity of nature's rhythm—the movement from day to night and the cycle of seasons. We can rely on this rhythm with ironclad confidence. It is more powerful than any human force. Nothing can break the rhythm or inherent movement that organically arises out of the expression of *yin* and *yang* in nature.

Taoism recognizes that any of us can show symptoms of disruption in the expression of this dynamic relationship—we can become too cold or too hot; we can be too agitated to sleep or too lethargic to get out of bed. However, it is also fundamentally true that the underlying dynamic and fluid nature of the *yin/yang* relationship cannot be broken.

No insult, threat, accident, or injury can destroy this fundamental rhythm. Those of us whose autonomic nervous systems have been overwhelmed and left dysregulated by life-threatening events can find our way back to this fluid movement. It is always there. In fact, we are hardwired to return to regulation after arousal.[5] We are part of the Tao—the same universal rhythm that causes tides to come and go, crocuses to emerge from the snow in spring, and leaves to fall off the trees in autumn. Healing is about finding our way back to our Tao, back to our essential nature, and restoring our place in this universal rhythm.

Many trauma survivors feel broken by their experience. They can't begin to imagine finding their way to equanimity or peace. The essential truth that the energy that arises from the fluid, life-giving movement of the Tao in nature is also and always available to help humans restore balance and regulation can be vitally important for providers to consider and hold for the sake of their clients. When clinicians embrace this notion, they can support survivors to imagine a new sense of possibility.

The promise of transformation from one state to another is all around us. Given the right time and circumstances, seeds that rest all winter will sprout, banana peels and eggshells in a compost pile will become rich fertilizer, and carbon molecules will become diamonds. Storms, including those with violent winds, come and go, as do the storms in our own lives. Our personal storms, when they unfold within the right circumstances—such as a sense of safety and relationship, support, and encouragement—can transform into powerful lessons that expand our consciousness and inform our life's journey in fundamental ways.

We can see the dynamic connection and interplay between apparently oppositional phenomena when we examine how the body regulates its survival functions. Of particular relevance to *The Tao of Trauma* is how the law of *yin* and *yang* is mirrored in the autonomic nervous system's division into its sympathetic and parasympathetic branches. In Chapters One and Two, we discussed these opposing roles from the Western neurophysiological perspective. AAM mirrors Western neurophysiology—it also embraces the dynamic interplay between these two opposing functions in our bodies.

The sympathetic branch is more *yang*—it prepares us for action and activity—while the parasympathetic is more *yin,* inhibiting and quieting its partner, so we can rest and find the stillness needed to restore our strength for the next action or activity. As with *yin* and *yang,* the SNS and the PNS function as opposing states in dynamic tension with one another—and yet are united in one system. Affirming this dynamic relationship offers hope to trauma survivors. These opposing yet connected states arise from each other and are in a perpetually fluid, moving relationship.

If we feel stuck in sympathetic hyperarousal, we can trust that parasympathetic restoration is—at the same time and in equal measure—available to support the transformation of our agitation, sleeplessness, anger, and volatility. While we may not be able *yet* to find this balance, it is not out of our reach forever. Similarly, if we feel stuck in parasympathetic numbing and collapse, or freeze, we can trust that sympathetic warmth and vitality is similarly available to help transform our passivity, fear, or isolation. We may need the support of a competent and caring provider to help us, but we can trust that balance and regulation between these states is always possible.

We will use this principle of connection between SNS and PNS—*yin* and *yang*—in all the clinical applications described in Part Three. We call it "tick-tock." Providers will begin by helping their client find a sense of safety—or at least neutrality. You will then gently guide your client's attention to the *outside edge* of a memory of arousal or anxiety. Allowing time for this arousal to rise modestly, you will then guide your client to return to his or her experience of safety. We are essentially supporting the organic movement and connection between the opposing yet connected states of PNS and SNS, *yin* and *yang*.

The principle of titration helps us to keep the swing of tick-tock within a manageable range for our clients. If the pendulum of tick-tock swings too far toward safety, it will necessarily swing an equal distance toward arousal—and we will risk an explosion instead of a good "sizzle" for our client.

Supporting this movement and connection taps into the life-giving wave inside their zone of resiliency. Witnessing waves of inner movement come alive as constriction in your client's digestive, musculoskeletal, respiratory or cardiac systems gives way—or watching tone return to collapsed, frozen body systems is downright magical! We will explore tick-tock more fully in Chapter Five and then in each Element's chapter in Part Three.

Qi (Energy)

Qi, pronounced "chee," is the most powerful concept in all of Chinese medicine. While it is impossible to accurately translate, "energy" is its closest English approximation. Physicists teach us that the tension between positive charges and negative charges creates the electromagnetic field out of which energy—manifesting as light, warmth, and movement—emerges. AAM similarly teaches that the tension between the opposing polarities of *yin* and *yang* create *qi*. Physics and AAM also both understand that by its very nature, energy has a dual expression—it exists as a more *yin*-like particle that is more substantial, and a more *yang*-like wave that is more etheric.[6]

Qi constantly moves between *yin* and *yang,* between states of condensation and dispersion. It is in a continuous state of flux, aggregating and taking on physical form and dissolving into etheric impulses. Like water that, depending on temperature and pressure, can be solid ice, liquid water, or immaterial steam, *qi* moves between its more *yin*-like condensed form and its more *yang*-like dispersed form. Every birth is an aggregation of *qi* into material form, and every death is a dispersal of *qi* into etheric or spiritual form.

Life is animated by the rhythm that arises from the dynamic connection between these opposing manifestations of *qi*/energy. This rhythm guides and contains our lives. When these forces are moving in equal tension, we experience homeostasis, or balance. This fundamental, unbreakable movement between *yin* and *yang* governs the rhythms that create the energetic basis for all expressions of life.[7]

Qi is the "fuel" for every action and function of our physiology. *Qi* transforms food and drink into the basic constituents of our body. *Qi* transports the energy from foods to where they are needed to ensure every body function. *Qi* holds our blood, fluids, and organs in place, protects us from infection, and warms us. We exhibit symptoms when our *qi* is deficient and when it collapses, becomes stagnant, or becomes rebellious and moves in the wrong direction.[8]

Qi/energy is not mysterious or exclusive to Eastern philosophy. It resides within us and all around us. Our *qi* serves us in innumerable ways, both subtle and gross, to help maintain health. It provides the energy or impulse to digest the gristle in both our food and our life experiences. *Qi* moves our muscles both consciously and impulsively. It performs every invisible metabolic or regulatory transformation and shapes both decisive thoughts and longing prayers. It is the energy that helps our bodies, minds, emotions, and spirits to cope, find comfort, and heal.

A central axiom of the Taoist school is that health is fostered and preserved by aligning with the laws of nature. Taoism understands *qi* as nature's fundamental building block and the energy inherent in all living things. Understanding the world from this *qi*/energy point of view offers an additional perspective that extends the lens of Western medical science, with its orientation toward biochemical function and physiological structure.

There is much to be hopeful about in the ongoing development of approaches to trauma treatment in Western medical settings. Western research has deepened our understanding of the nuance and complexity of trauma and its impact on the lives of survivors and their family members and communities. Suggestions as simple as using smartphones to remember appointments can fill in for some of the functions that traumatic stress may have disturbed. However, because of modern Western medicine's focus on providing high levels of specialized care to discrete symptoms in particular locations or functions of the body, it risks missing the essential disturbance to whole-body regulation caused by traumatic stress.[9]

Approaches such as AAM that focus on restoring fundamental balance and regulation, rather than parsing out discrete symptoms, offer a different perspective from which providers can approach their work with trauma survivors. Integrative medicine holds promise for unleashing multi-system healing responses that attend to the underlying cause of the complex, multi-system impact of overwhelming life threat. Restoring regulation and balance to the energetic infrastructure in our bodies is fundamental to bringing trauma survivors back "home" to themselves.[10]

Seen through this Taoist lens, traumatic stress is a vibrational (or energetic) disturbance, and AAM, as vibrational (or energetic) medicine, speaks its language fluently. Restoring balance and regulation to the inherent rhythm and relationship between *yin*'s rest-and-digest state and *yang*'s awake-and-alert state is crucial to helping trauma survivors find healing. Since this fundamental regulation resides in the body, the remedies we present in Part Three are all rooted in body-based, energetic approaches.

Qi is AAM's unique contribution to the treatment of trauma and traumatic stress. *Qi* is primordial—it powers the impulses that drive the fight, flight, and freeze functions expressed by our most primal instinct for self-preservation. Through this lens, when our self-protective responses are interrupted or thwarted, we see a disruption of the movement and organization of *qi*. An incomplete survival response prevents our *qi* from moving through the natural rise and fall that typically restores the regulation and relationship between *yin* and *yang*. Instead, energy is blocked, backed up, or distorted. This distorted *qi* then wreaks havoc in our tissues, dominates our mind and emotions, and holds our spirit hostage.

Our health is influenced by the quality, quantity, and balance of our *qi*/energy. Our *qi* can become depleted. It can become stuck or disorganized. But no matter how depleted, stuck, or disorganized we may feel—we can always work with *qi* to restore, release, or reorder the body's energy and support our innate capacity for healing. So long as we are alive, *qi* is available to support us.

The Law of the Five Elements

The ancient Chinese lived an agrarian lifestyle. Their lives were governed by and organized around the rise and fall of the agricultural calendar—the time for the planting, growth, flowering, harvest, and decline of crops separated the annual cycle into five identifiable phases. These Taoist farmers and philosophers divided the same "seasonal pie" that the West divides into four seasons into five, adding late summer to autumn, winter, spring, and summer.

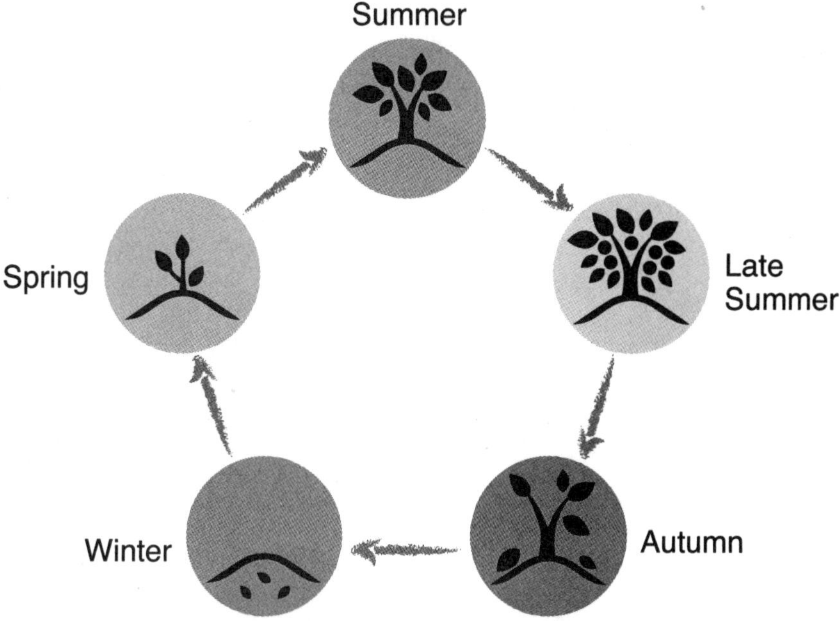

FIGURE 3.1. Five Element Cycle by Seasons

The Taoists identified an association between their experience of each of these five seasonal phases with a corresponding Element: Metal (autumn), Water (winter), Wood (spring), Fire (summer), and Earth (late summer). These Elements are not static constituents of life—as might be embraced in a Western framework—but are expressions of movement and relationship. Each of these Elements helps to generate vitality for the functions of the next Element around this cycle. Metal creates Water, Water creates Wood, Wood creates Fire, Fire creates Earth, and Earth creates Metal. Just as spring precedes and gives rise to summer, the Wood Element precedes and gives rise to Fire. In an agricultural sense, we can see that an unusually cold or dry spring will not give rise to the same quality or quantity of apples on the trees in the following summer as a more typical spring might.[11]

Just as each season brings essential qualities for the success of the entire agricultural cycle, each of these Elements is similarly essential for all living things. In a metaphoric sense, we too need quality minerals, water, support to sprout, the sun's warmth and light, and the right soil for our growth. When any one of these Elements is deficient or dysregulated, we feel unbalanced, and symptoms may arise. This differentiation became the foundation for Taoism's Law of the Five Elements.

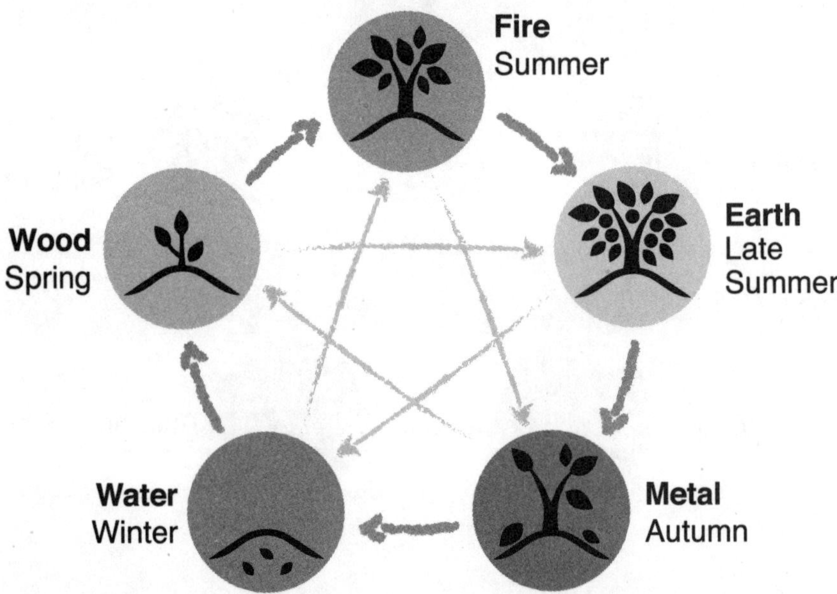

FIGURE 3.2. The Five Element Cycle with Seasons and Elements

The Taoists also recognized nature's gift of containment and the limits it places on growth. The generation of life expressed in this cycle of seasons and Elements risks turning into its opposite without balancing controls. Every sprout needs water, but too much water will rot its roots. Every fire needs wood, but too much wood will snuff it out. Every compost pile needs heat, but too much heat will kill the bacteria and insects that break down vegetable peels and create rich soil. Carbon needs the pressure of the earth to produce diamonds, but that same pressure will obstruct tender roots trying to penetrate the soil in search of trace minerals. We too can be given too many minerals, too much water; we can be pushed to sprout too soon, be exposed to too much sun, or be planted in the wrong soil—all of which will disturb our healing journey.

These wise Taoists acknowledged that nature also provides a "control cycle" that exists alongside the "generative cycle" and creates life-giving tension. Each Element both generates the subsequent Element in the cycle and controls or inhibits the growth of the Element across from it. Metal prunes Wood, Water extinguishes Fire, Wood stabilizes Earth, Fire melts Metal, and Earth contains Water.

The model of the Five Elements provides a framework for working with the tension between the generation of life (expressed in the movement from season to season around the outside of this circle) and the control of that generation (expressed in the arrows that reach across its center).

The Taoists' instruction to live in harmony with nature, together with their agrarian lifestyle, made them keen observers of the movements and relationships inherent in the agricultural cycle. They took direction from each season's characteristic tasks and considered how each phase could guide choices about their own daily activities, their health, and even their spiritual journey.

Lessons were found in each phase of the year. For example, they noted that in winter, while the fields lay fallow and animals hibernated, humans too felt the need for deep rest and a calling to engage in quiet contemplation. With the increasing light of spring came a surge of energy and vitality that supported the preparation of the fields for planting and created a sense of hope for the coming year. Maturing fruit on the vines in summer gave them a carefree sense of fullness that supported playfulness and heartfelt connections. The ripening of grain in late summer called them to harvest and store nature's bounty and supported an appreciation of the sweetness of life. The dying of the growing season in autumn required the collection of dead plant matter to compost to create fertilizer for the season to come, leaving them melancholy and in thoughtful preparation for their own eventual death.

Beyond agriculture, Taoist scholars reflected on a wide range of phenomena that appeared to share similar metaphoric affinities—those they resonated with—the five energetic expressions or phases of the agricultural cycle. Everything, in its own time, is conceived, born, matures, declines, and dies.

The movement through the cycle of seasons is also mirrored in our daily cycle. In balance, we rest in the night, make plans and engage in activities during the day, complete our daily tasks, harvest the lessons of our day, and let go of its imperfections at day's end. People, organizations, ideas, experiences, and even governmental dynasties seem to mirror nature in their evolution. The rise and fall of each phase shares metaphoric correlations that can inform how we plan our days, relate to the institutions we create, and reflect on the movement of our thoughts, dreams, and aspirations.

The phases of the agricultural cycle also exist as metaphors in every day, every experience, and every life. Nature is our constant teacher—revealing insights in all of life's cycles, in addition to the seasonal one.

Taoist scholarship developed over many hundreds of years. It came to include patterns and associations in health and illness that were codified through the Five Elements into a system that includes the organs, emotions, senses, body tissues, psychological challenges, and spiritual gifts. These phenomena correlate with one another at the interface of body, mind, emotions, and spirit.

Later chapters will explore this correlative thinking, or resonance, between what appear to be disparate phenomena and how those correlations can inform our understanding of the impact of traumatic stress. (See Appendix 1 for a more comprehensive description of the Five Element correspondences in the context of the self-protective response).

For the ancient Chinese, the Law of the Five Elements provided the beginning of a coherent, scientific understanding of the nature of being. It replaced earlier concepts of health and illness that were rooted in shamanic practice and supernatural influences. Manfred Porkert, a German sinologist, credits the theoretical framework of the Law of the Five Elements for the formation of AAM's systematic and scientific basis.[12]

THE SELF-PROTECTIVE RESPONSE AND THE FIVE ELEMENTS

Our approach builds on the work of Dr. Peter Levine, who developed the Somatic Experiencing model of trauma treatment. His exploration of the threat response cycle, which manifests in predator-prey relationships in the animal kingdom, gave rise to his recognition that humans share similar responses to threat. While human beings are most often predators, we are sometimes also prey. As part of the universal Tao, we experience the same responses to threat that all animals do. We may respond by fighting, as would a lion; by fleeing, as might a deer; or freezing, as a rabbit might.

Levine's seminal work outlined five distinct and universal steps animals (and humans) move through as they detect and survive danger or life threat. He named these phases *arrest/startle, defensive orienting, specific self-protective response* (fight, flight, or freeze), *completion,* and *integration.*[13] While various models articulate how humans carry out self-protection in response to threat, Levine's version has been the most informative for us in our integration of the self-protective response with the theories of AAM.

Threat response is the common term used to describe how we react to threat. However, we have chosen the term *self-protective response* as a way of describing the entire sequence of response to potential threat. We find it to be a more affirming, empowering, and descriptive term, particularly with trauma survivors, who may still be living with a sense of threat every day—and who may have highly charged reactions to the word *threat.* We use *5-SPR* as shorthand for these five steps of self-protection. The identifiable phases of this self-protective response—those that typically occur when we are successful in our response—are as follows:

1. Arrest/startle: In response to something new in the environment—a sound, smell, or movement—we pause to assess the change and judge whether it might be potentially threatening. There is a slight arousal in the SNS.
2. Defensive orienting: We work to evaluate the source of the possible threat, assess the magnitude of the potential encounter, and seek escape routes. Arousal increases in the SNS.
3. Specific self-protective response: We fight, flee, freeze, submit, or move toward help and support. SNS arousal increases in fight or flight; if our efforts are unsuccessful, our PNS overwhelms it in a freeze response.

4. Completion: Our self-protective efforts prove successful. Balance between SNS and PNS returns, manifesting with a relaxed and rhythmic heartbeat and breath.
5. Integration: We integrate our experience of success, assimilating lessons learned to help us manage future similar circumstances. After this stage, we can begin a return to curiosity and exploration of our environment.

One of the core concepts in Levine's Somatic Experiencing model of trauma resolution is that interruption at any step of this self-protection effort leads to an incomplete survival response, which, in turn, shapes and alters how we respond to future situations and environments. Levine postulated that successful completion of all five phases is ideal for diminishing the negative effects of trauma. Significantly, he also found that disruptions at different phases of the survival response left different physiological imprints on the survivor.

He noted, for example, that someone whose survival response was thwarted at the first awareness of threat has a distinctly different experience and physiological imprint than someone whose response was interrupted in the midst of mobilizing a response. Each step of the threat response holds a different type of physiological survival demand—locating the source of the threat requires all our sensory systems to go on high alert, while fighting against that threat requires active mobilization of our physical protective responses. These demands provoke specific types of physiological and behavioral activity that may persist after the threat has passed—we may, for example, feel compelled to continually scan our environment for potential threat, or may remain chronically braced (that is, tensed in constant anticipation of some kind of threat) in our muscle system.

Understanding the neurophysiological changes in the body that occur in each of the five steps of the self-protective response helps us better comprehend the puzzling physical symptoms or behavioral expressions in someone who experienced an incomplete survival effort or unresolved traumatic stress. Note how this movement reflects rising into *yang* (activity) and falling into *yin* (closure). Within this fluid rise and fall, the Five Elements mirror Levine's articulation. Everything, including our 5-SPR, begins as an impulse, takes shape, becomes an action, comes to completion, and finds closure.

The movement through the Five Elements moves in parallel with Levine's model for the steps animals and humans use when navigating a threat. By overlaying the five steps of the self-protective response with the Five Elements (see chart below), we can deepen our understanding of both the neurophysiology of trauma and the energetics of AAM.

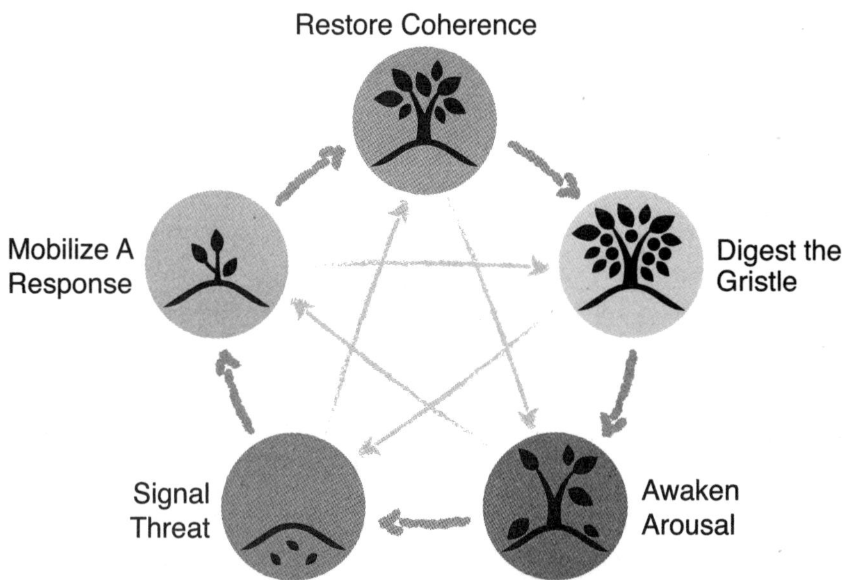

FIGURE 3.3. The Five Elements and the Five Steps of the 5-SPR

Both the Western bio-behavioral perspective and AAM's energetic view provide useful information for understanding how dysregulation and imbalance can manifest when efforts at self-protection are interrupted or thwarted. Each perspective informs the other and further reveals how traumatic stress impacts our health and vitality and can support the creation of integrative approaches that better serve the restoration of balance and regulation in trauma survivors.

THE SELF-PROTECTIVE RESPONSE

SELF-PROTECTIVE RESPONSE		SEASON	ELEMENT
In 5-SPR terms	In AAM terms		
Arrest/Startle	*Awaken Arousal*	*Autumn*	*Metal*
Defensive Orienting	*Signal Threat*	*Winter*	*Water*
Specific Self-Protective Response	*Mobilize a Response*	*Spring*	*Wood*
Completion	*Restore Coherence*	*Summer*	*Fire*
Integration	*Digest the Gristle*	*Late Summer*	*Earth*

In the section below, we present in greater detail the intriguing parallel between Levine's observations of the self-protective response from the perspective of bio-behavioral science and the ancient Taoist understanding of the cycle of life, as applied to the same self-protective response.

FROM AAM: AWAKEN AROUSAL; CORRESPONDS WITH METAL/AUTUMN

The growing season is over. We take time to pause and reflect on its success. If nothing breaks our pause, we simply enjoy the clearer, fresher air and the inspiration that comes with autumn's beauty. Our system finds regulation in its easy inhale and exhale. All our sense organs are relaxed, curious, and available, but not "activated."

If this pause is broken by a sense that something is amiss, arousal is awakened—our senses become alert and focused on this phenomenon so we can assess whether it is threatening.

In contrast to the Western view of a linear response cycle with a beginning, middle, and end, AAM holds that each phase is part of a continuous and ongoing cycle. The awakening arousal function of the Metal Element arises out of the clarity that comes from having returned to an easy inhale and exhale via the full integration of any previous experiences of threat.

Our capacity to experience this arousal rests in our ability to pause and reflect on our previous success. Like the dead leaves that break down and add critical trace minerals to a compost pile for next year's garden, our previous life lessons are broken down to help us prepare for our next growing season. Extracting our own "trace minerals" and eliminating any remaining waste from our experiences helps us start fresh the next time we need to respond to a potential threat.

Like the agricultural calendar, which finds both its first and last breath in the autumn, the 5-SPR comes full circle in autumn's Metal Element. From the AAM perspective, this is both the beginning and the ending of a cycle.

FROM THE WEST: ARREST/STARTLE

We move from a platform of open and curious exploration to note novelty in our environment. We stop and make use of our sense organs to gather information. Alertness increases, our body begins to prepare a response to a potential threat to help ensure survival. Our focus narrows, goose bumps may rise or body hair may stand on end. Our breath catches, and we experience a pervading sense that something is amiss, often experienced in our guts.

FROM AAM: SIGNAL THREAT; CORRESPONDS WITH WATER/WINTER

All of nature is resting deeply. Fields lie fallow, animals hibernate, and we too are called to profound quiet and contemplation. Wisdom emerges in a time of reflection that echoes winter's icy ponds.

Winter is the harshest of all seasons. Our quiet contemplation can easily become its paired opposite—a consuming fear arising from questions about the future: How long will this winter last? Is the year's harvest sufficient to carry me through until spring? Am I hearty enough to weather winter's severity?

In the 5-SPR, it is the Water Element's vulnerability and capacity to communicate fear that signals life threat. The Water Element's association with the Kidney/adrenal system provides both the energetic and biochemical signaling of the presence of life threat. Fear is a consuming messenger. It alarms the entire body-mind-spirit.

FROM THE WEST: DEFENSIVE ORIENTING

We gather information about our environment in a focused, survival-oriented way. We are no longer open and curious; instead, we are focused on identifying the threat, assessing the magnitude of a potential encounter, looking for safe social connections, means of escaping, or weapons. We gather the information necessary to make critical choices for our survival.

FROM AAM: MOBILIZE A RESPONSE; CORRESPONDS WITH WOOD/SPRING

Spring is characterized by the return of light. It wakes up dormant seeds, trees, and all of life to a new growing season. Nature's surge of energy and vitality supports us to make plans for this year's growth and restores a sense of hope for the future that may have been lost in winter's darkness.

Like the bulbs bursting through winter's packed-down soil, we feel able to push through or break down obstacles in our path and find our way forward toward new growth opportunities.

In terms of the 5-SPR, the energy of spring, mirrored in the Wood Element, is reflected in the sympathetic nervous system. It supports us to orient to threatening circumstances, plan our escape, and feel empowered to mobilize a fight-or-flight response for our protection.

FROM THE WEST: SPECIFIC SELF-PROTECTIVE RESPONSE

We are compelled into specific self-protective actions—fight, flight, or freeze. We may also seek social connection or utilize submission. Our focus turns exclusively to whatever may support our survival.

FROM AAM: RESTORE COHERENCE; CORRESPONDS WITH FIRE/SUMMER

The sun is at its peak. Summer's days are long and warm. Fruit is set on the vines. The harshness of winter and the struggle to till soil and plant seeds in spring is over—our garden is mature, vibrant, and vital.

In terms of the 5-SPR, the Fire Element can give us a heartfelt recognition that we moved through the awaken arousal, signal threat, and mobilize a response phases successfully. Like our garden, we too feel more mature, vibrant, and vital. Our regulated, peaceful, and invisible heartbeat creates a sense of peace and propriety in the entire kingdom of the body.

The Fire can help us embrace a sense of fullness that gives rise to qualities of playfulness and heartfelt connection. There are sufficient resources and bounty "on the vine" to support the community to relax, celebrate, and enjoy the vibrancy we have cultivated.

FROM THE WEST: COMPLETION

We complete the act of self-protection and recognize our success and survival. We experience a sense of whole-body coherence, coming into alignment with our now-regulated heartbeat.

FROM AAM: DIGEST THE GRISTLE; CORRESPONDS WITH EARTH/LATE SUMMER

The energies of all the previous seasons have created the bounty of late summer. The produce in the fields is ripe, sweet, and nurturing. We can now harvest and store this abundance for the coming year—and enjoy the sweetness of life.

In terms of the 5-SPR, the Earth Element signals our body to restore peristalsis—the contractions in the walls of the digestive organs that push digested food onward. We are able now to "digest the gristle" in both our food and our experiences of traumatic stress. We break down and harvest the lessons that can nurture us in future challenges, should they arise in any one of these phases. The Earth Element helps us to integrate these lessons into the flesh of our existence.

As noted in the first step of the AAM-informed 5-SPR, we are immersed in the continuous flow of the seasons and their elemental relationships in the natural world. As we flow naturally through the integration of our experiences, so too do we return to the open, sensate curiosity associated with the Metal and the potential held within the awaken arousal phase. We take time to savor the feeling of success, victory, and pride in overcoming obstacles and proving ourselves strong enough to survive a challenge. We acknowledge the self-confidence we have earned. We can now return to curiosity and exploration—of our environment, of other people, and of the beauty we find in our perfect world.

FROM THE WEST: INTEGRATION

We integrate our experience and harvest insights about how to respond to similar experiences in the future. The easy rise and fall between sympathetic arousal and parasympathetic restoration is restored. Peristalsis returns to our digestive organs. We are grateful for the new skills we have learned.

This integration of the Western bio-behavioral perspective with the Five Element theory of AAM serves as the foundation for our East-meets-West orientation for exploring and working with the impact of traumatic stress.

THE FIVE SURVIVOR TYPES

Our concept of survivor types grows out of the Five Element school of AAM and its concept of *constitutional focus* (or *factor*) as an approach to diagnosis and treatment. By drawing a connection between a thwarted step of the 5-SPR and its corresponding element in AAM, a new diagnostic framework opens, one that distinguishes a constellation of symptoms or phenomena that share an affiliation with the disrupted step in the 5-SPR.

The idea that we are born with a particular constitution is widespread in the foundations of AAM. At various times, the concept of a *constitutional type* has been presented as a four-fold, five-fold, or six-fold construct. We are using the Five Element style, developed and refined for the West by Dr. J. R. Worsley,[14] whose model focuses on the physical body, as well as the mind and spirit, and embraces both the strengths and challenges inherent in each type. For purposes of this discussion, we will set aside the unanswerable question of whether this constitutional type is inherited or the result of early life experience.[15] Any of us who either has a sibling or has more than one child will easily recognize that in spite of similar genetic backgrounds, we are all born with a distinct and unique nature.

Our constitutional type can be thought of as an expression of our personality or our nature. Our type informs how we harvest life's gifts, as well as how we navigate life's challenges. As we go through life, we tend to get "snagged" in the Element (Metal, Water, etc.) most closely reflecting our true nature. In most circumstances, we will repair the snag and continue around the cycle of life. However, if we get snagged too deeply or too often, a more permanent wound will open in our psyche and our tissues.

Are we missing certain minerals? Do we need more water, a sturdier sprout, warmer sun, or better soil in order to truly flourish? Which of these essential Elements, when provided in the exact right proportion, would support our whole "plant" to grow? The answer to this question can influence every aspect of our lives—including how we respond to danger or life threat.

The Worsley Five Element model posits that focusing support or resolving dysregulation in the particular Element that most reflects our nature—and the organ systems that Element includes—will simultaneously help bring regulation to our whole being,[16] and each of these five requirements for life.[17]

Our "type" is an expression of the duality between our greatest strengths and our greatest weaknesses. While all Five Elements exist in dynamic relationship with each other for all of us, and each may be impacted in a traumatic experience, this one particular Element—the one that is most reflective of our constitutional nature—is often an indication of where we are most likely to have been challenged in the 5-SPR. This is most likely where and how the incomplete stress response will be stored in our body-mind-spirit. Thus, our embodied experience, or the meaning we make of our experience, is a deeper reflection of trauma's impact than the circumstances or facts relating to it.

It is important to note that while the Five Element model provides a helpful construct, in no way should it be understood to categorize people who have experienced trauma. We each have a certain constitutional affinity for one of the Five Elements, but we contain and embody all of these Elements, in varying proportions. All Five Elements function in dynamic relationship with each other inside us and affect how we relate with others. As in an orchestra, sometimes the wind instruments come forward, and sometimes the strings, the horns, or the percussion section. All the instruments are there, but one section is speaking the loudest during a particular movement. Each person has his or her own unique experience and way of responding to circumstances. Similarly, when we use the term *survivor,* we do so with the utmost respect for the deep strength and courage that underlies any individual's efforts to continue on in the face of sometimes overwhelming challenge.

We have restricted our exploration of the diagnostic framework of the Five Elements to our client's experience in the 5-SPR, leaving its other and more complex diagnostic information for providers who are trained to provide other and more unique treatments within the scope of AAM with this information. We trust that this exploration will help providers identify which of these five survivor types describes the impact and experience of traumatic stress in their client most accurately. The Five Elements provide a framework for understanding the connection between apparently disparate symptoms that cluster together in resonant relationship with each other. They provide a sense of order to the often complex, overlapping, and overwhelming symptoms many trauma survivors experience—symptoms that may appear to be random or disconnected when looked at from an exclusively Western paradigm. And they can inform helpful interventions for complex clients.[18]

Each survivor type will be explored in its own chapter in Part Three. Here we provide a simple overview of the interplay between the survivor types and the 5-SPR. This summary also provides a sense of the basic structure of the Five Element model. As you read, notice how the imagery, metaphors, and meaning these ancient scholars developed continues to speak to us today, deepening our understanding of the impact of traumatic stress—and of how we heal.

The Metal Type: The Arrest/Startle Phase—Awaken Arousal

If we are a Metal type, we are more likely to have been interrupted in the arrest/startle or awaken arousal phase of the 5-SPR. As a result, we may have a tendency to be overly responsive to novelty in the environment—voices in the hallway or a slamming door may cause us to startle and feel jumpy. It will be difficult for us to settle. Once our arousal has been awakened, it will be hard to soothe and quiet that arousal.

In the Metal element, the Lungs are paired with the Colon. Together, they support balance and connection between our taking in and letting go, our inhaling and exhaling. When our Metal is healthy, our Lungs regulate the rhythm of our breath and help us receive "*qi* from the heavens."[19] At the same time, our Colon helps us "let go of life's imperfections."[20] Our Metal helps us hold life's tragedies in a broad context. Just as each exhale is connected to each inhale, the Metal element reminds us that imperfection is necessarily part and parcel of an essentially perfect world. Our Metal supports our capacity to make connections with others, despite the toll that loss and grief can extract as a cost of loving.

If our capacity to receive inspiration and let go of imperfections has been wounded, we may find ourselves full of grief. Anyone who's experienced grief knows it can be one of the most debilitating emotional states to live with. We may struggle to find a fresh breath to inspire a new chapter in our lives. It becomes difficult to inhale—to receive life and the gifts available in the present moment—or to exhale and let go of the past. We lose sight of our own value and our vital connection with others. It becomes difficult to allow a new reality to take the place of what's been lost—and to let go of challenging experiences, circumstances, or people.

The task of transforming grief and loss, receiving inspiration, and letting go of waste often calls us to ethereal or spiritual realms. Deeply existential questions, like, "How can a loving God allow bad things to happen to good people?" can plague us.

The Water Type: Defensive Orienting Phase—Signal Threat

If we are a Water survivor type, we are more likely to have been interrupted in the defensive orienting or signal threat phase of the 5-SPR. Our whole body-mind-spirit becomes alarmed when fear in the Kidney/adrenal system signals threat. Loss of the ability to regulate this function leaves us unable to turn off the signal of imminent danger, and we may be at a greater risk for over-response when encountering threats in the future. Fear, or the lack of fear, predominates and may consume our worldview.

In its healthiest and most balanced state, the Water element is a source of deep wisdom, of deep listening to our own inner knowing and that of others. We are able to hear, receive, and reflect upon information that may be uncomfortable or frightening to acknowledge. Water types draw on their considerable emotional and physical reserves to meet the challenges of life. They have copious will, ambition, and determination to survive and prosper. This power to overcome fear and surmount obstacles originates in the Water element.

When our Water element is unbalanced, we can't utilize our fear effectively or productively. We may struggle to differentiate safety from threat. Our eyes scan constantly in anxious and fearful attention, and we may not sleep, out of fear of what may come in the night. We are either hypervigilant and fearful or completely fearless, putting ourselves in dangerous situations without noticing the risks around us. At one end, we are agoraphobic and unable to leave our homes; at the other, we can't sit or be still. We constantly thrash at the surface, unable to dive deeply and find the pearls created by the grit in our deep, dark life experiences. It is difficult for us to receive sincere expressions of reassurance from others, and we find it difficult to find secure boundaries around us or to recognize a boundary between ourselves and others.

The Kidneys and the Bladder are the organs associated with the Water. Physically, they manage the storage and movement of urine and other fluids. Mentally, they help us find anchors for our own truth, helping us avoid anxious and fearful states. Emotionally, they help us create a container for the fear that would otherwise leave us scared speechless. Spiritually, they help us find the faith needed to imagine spring's return.

The Wood Type: Specific Self-Protection Response Phase—Mobilize a Response

If we are a Wood survivor type, we are more likely to have been interrupted in the specific self-protective response or mobilize a response phase of the 5-SPR. The Wood Element's essential nature is benevolence. When our efforts to actively protect or defend ourselves or others—by fighting or fleeing—are thwarted, we can become angry (fight) or lose our capacity for assertion (flight). We will see obstacles rather than openings. We may live with constant frustration, anger, and resentment disproportionate to our circumstances. Or the opposite may be true—we may be excessively timid and unable to mobilize defenses to protect ourselves. We suffer from threats that others might navigate with ease. Over time, we may lose our sense of direction or purpose.

The Liver and Gall Bladder are the organ systems of the Wood Element. In AAM, the Liver is responsible for strategic planning, long-range vision, the forceful execution of actions, and protection of the body. The Gall Bladder supports regulation of body systems. The Liver helps us create long-term, strategic plans, while the Gall Bladder carries them out, step-by-step and moment by moment.

In its most balanced and healthy state, our Wood Element helps us chart new beginnings, imagine our future, make good decisions, mobilize strategic responses to threats, and flow smoothly around obstacles and through life. When our Wood Element is out of balance, we can become blinded by anger. On the mental and emotional plane, we can't find hope for the future—our metaphorical growing season. We are depressed, immobilized, and unable to find our way around obstacles. We can become excessively tight, angry, and resentful. We may not check to see if the door is unlocked before we break it down.

The Fire Type: Completion Phase—Restore Coherence

If we are a Fire type, we are more likely to have been interrupted during the completion or restore coherence phase of the 5-SPR. We have difficulty integrating an embodied experience of our successful survival. We struggle to trust our instincts and abilities. We constantly feel we got something wrong. A pervasive sense of failure is the hallmark of interruption of this phase in the 5-SPR. Joy becomes illusive, and we can be overcome by a sense of panic.

While all the other Elements are composed of two organs, the Fire Element is composed of four. Together they function as a team that manages all the matters of the Heart. In AAM, the regulation of the Heart critically influences all other organ systems.

In classical AAM literature, the Heart is called the *Supreme Controller.* AAM posits that the welfare of the entire "kingdom" of the body depends on the health of the Heart. The Heart corresponds to the mind in AAM. Its functions mirror those of the neocortex. The Heart, along with its partner, the Small Intestine, supports our capacity for an expansive mind. Together, they call us to high consciousness—a sense of one heart beating in all of humanity.

The Pericardium, or Heart Protector, and its partner, the Triple Heater are two "organs" in AAM that do not correspond to any in Western medicine and will be discussed in greater depth in Chapter Nine. They relate to our connections with others and to our ability to find joy and pleasure in our relationships, especially with our most vulnerable and intimate expressions. When our Fire is most balanced and healthy, we experience joy and readily find peace. These two "organs" support our capacity to have open-hearted relationships with others and compassion for those who suffer, to enjoy our sexual expression, and to find pleasure in life.

If we are successful in our response to threat, the Heart signals our success by sending a message of regulation to the body-mind-spirit in the form of a regular heartbeat. Balance between *yin* and *yang* is restored, which is expressed by the even and steady rhythm of the heart.

When our Fire is out of balance, we face extreme difficulty relating to others. Our eyes and emotions feel flat. We can't connect with ourselves—we might be agitated and jumpy, or we may lack a sense of vitality and sparkle. We can't connect with others; we feel socially awkward and can't embrace play. Feeling vulnerable and safe in relationships is challenging. We may choose untrustworthy people as friends. We may have little sexual interest. Or, conversely, we may feel manic, vivacious, and overly interested in sexual contact, but the connection is mechanical or abusive, lacking intimacy and heart. We are prone to panic attacks, may experience heart irregularities or impaired memory and cognition, or may find it challenging to take control in situations that require nuanced discrimination between safety and threat.

The Earth Type: Integration Phase—Digest the Gristle

If we are an Earth survivor type, we are more likely to have been interrupted in the integration or digest-the-gristle phase of the 5-SPR. We may struggle to integrate the lessons inherent in life-threatening experiences. We may feel compelled to relive such experiences again and again, trying desperately to extract meaning and significance from them. Not metabolizing lessons from life's hard knocks leaves us more vulnerable to future threats. If we are unable to integrate the lesson of burning our fingers on a hot stove or failing to look both ways before crossing a street, we will have trouble navigating life. We may crave sympathetic nurturance and long to feel understood. Or, conversely, we may reject offers of support. We see ourselves as the victim.

The Spleen and Stomach are the organ systems of the Earth Element. The Stomach receives nourishment, and the Spleen transforms it into *qi* and blood and distributes it to the community of our body. Together, they create a dynamic balance between receiving and giving. In a successful 5-SPR, the Spleen and Stomach break down the experience of life threat; transform it into manageable, bite-sized pieces; and help us assimilate or metabolize the lessons inherent in our experience. They "digest the gristle" in the stew of life and harvest the nourishment inherent in that stew. The Earth Element helps us find our ground and stability.

THE FIVE ELEMENT CORRESPONDENCES AS A RESONANT FRAMEWORK

Part Three of the *Tao of Trauma* explores the network of Five Element correspondences—clusters of phenomena that include organs, tissues, emotions, psychological themes, spiritual challenges, *and phases in the 5-SPR* that share a resonant or energetic relationship with each other. While they may seem unrelated in a Western paradigm, they are connected in dynamic and nuanced relationship through the AAM understanding of *qi.* These correspondences can help guide clinicians to access and support the completion of a particular phase of the 5-SPR that may be hidden from view but remains in embodied memory. Restoring normal regulation in one aspect of the network of correspondences associated with a particular 5-SPR phase will free up valuable inner resources in our client—physiological, psychological, and spiritual.

In the conceptual framework of this ancient healing tradition, the correspondences provide an important framework for understanding how *qi,* the energy inherent in all living things, expresses itself and can be worked with to support optimal health. Below you will find a classic Five Element chart showing each element, its role in the 5-SPR, and its corresponding emotion and organ systems.

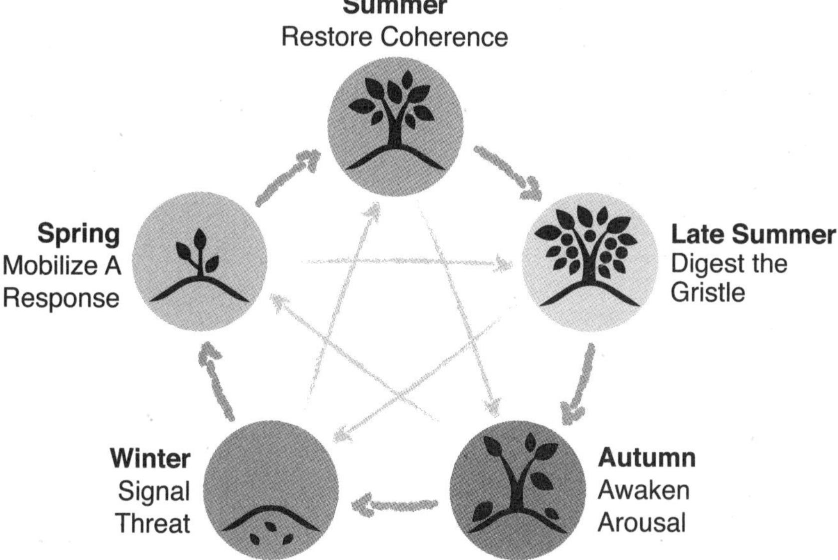

FIGURE 3.4. The Five Element Cycle with Correspondences of the 5-SPR

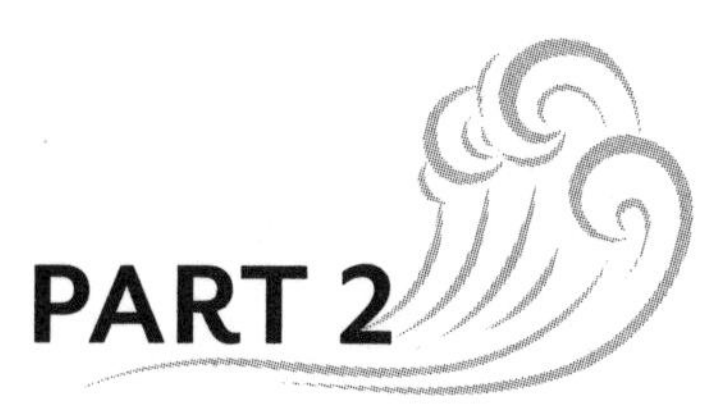

PART 2

PREPARING FOR CARING

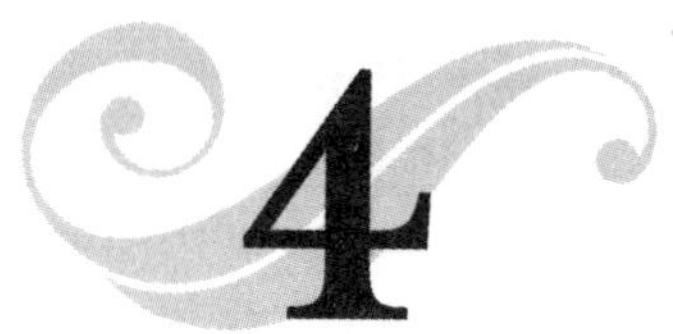

Touch, Coherence, and Resonance

THIS CHAPTER AND the one that follows present theoretical and practical guidance for working with all survivor types. Readers who already have extensive experience with touch may choose to skim these two chapters and move on to Part Three, where specific remedies appropriate to each survivor type are presented.

We begin with a theoretical orientation and conceptual framework for our bottom-up, energetic orientation to treating trauma survivors, and we also explore the nature of various body tissues and their role in the 5-SPR. Chapter Five focuses on how we can incorporate these principles into the more practical considerations of our work with clients—how to frame a session, pace treatment, and find ways to safely and ethically incorporate touch into your practice. It also explores how this approach might be incorporated into various disciplines, the scope of practice concerns, and the many ways integrative medicine is already providing hope for trauma survivors.

Many of the remedies we present in this book involve touch. Touch is as vital to our existence as food.[1] It is the first sense we develop, our first and most primal communication, and the only sense without which we cannot survive.[2] Many trauma survivors are starving for safe and nourishing touch, even if the idea of touch or physical closeness may also leave them feeling uncomfortable.

Touch has the power to reach beyond language to cultivate experience-dependent maturation of brain functions that were delayed or stunted by the lack of touch, wrong touch, or other traumatic experiences from infancy or childhood.[3] Those who find sexual intimacy, physical proximity, or emotional closeness challenging as a result of trauma may not have a safe person with whom they can experience nourishing touch. Providing survivors with safe touch and safe relationship can restore their capacity to access this primal human communication and repair the developmental functions that may have been waylaid by an overwhelming demand for survival long ago.[4]

We use the term *touch* to imply a range of clinical interventions. Physical touch is one—using various types of physical contact that include purposeful placement of hands, as well as the conscientious calibration of touch when working with trapped and disrupted energies in the body. *Somatic mindfulness* is another type of touch, even though it does not involve actual physical contact. In this, clinicians utilize body awareness and guided attention to enhance their observations and understanding of a client's inner process. Using this awareness, providers can help clients increase the embodiment of their experience.

Touch can support the creation of a safe, secure, and respectful "relational field" for trauma survivors. This relational field is critical for those whose first trauma occurred before language developed[5] and for those who experienced overwhelming and repeated trauma as adults.[6]

The context within which a provider works may prevent the use of physical touch. With that in mind, we also present several body-oriented methods that don't include physical touch. There are some providers who do not plan to use touch with their clients. We encourage them to read the discussion of touch anyway, as they will benefit from a deeper understanding and awareness of the bio-physiology of traumatic stress, how healing happens in the body, how it's experienced by a survivor, and when a referral to a provider who does incorporate touch would enhance or facilitate their client's process.

TOUCH AND THE HUMAN EXPERIENCE

As we explained in Chapter Two—and will discuss more deeply in Chapters Nine and Ten—infants need a caregiver to serve as an external parasympathetic nervous system until they are older and their capacity to self-soothe is more fully available.[7] Infants' ventral vagus nerve, which helps them mitigate unnecessary sympathetic hyperarousal, is not fully myelinated at birth, and while its myelination happens rapidly in the first year of life, it is not fully functional until late adolescence. Infants therefore lack the physiological capacity to self-soothe, self-regulate, or enter into parasympathetic rest-and-digest states on their own. They learn to regulate themselves by co-regulating with their caregivers, largely through loving and safe touch.

Touch is the primary communication between infants and their caregivers. John Bowlby's classic work on the dynamics of infant attachment describes the long-term impact on people who did not receive sufficient touch and loving attention as infants. His theory suggests that children have an instinctive, biological need to form a safe attachment, and it asserts that both infants and their caregivers are physiologically hardwired for touch. From an evolutionary point of view, babies whose crying and smiling helped ensure proximity and contact with their caregiver were more likely to survive and thus have children of their own. An attached and attentive caregiver is protective and watchful, and offers a child comfort in times of distress and arousal. Bowlby further asserts that attachment to a primary caregiver influences all future attachments and that disruptions to this attachment can have significant consequences—particularly for the development of sociable behaviors and healthy relationships in adulthood.[8]

Conscious and safe touch communicates a wide range of emotions across cultures. It sends a cascade of chemical reactions into motion. Research has demonstrated the helpful impact touch therapies can have on cortisol, dopamine, oxytocin, and serotonin levels, resulting in similarly positive effects on parent-infant bonding, relational satisfaction,[9] and depression.[10] It can also help bring awareness to processing interoceptive messages, such as those arising from phobias, sensory integration disturbances, and boundary ruptures.[11] The term *interoception* refers to our subjective perception of body states.[12]

Likely because of its deep physiological and relational impact, touch can be a double-edged sword for trauma survivors. It can both trigger the perception of threat and provide a critical container for safety. Using touch with trauma survivors is similar to early humans harnessing fire—it is a potent force, with potential to inflict harm if used inappropriately, but it is also life sustaining and nourishing when understood and used appropriately. Like our ancestors who, over time, learned to manage fire, survive cold winters, cook food, and advance society, we can learn to use touch as a life-sustaining and coherence-building tool.

Touching survivors who experienced a lack of touch or an "unsafe" touch can trigger flashbacks, bracing, or collapse in the body and mind of survivors. It is not always appropriate to use touch, at least in the early part of treatment. At the same time, when used correctly, touch can reach beyond words to support the creation of primal and embodied states of safety and connection. This is why it is so important to learn to touch intelligently, judiciously, and intentionally.

The use of touch, as with all interventions with this population, must be done with a keen understanding of how it may be experienced by its recipient. Many survivors of trauma have negative associations with touch. It may have been used to abuse them, may have been part of a painful medical procedure, or may have overwhelmed their processing capacity for tactile information at a time when their physiology was already overstimulated. Be mindful when you touch, and remain curious about how touch is received by clients moment by moment.

COHERENCE IS CARDIAC REGULATION IN OUR ORGANS AND TISSUES

When fear signals an imminent life threat, the Heart rings all its alarm bells to communicate this threat to every organ and cell. This highly discordant vibration, which is explored more fully in Chapter Nine, has a profound impact on our body, mind, and spirit. Every organ, cell, and body function operates from the same message of alarm, communicated by the heart's increasingly rapid beat. Access to the regulated wave that is our Tao, our true nature, becomes obstructed.

A provider's job is to help clients reconnect with this essential wave. It is always available to support restoration of balance and regulation. Nothing one human being does to another can impact the fundamental, coherent, and dynamic tension between PNS and SNS, *yin* and *yang,* that is found in nature. The rising and setting of the sun, the waxing and waning of the moon, and the movement from winter to summer and back to winter are unbreakable.

When we are safely inside the zone of resiliency described in Chapter One (and which will also be discussed in Chapters Six and Eight) all of our body's systems are working as they are designed to and are communicating effortlessly with one another. The dynamic movement between *yin* and *yang*, PNS and SNS, is functioning as a balanced, fluid, and harmonious wave. There is a sense of wholeness, integration, and connection across all aspects of our body, mind, emotions, and spirit. We feel coherent and cohesive.

Traumatic stress necessarily takes us out of our zone of normal, balanced function and into extra-normal responses that support a variety of survival and management strategies. If we are unable to return to our zone of resiliency after a threat has receded, but instead become habituated to a hyperaroused or hypoaroused state, we will experience an increasing lack of coherence in our whole system.

The term *coherence* originated in physics to describe the ordered distribution of power in a wave, such as a sine wave.[13] Our organs and tissues communicate with each other via rhythms and patterns of *qi*/energy similar to the sine waves studied by physicists. These waves, such as those of the heartbeat or the rise and fall of our breath, arise out of our neurophysiology, impact our biochemistry, and inform our physiological and psychological function. They are the basis for the systems of feedback and interaction from which allostasis—how we distribute stress across multiple body systems in order to maintain stability, which is also discussed in Chapter Three—arises.

Our clinical experience affirms this law of physics: when any system—whether human, automobile, or workplace—is highly coherent, there is less internal conflict and more efficient functioning.[14] We feel better when we experience coherent order and regulation in our bodies, as we do in our communities.

Our bodies are in constant, system-wide, and highly interactive vibratory communication. This communication allows us to adapt to complex and constantly changing social and environmental demands while maintaining our inner balance and stability. The more ordered and harmonious these waves are, the more they contribute to flexibility in our response to stress and the greater our clarity of cognitive function and fluidity in our emotional state. For example, the rhythm of our breath regulates the levels of carbon dioxide and oxygen in our blood, which, in turn, affects our blood pressure, cardiac output, and nerve and muscle excitability, and it can also influence our mental function and focus.

The heart is the primary generator of our vibrational interactions. Beat-to-beat variability in its rhythm communicates everything from peace of mind to abject terror. These vibrations of *qi* have a particular line of communication with our brain's frontal cortex, thalamus, amygdala, and other brain structures, and thus they influence the regulation of our entire body, including our immune, endocrine, neurological, and metabolic systems, as well as fear conditioning and other functions. A coherent heartbeat is one characterized by order, stability, and harmony in its rhythm. It has a positive influence on cognitive performance, emotional experience, and our capacity to regulate or inhibit those primal impulses that, in the wrong context, could be antisocial—such as rage or terror.

While the heart is the organ with the largest and most impactful vibration, all of our organs and tissues use systems of vibrational communication and collaboration to keep each other informed and harmonious. The more coherent or regulated our heart rhythm, the greater the synchrony and message of coherence, or *entrainment,* between all other organs. Physicists describe this as *cross-coherence*—the way in which two or more waves can, over time, cause another rhythm to fall into a synchrony. Our respiratory and heart rhythms, for example, harmonize with each other and then support other body systems, such as our blood pressure and brain or encephalographic rhythms, to join in coherent, system-wide function.

The more coherence we experience in any one tissue or organ, the greater the possibility for cross-coherence between all our tissues and organs—or, we could say, the greater the resonance between that tissue or organ and all other body tissues and functions. In particular, the more coherence we have in our cardiac system, the greater capacity we have to create a coherent, regulated state between our heart and the rest of our body. For our purposes, the more coherent our heart rhythm, the greater capacity we have to bring regulation to patterns of traumatic stress embedded in tissue memory.

The same is true on an interpersonal level. Regulation anywhere supports greater regulation everywhere. The more coherent we are, the easier it is to create states of resonance in our relationships with others. And when we are in resonance with others, we can offer greater empathy, understanding, and compassion—and will be less likely to engage in conflict.[15]

As described in Chapter Nine, AAM mirrors Western research on the central role of the heart in physiological coherence and in the heart's dynamic role in the function of the brain and mind. In fact, the Heart and mind are represented by the same Chinese character—and are thus tied to one another in the language of this culture. AAM understands that when we are troubled in our Hearts, our minds are also troubled, and vice versa. Like Western research on cardiac coherence, AAM affirms that when the Supreme Controller is peaceful, our body—or "kingdom"—is also at peace.

When we experience a felt sense of safety in our tissues, this vibration communicates a sense of coherence that influences the kingdom of our body. Coherence is cardiac regulation in our tissues and organs.

COHERENCE BUILDS RESONANCE BETWEEN SYSTEMS

Coherence and *resonance* are related terms. *Coherence* refers to order or unity within a system. *Resonance* (from Latin *resonantia,* "echo," or *resonare,* "to resound") refers to how one system vibrates with another system.[16] On an inner (personal) level, or micro-level, *resonance* describes how the vibration of various organs or tissues influences others. On a social or macro-level, *resonance* describes how the coherent vibration of an individual influences interpersonal relationships and, by extension, families, communities, or workplaces.

The term *resonance* originated in the field of acoustics. Musicians observed that when a violin string was plucked, it stimulated nearby strings to also vibrate and produce sound.[17] Physicists speak of resonance as a vibration that appears in response to an external stimulus whose vibrational frequency is identical or nearly identical to its own.[18] Thus, resonance is an expression of coherence between systems that have the capacity to respond to one another. Coherence within a system allows the possibility for resonance between similar coherent systems.

Richard Lannon, Fari Amini, and Thomas B. Lewis write eloquently about the function of resonance in human beings in their book *A General Theory of Love.* They explore how our brain chemistry and nervous systems are affected by our close relationships, how we synchronize with each other in ways that influence our emotional health and personality development, and how negative patterns can be transformed and healed. They are clear: "Our nervous systems are not self-contained, but rather demonstrably attuned to those around us with whom we share a close connection." They have a name for this unique capacity in mammals to attune to and exchange with another's inner state: *limbic resonance.*[19]

In *The Wise Heart,* Buddhist teacher Jack Kornfield correlates these findings of Western psychology with Buddhist thought: "Each time we meet another human being and honor their dignity, we help those around us. Their hearts resonate with ours in exactly the same way the strings of an unplucked violin vibrate with the sounds of a violin played nearby. When we meet others with love and respect, it produces a state of heightened resonance in both of us."[20]

Humans are programmed to function as a herd, as if we were one coherent body.[21] Our survival depends on knowing and accurately interpreting how others in our tribe are responding to current conditions. Evolution selected for those ancestors who could discern a saber-toothed tiger in the bush and communicate their fear to other tribe members who were also able to resonate with this signal. Everyone's survival was at stake in both giving and receiving messages of safety and threat. This capacity for constant, nonverbal, resonant connection with one another is an evolutionary gift from our ancestors.

We communicate our sense of safety and threat in our modern-day tribes with this same capacity for interpersonal resonance. Providers can use this interpersonal energetic communication in their treatment rooms by bringing their own coherence to their sessions, thereby helping to create an embodied experience of greater regulation for their clients.

You will notice coherence in your clients when you sense that they are present, peaceful, engaged, and relational, with a regular rhythm in their heart and breath. It is important to observe movement to or from greater coherence in order to appropriately pace your interventions and titrate your work.

Providers who have their own trauma histories may be programmed to resonate or join their clients' expression of threat. The task for clinicians is to develop the ability to *not* join clients in their arousal and activation—to remain in relationship with their clients and to resonate coherence and calm in response to their activation. This is an important treatment-room skill. When we don't join an unhealthy expression, but stay in relationship, we can help clients restore their sense of belonging to a tribe and affirm their fundamental humanity.

A clinician who can recognize when his or her own system is out of coherence and can return to equanimity is a highly valuable resource for any client. An anxious, agitated person will join, resonate, and calm when accompanied by someone who is in a peaceful state. Knowing when we are activated or triggered by our client's story or experience—and cultivating resource states to help us manage our activation—is a critical tool in any clinician's toolbox. Colleagues report a number of ways to support their return to greater inner coherence when they feel themselves going into arousal—grounding themselves with feet on the floor, taking a few mindful breaths, saying a prayer, inviting the presence of a spiritual teacher, or bringing to mind the people who love and support them and their work. Ongoing mindfulness practices such as meditation, *Qigong, Taiji,* or yoga, as well as personal acupuncture, bodywork, or psychotherapy will deepen both your personal experience of life and the professional contributions you are able to offer.

MINDFUL TOUCH SUPPORTS COHERENCE IN AND RESONANCE BETWEEN SYSTEMS

Mindful touch—touch that is considered, purposeful, respectful, engaged, and applied with a sense of presence—will support the development of internal coherence and the capacity for interpersonal resonance with others. Building coherence in any individual also builds the possibility for resonant relationships with family, neighbors, and coworkers—relationships characterized by greater empathy, compassion, and understanding. These resonant relationships, in turn, support the intrapersonal coherence of all parties.[22] Nothing else plays a more vital and important role in our social health and community vitality.

As we pay attention—with our eyes and our hands—to our clients' process of restoring regulation and balance, we support their change process. Co-regulation with a client's inner state will enhance his ability to focus attention on his physical, embodied experience as he moves toward restoration of regulation. This attention and awareness can also help him understand his somatic state, learn how to support his own regulation in various circumstances, and gain a greater sense of harmony within himself.

THE ENERGETIC NATURE OF BODY TISSUES

But how do we know where to place our focus? Which organ or tissue needs attention? What quality of touch will support the greatest return to coherence for a particular and unique client? Put on your Five Elements glasses and evaluate your client's presenting symptoms and energetic presentation, together with her story—and your instincts—to help you choose.

Identifying the organ or tissue that most clearly holds a client's stress pattern will depend on her survival type, the management strategy she makes use of, and the nature of her trauma, as we've discussed in the previous chapters. The chart of correspondences (see Appendix 1) will help you discern the tissue to focus on and where your touch will likely be most potent for each survivor type.

Traumatic stress responses are held in body or tissue memory. When we relive a traumatic memory, our skin, gut, or muscles awaken the sensations we experienced in the original event—and send their message of alarm to our brain.[23] Making physical contact with different tissues can help you access the traumatic stress responses held in body memory and support the release of a brace response or bring tone to a flaccid or collapsed response. Different body tissues have different inherent natures. Survivors will unconsciously use these various tissues to help them manage, contain, or control widely divergent experiences. By making contact with different tissues, clinicians can access the traumatic stress responses held in their client's body memory.

Understanding the nature of various tissues will allow you to use these differences purposefully. For example, skin, fluids, and connective tissues are whole-body, global tissues, whereas bones have a clear beginning and end. Muscles, like bones, have a localized nature, but unlike bones, muscles also serve a connecting function—from one bone to another or across a joint. The same goes for tendons and ligaments.

If your client becomes highly aroused and anxious as you work with a global tissue, shifting your attention to a muscle or bone may help the client find a more anchored, dense, and stable feeling. Moving your attention from a global tissue to local tissue and then back again can support a return to the dynamic wave inside the client's zone of resiliency.

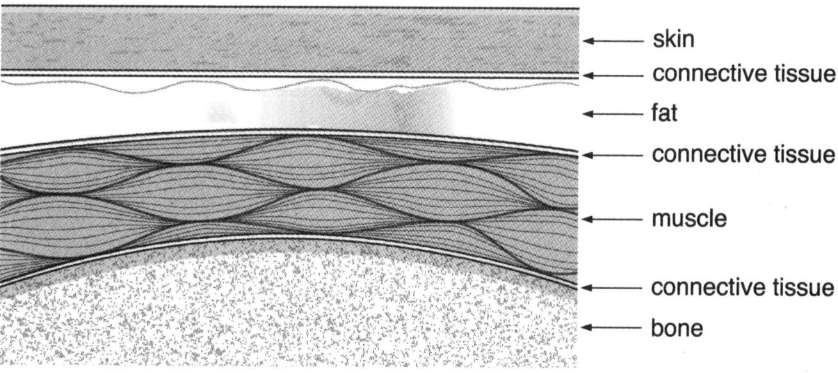

FIGURE 4.1. Body Layers

Skin is relatively global. It is our largest organ and serves as a container for our entire body. It is an intelligent boundary system that helps us make the distinction between "me" and "not me." Skin communicates sensations from the outside world. It wisely discriminates between excitement and activation and will know the moment that, for example, the pleasure of a tickle turns into a feeling of invasion or encroachment. As a clinician, your intention when you make contact with a client's skin will create a distinction between engaging the skin as a boundary structure or as a global structure. Sometimes you will want to help your client restore her sense of protective and contained "armor" in her skin, and sometimes you will want to bring regulation to an expansive and global experience of threat that is stored in her skin. This can be a critically important distinction if your client does not yet have adequate foundational regulation on board to integrate a global experience of threat without causing hyperarousal and overwhelm. Skin corresponds with the Metal Element and supports interoception. It is explored in greater depth in Chapter Six.

Muscles have clear beginnings and ends. They also form connections across joints, so they can play a role in how survivors connect with themselves or others. They carry the experience of thwarted self-protection and tend to have strong feelings about experiences involving failure to provide protection for the self or others. They communicate sensations from our inner experience. More contained than skin, fluids, or connective tissue, muscles aren't as likely to disburse energy throughout our body, as more global tissues would. Muscles correspond with the Earth Element. Their tone and vitality can inform us about the health of the Spleen, and its capacity to build flesh from food and drink. Muscles are explored in greater depth in Chapter Ten.

Like muscles, **ligaments** and **tendons** have clear beginnings and ends, and they connect muscles to bones and bones to bones. They too may play a role in how survivors of relational or interpersonal traumatic experience recover their ability to connect with themselves or others. Proprioceptive nerves are embedded in tendons, and these provide us with kinesthetic and proprioceptive information to support navigation around obstacles or threats. Tendons and ligaments correspond with the Wood Element. Their function can be disturbed by physical injury in the midst of an active self-protective response—and they can carry the memory of such experiences as well. We will explore them in greater depth in Chapter Eight.

Connective tissue is a global tissue. It covers every cell, muscle, bone, organ, and vascular structure. If everything comprising your physical body *except for your connective tissue* were removed, you would still look absolutely like yourself; it is everywhere within the body. Connective tissue has a strong correlation to body fluids. It creates a container for these fluids, and the fluid system, in turn, carries messages across membranes created by connective tissue. Its global nature includes its capacity to carry high-intensity, whole-body traumatic stress. At the right time, and with the right pacing, mindful touch of connective tissue has the power to restore whole-body balance and regulation to survivors of overwhelming life threat. Connective tissue corresponds with the Fire Element. We will explore it in greater depth in Chapter Nine.

Bones are the most local of all the tissues. Bones have clear beginnings and ends. They float as distinct elements, held in place by the dynamics of tension and pressure between their connecting muscles, fluids, and tendons.[24] While we think of the skeleton as one structure, it is actually made up of individual bones that, when healthy, never touch each other. Bone is our densest body tissue. Touching bone can be an important anchor or resource when fear becomes overwhelming. Bone corresponds with the Water Element. We explore this in greater depth in Chapter Seven.

Fluids are the most global of all tissues. Fluids serve every cell and every function. Reflecting their global nature, all Five Elements play unique and distinct roles in fluid metabolism, movement, and service. Our fluid system is profoundly impacted by the ingestion of toxic substances or the exposure to excessive electrical currents. We explore this in detail in Chapter Ten.

The correspondences of the Five Elements create a coherence-based paradigm. For example, the Liver, whose function is described in detail in Chapter Eight, is associated with the Wood Element, the mobilization response, and the presence or absence of the emotion of anger. In addition to these associations, it also relates to the tendons and ligaments, the eyes, the blood, and our ability to find hope and feel benevolent. Mindful touch over the proprioceptive beds in the tendons and ligaments is one way to help a survivor whose active mobilization response was thwarted. Helping them complete this impulse will support the physical function of their tendons and ligaments, and help them release the anger that is stored in these tissues and may be blinding them to a more hopeful future. It will support all the functions of the Liver.

5

Principles of Practice

THE FOCUS OF our clinical engagement with clients is the restoration of system-wide coherence. Although a high level of inner chaos within a client has created many symptoms and specific complaints to choose from, our most effective interventions will be those oriented toward the completion of thwarted or incomplete phases of the self-protective response, thereby supporting a return to cardiac coherence and whole-body regulation.

A survivor's many symptoms tend to be intertwined and nearly impossible to tease apart as discrete phenomena. Treating trauma survivors is a bit like a game of pick-up sticks—it's difficult to work with one symptom without disturbing the rest. With much pandemonium, how and where do we focus an intervention and get the best results? Providers who specialize in a single-body system or category of symptoms risk overlooking the dynamics between systems, as well as the underlying dysregulation that may be critical to understanding the client's whole-body, whole-person experience.

Using our pick-up sticks analogy, we need to choose the stick that most closely relates to a particular client's incomplete step in the 5-SPR. Choosing this stick will bring greater coherency, rather than more turmoil, to the client's entire system. The Five Element model allows providers to locate and work with the tissue, organ, or function where a thwarted or incomplete step in the 5-SPR has left a powerful imprint in the client's body memory.

The "faux window," named by Kathy Kain and Stephen Terrell,[1] is a helpful construct to understand the challenges of understanding and working with survivors of developmental or complex trauma. This faux window is supported by a highly developed, and often invisible (to both the survivor and his community), set of coping or management strategies that allow him to feel functional or regulated—in spite of his extreme dysregulation. It allows him to have the external appearance that he is managing life easily and well, but internally, he is functioning outside his zone of resiliency.

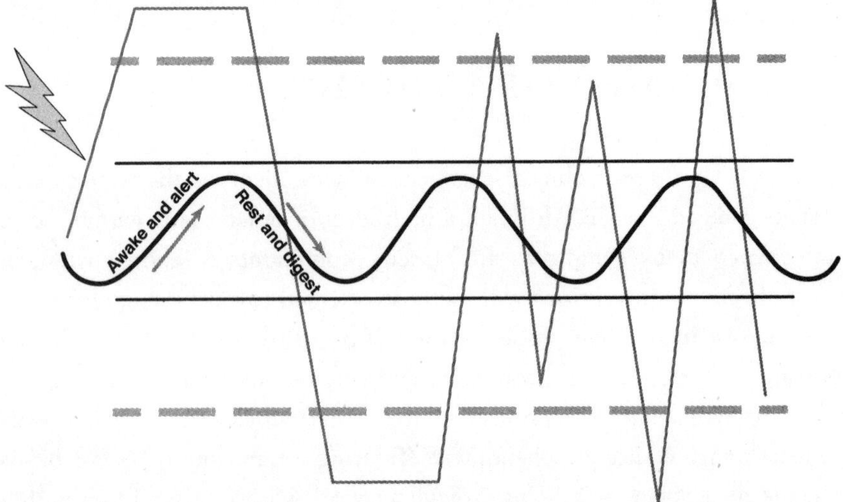

FIGURE 5.1. Faux Window of Tolerance

Note that while only the extreme ends of dysregulation are visible outside the faux window, significant chaos remains inside the dotted lines of this window. Perhaps a shot of bourbon helps us manage a job interview or social event, or isolating ourselves all weekend allows us to manage interactions at the office on Monday, or we come home after a stressful interaction with our boss and eat a half gallon of ice cream. These behaviors or activities help us manage our anxiety, but the cost to our health and wellness is quite high, and the relief is only temporary.

Managing our life inside the faux window gives our families and coworkers the sense that we are doing pretty well—and our appearance of regulation can also mislead our health care providers. Ask yourself, *How hard are your clients working to maintain an appearance of regulation?*

This faux window, discussed more in Chapters Six and Eight, provides a conceptual framework for working with the management strategies that trauma survivors unconsciously develop to help them cope. These strategies can be so effective in disguising dysregulation that providers can be easily misled. Providers may incorrectly assess their clients as having more stability than they truly do—resulting in mis-attunement, overtreatment, and the creation of even more chaos. Alternatively, a provider can miss underlying and hidden dysregulation and overlook critical opportunities for meaningful intervention.

Even for the most skilled clinicians, the distortions of the faux window can obscure diagnosis and treatment planning. When treating trauma survivors, the nature of the trauma response and its residual effects are easy to miss and difficult to pin down, which is why it's also easy to exacerbate symptoms. A survivor's entire physiology can become distorted by traumatic stress.

The Western medical model has developed along a trajectory of increasing specialization. While specialization is meant to provide better and more attuned answers, it can also have a blinding or narrowing effect, causing knowledgeable practitioners in one specialty to develop a kind of tunnel vision and neglect to consider the multi-symptom impact and multidimensional healing responses appropriate to disruptions manifesting in the trauma spectrum response.[2]

The complex nature of the trauma spectrum response requires approaches that treat the central and underlying dysregulation rather than focusing on discrete symptoms or body systems. Treating a discrete symptom without considering the whole person risks undermining what may be a fragile balance in a survivor. For example, using opioids to treat chronic pain outside of a multidisciplinary pain program can create dynamics that actually disturb overall regulation. The pain may be alleviated, but already fragile systems and functions now risk further dysregulation—opioids are known to negatively affect digestion and elimination, as well as cognition and memory. They also put survivors at great risk of addiction, exacerbating their sense of isolation and challenging their social engagement system—all critical elements for restoring balance and regulation.[3]

FRAMING A SESSION

Like all good farmers, providers must prepare the field before we plant our seeds. Traumatic stress, by its nature, is often experienced as "too much, too fast." Slowing down the pace of our engagement is our first step. Taking time to establish a solid footing in safety and relationship with our clients—and framing our interventions in a way that clients both understand and can embrace—will help prepare them to make use of what we have to offer. The following principles can guide clinicians working with survivors of all five survivor types.

Build Capacity in the Kidney/Adrenal System to Recognize Safety versus Threat

Building capacity in the Kidney/adrenal system to support a client's ability to differentiate safety and threat is the first step for all trauma survivors. In Chapter Three, we explored the five steps of the self-protective response, noting that the signal for life threat arises from the Kidney/adrenal system. The emotion associated with the Kidney/adrenal system, as well as the signal that initiates our threat response, is fear. Some of our clients may have become so habituated to threat that the neurological platform from which they live is consistently colored by fear.

Our first step, then, is to support our clients to find a sense of safety. Because of fear's primary role to signal threat, cultivating a sense of safety will be the foundation for work with all five types of survivors. The specific content of their story is not fully relevant until experiences of safety, relationship, regulation, and capacity are established. Inviting clients to choose where they sit in the room and the distance between your chairs, and helping them note, explore, and embody any experiences of safety, even small ones—and especially safety in the context of relationship—is a critical place to start. This is explored in greater detail in Chapter Seven.

Building capacity in the Kidney/adrenal system will help survivors recognize safety and respond to threat more clearly and competently. It will enhance their whole-body, multi-system capacity to manage threats and broaden their zone of resiliency. It will also create an opportunity to access a neurological platform that includes the ventral vagus nerve—and with it, a life that includes meaningful relationships, playfulness, improved cognition, and thoughtful consideration of choices—as well as significantly improved morbidity and mortality outcomes. The Kidneys and the Heart, the Water and the Fire will again find relationship.

Remember that while the Kidneys signal threat, it is the Heart that gives the command to the body to respond. We need to build capacity in the Kidney/adrenal system so that accurate messages of safety—as well as threat—are conveyed to the Heart. Whole-body coherence arises from a Heart that beats within our zone of resiliency—our Heart needs to know when it is safe. This is explored in greater detail in Chapter Nine.

Assess Your Client According to the Five Survivor Types

As you cultivate safety and relationship, use your engagement with your client to explore his presence, affect, story, and symptoms to help you decide which of the five survivor types best describes him. Discerning his survivor type will help you choose the approach that is most accessible and meaningful to him, as well as the most appropriate for your skill set and scope of practice.

Invite him to report what he notices between sessions—both cognitively and with his interoception. Look for movement toward coherence in any or all dimensions, but also for regressions or continued disruption. It is possible to work with the correct Element, but overtreat or undertreat your client, giving rise to a negative treatment response. With practice, you will develop a sense for interpreting your client's response to your work and calibrating your treatments accordingly. You may move to another Element as you get to know your client better and as his increased regulation allows his true nature to be revealed in a clearer way.

Engage in an Ongoing Consent Process

Ongoing consent will build a sense of safety and relationship. As your client shares her experience, confirm that you understand her. Explaining the intervention you are considering and why you have chosen it and then asking if it makes sense to her is a good way to determine if you truly understand what she has shared. Engage her consent at every turn. While signing a consent form at the initiation of treatment may be a legal requirement of your licensure board, the ethics of treating trauma survivors requires that you hold consent as an ongoing process. Toxic shame, cognitive confusion, and dissociation are predictable in survivors of complex trauma and will confound genuine, engaged, and informed consent. Moreover, as the "expert" in the room, it is easy to override a survivor in the consent process. The loss of what may be a tenuous experience of safety and the breach of trust that occurs by overriding consent will put your treatment relationship at significant risk. Go slow, educate, inform, listen, and secure your client's engagement before you begin any intervention.

Practice Tick-Tock to Restore the Wave inside the Zone of Resiliency

As your session progresses, use a tick-tock approach. First help your client find a felt sense of safety and security. As appropriate to your client, use either the touch or non-touch approaches in Chapter Seven, and begin with cultivating an anchor of safety. This may take a few minutes or several sessions. From here, you can tick-tock into the outside edge of an experience or memory that contains modest arousal. Gently guide your client's attention between his embodied experience of safety and this mild arousal. Move between these two states, giving any arousal time to rise and resolve before inviting another round of tick-tock. The pendulum of your tick-tock should swing in a fairly narrow and manageable range. You want to help his body restore the regulated rise and fall of the wave inside his zone of resiliency. You are restoring the dynamic and life-giving movement, relationship, and tension between *yin* and *yang*.

Continue to support and observe the natural ebb and flow between the rest-and-digest and awake-and-alert states that reside inside his zone of resiliency. This ebb and flow is the movement of *qi* and life itself. Sympathetic arousal provides the power to thaw parasympathetic collapse. Both arousal and safety must be allowed and supported in the room in order to transform dysregulation in the traumatic stress response.

Look for movement to or from coherence, and adjust your interventions accordingly. If your client moves toward sympathetically driven hyperarousal, invite a shift in her attention toward an experience of safety. For example, you might say, "From the outside, it appears your jaw is getting tight. I wonder—if you brought your attention to wherever the chair you're sitting in feels the most comfortable or supportive, what would happen in your jaw?" Alternatively, if she moves toward parasympathetic collapse, invite curiosity: "I'm noticing a faraway look in your eyes. I wonder—if you brought your attention back to this room and the color green, how many things you would find that are green? What happens as you look for green?"

The most effective treatment comes when modest safety is paired in *yin/yang* fashion with modest arousal. In this pairing, the regulated wave inside the zone of resiliency is supported; dysregulation is transformed into regulation, and coherence returns. Overwhelm, or hyperarousal, is similarly paired in *yin/yang* fashion with collapse and freeze. If hyperarousal is provoked, it can only transform into a deep collapse. We want to work with modest arousal to support modest restoration. Use the tick-tock approach to build regulation one step at a time, working in a narrow, modest range.

Note that while all things emerge out of the Tao, not all things are paired—that is, not all things will naturally transform. At the proper time and with the proper conditions, an egg becomes a chick, but a stone can never become a chick, no matter how perfect the conditions. Things that are not naturally paired cannot be transformed. For example, a trauma survivor who pairs all bright headlights with his automobile accident will be unable to transform his sense of alarm while driving at night. He has made a connection between things that are not naturally linked but are, instead, linked by his residual fear and trauma from the accident. They feel connected, but they are not actually paired. Without disconnecting tonight's headlights from the headlights from the accident, the interrupted survival responses cannot be fully completed and integrated.

Conversely, another trauma survivor may have trouble seeing the natural links and connections—the pairing—between circumstances that are, in fact, quite similar. Even though she may have had other experiences of aggressive and dangerous dogs, this dog looks nothing like those biting dogs, so its aggressive behavior isn't clear to her. In terms of risk assessment, the natural pairing between the dog's aggressive behavior and the potential for a dog bite has become invisible. She continues to put herself at risk and needs help pairing these experiences in order to change the choices she makes to keep herself safe in the future.

Like the egg that, with the right conditions and the right timing, becomes a chick, our inner states can also transform into their natural and healthy expression once the interruptions in these dynamics of pairing are resolved. This reestablishment of patterns is discussed more fully in Chapter Eight.

Use Interoception to Harvest Embodiment of Qi in Tissues and Organs

Guide your client—using the tick-tock method to move between states of relative safety and modest arousal—and anchor the movement toward regulation that emerges with somatically mindful, or interoceptive, awareness in your client. Interoception helps us accurately evaluate the physical sensations and perceptions that come with every experience. It supports us to decipher what the somatic voice inside each of us has to say about how we are and even who we are. This capacity is at the foundation of many mind-body approaches to healing traumatic stress, including Somatic Experiencing, Body-Mind Centering, Sensory-Motor Psychotherapy, Hakomi, and Eye Movement Desensitization and Recovery (EMDR). It is also called *somatic mindfulness*[4] or *felt sense*[5] in some traditions. It provides us with life-giving signals about the current state of the body.[6] For example: If we were raised in a highly rigid or autocratic household and not given time or support to recognize our own inner beliefs and impulses, we may be vulnerable to abuses of power later in life. We can lose our moral compass if we see that a superior is abusing a coworker and later be plagued by a deep sense of moral injury for not speaking up or defending our colleague.

Many of us who have experienced traumatic stress may be challenged in our capacity for interoceptive awareness.[7] Misrepresentations of our internal state or disconnect between the body's signals and the brain's assessment, interpretation, and predictive meaning of those signals is strongly correlated with a wide range of mental health diagnoses, including anxiety and depression.[8]

In this way, a lack of interoceptive capacity can put our very survival at risk. Conversely, the greater our interoceptive capacity, the more successful we will be at navigating life. Stephen Porges refers to interoception as our sixth sense and asserts that it is "the foundation of physical, psychological, and social development."[9]

If, at some point in our past, we had to engage our dorsal vagus system to stop hyperarousal in our heart, we would have necessarily become numbed to our body sensations as a result. This massive brake on our heart includes a brake on our sensate awareness (and we secrete endorphins and other substances that also numb us to pain and contribute to a sense of disconnection from self and body). In terms of AAM, we would say that our *qi* has become so disturbed as to be virtually inaccessible.

However, our long-term health requires our *qi*, embodied in our interoceptive awareness, to provide regulation to our tissues. During trauma and its aftermath, we are much too overwhelmed to remain fully aware of what's happening. But now, with an embodied experience of safety, we can cultivate and restore somatic awareness without leaving us vulnerable to major distress. We can begin to differentiate between two realities, rather than collapsing all experiences into one—that was "there and then," and this is "here and now." We desperately need our capacity to recognize the embodied signals that arise from our inner knowing, the signals that indicate we need to eat or sleep, trust or not trust, speak up or remain silent. A clinician's job is to support the return of ordered and coherent *qi* to the body-mind.

As you engage in a guided tick-tock exploration with a client, help him track the interoceptive experience that rides alongside the experience of what brought him in for treatment. As your client shares his experience, a helpful question to promote interoception may be: "Where do you notice that in your body?" Listen with your most thoughtful ears, and go to this location with your attention, intention, and perhaps your touch. Invite observation of the release of braced tissues or the enhanced tone in collapsed tissues. Supporting this embodied awareness helps support overall capacity for interoception. It will restore a regulated and coherent movement of *qi*.

Titration—Build a Solid Foundation, One Brick at a Time

Titration—a concept borrowed from chemistry—is a critically important concept in treatment planning for clients with high arousal states. Chemically speaking, when a caustic acid is combined with an equally caustic base all at once, an explosion will occur. However, if we titrate—or introduce the base drop-by-drop into the acid—it will briefly sizzle but won't explode—and, in fact, will transform into a salt. Similarly, our clients can experience transformation of their highly caustic states when we take them through treatment "one drop at a time."

Consider a gumball machine. When one gumball falls down the chute, every other gumball adjusts its location ever so slightly. Similarly, every time a client experiences a subtle movement toward regulation in one organ or one tissue, the whole body will adjust to this newfound regulation. We don't want all the gumballs to race down the chute at the same time—it will be too overwhelming to integrate. We can't possibly catch them all, and they'll create a tripping hazard as they scatter across the floor! Therefore, it's important to move just one "gumball" of experience at a time. This also leaves space for you to help your client integrate the experience of each gumball as it is released and the others all shift. Helpful things to say might include: "Notice what happens in the rest of you as you take that breath," or "As your stomach lets that belch go, what do you notice?"

Titration allows us to keep the swing of tick-tock within a manageable range for our clients. If the pendulum of tick-tock swings too far toward safety, it will necessarily swing an equal distance toward arousal—and we will risk an explosion instead of a good "sizzle" for our client.

It's important that we support integration of the balance and regulation that emerges as the wave of *qi* returns to the zone of resiliency and is restored. Allowing spaciousness between your tick-tocks will help to build a solid foundation, one brick at a time. If we put another layer of bricks in place before the first layer of mortar has cured and dried, we risk creating overwhelm or collapse. Look for movement toward or away from coherence, and adjust your interventions accordingly.

WHEN THERE IS AN "OOPS"

The fragile and highly dysregulated energy body of survivors makes them highly volatile. Their systems can move quickly, produce strong reactions, and cause unusual symptoms to emerge with treatment. Helping a client learn how to interpret her response to treatment is critical to helping her engage more deeply in her healing process.

The father of American homeopathy, Constantine Hering, developed his Law of Cure in the 1830s. Beyond homeopathy, this law has been applied to diverse healing modalities to help with interpreting the meaning of symptoms that may arise with treatment. The law states that as healing proceeds, symptoms will naturally arise and be released from the body-mind. These Law of Cure symptoms are actually manifestations of healing, not exacerbations or abreactions. They typically last for twenty-four to forty-eight hours and are accompanied by a sensation of "I'm okay" on the inside in spite of their uncomfortable presence. They should be allowed to emerge without blocking them with medications, such as cortisone creams for skin rashes, unless they are intolerable.[10]

His law states that as healing progresses, symptoms will emerge according to these three principles:

- The symptoms will move from the inner to the outer experience of the client. Thus, if a client feels emotionally better but develops joint pain, or if his asthma clears, but he develops a skin rash, we can affirm for him that this is the natural direction of healing, these symptoms are not problems, but causes for celebration.
- From more recent to older symptoms. More recent symptoms will resolve first, and the longer a symptom has been experienced, the more time it will take to heal. The headache that came on yesterday due to dehydration will resolve before the eczema that developed during childhood. Later in treatment if mild eczema emerges for twenty-four hours and then clears, we can interpret that deep healing has occurred.
- From the uppermost part of the body to the lower. If a client presents with knee pain and reports having ankle pain after your treatment, this is the direction of healing and not a cause for concern. Alternatively, if he reports having hip pain, this is an abreaction and is a cause for concern.[11]

It is also true that the highly dysregulated energy body of trauma survivors makes them vulnerable to overtreatment or inaccurate treatment. It is inevitable that some of your clients will experience an abreaction. They may experience a return or exacerbation of previous symptoms—or even develop some totally new symptoms. It is always right to say, "That was an 'oops'; it is never my intention for you to suffer." Many survivors have been to many providers over many years. They have experienced many abreactions. Yours is not their first. However, your acknowledgment that you made an error may be their first—and your honesty and sincerity will go a long way to building lasting trust.

Come back to the core principles of titration of treatment and the importance of establishing a core sense of safety in the Kidney/adrenal system. Slow down your pace of engagement, come back to restoring regulation in the signaling center for threat in the Kidney/adrenal system, and reconsider your impression of their survivor type. Using remedies that reflect your most accurate assessment of the missing step in their self-protective response and offering them at a titrated and useful pace is our overarching clinical advice.

GUIDANCE FOR THE USE OF TOUCH

The use of touch, as with all interventions with this population, must be done with a keen understanding of how it may be experienced by its recipient. Many survivors of trauma have primarily negative associations with touch: it may have been used to abuse them, it may have been part of a painful medical procedure, or it may have overwhelmed their processing capacity for tactile information at a time when their physiology was already overstimulated. This is why we must always maintain awareness of how and where we use touch.

Begin any touch intervention by explaining where you plan to touch your client and what you hope to achieve with your touch. Secure her complete buy-in and consent, but only as she is willing to give it. It is critically important for her to not override her own sense of safety by giving consent to please you or avoid any shame that may come with saying no.

Begin your touch intervention by bringing your attention to the area in your own body where you anticipate touching your client. This can help quiet and focus your mind. Then, imagine the location in your client's body that you anticipate touching. This will deepen an experience of a resonant connection between you and your client and help establish an intention or focus for your treatment. Notice your client's response—is there bracing, relaxation, or a change in facial expression or the nature of her breathing? Is there a sense of welcome for your touch? Wait for a sense of invitation to emerge. Only then is it right to touch her—mindfully and respectfully.

Your touch will most often be a "still" one. It may take some time, focus, and quiet for your fingers to "see" or "hear" what is inside your client. Bring kindness to your hand. She may sink and settle with your touch. On the other hand, she may brace, tighten up, or "go away." Adjust your touch appropriately—use the principles of tick-tock and strategies for enhancing interoceptive awareness as you explore touch together.

The use of touch, when applied appropriately, safely, and ethically, can be useful to repair attachment ruptures, promote healthier and more accurate interoception, create a sense of safety and connection, and support better access to both co-regulation and self-regulation. Touch can help clients identify and more fully develop appropriate boundaries and experience a sense of agency when determining how, when, and what type of touch occurs. If healthy touch was not provided during early developmental phases, therapeutic touch can begin to repair some of what was lost in earlier developmental phases.

While non-somatic therapists sometimes express concern that working somatically, with or without touch, can produce impossibly complex dynamics of transference, research does not bear this out. Studies about the inclusion of touch in the psychotherapeutic environment indicate that clients experience their therapists as skillful in their interventions and more understanding of their history and needs. A somatic approach does not inherently bring more complexity to transference and countertransference, but it does require heightened awareness and attention on the part of the clinician.[12]

As you titrate your touch with clients, it may be helpful to know that the back of our body tends to be less vulnerable than the front. You may want to begin your touch with very sensitive clients on the back of their arm or hand rather than the front. You may even use the back of your hand rather than its front. You will want to begin with the least sensitive parts of the body—the back or shoulder—before you touch softer and more vulnerable areas, like the chest or abdomen. Invite the client's awareness: "How is it for you when I touch here?"

SCOPE OF PRACTICE

The principles and practices of *The Tao of Trauma* can be applied in a variety of treatment settings.[13] Our goal is not to turn mental health providers into physical care providers, nor physical care providers into mental health providers. Providers with a variety of licensure can use this material within the scope of their own practice guidelines. Psychotherapists are advised to consult with their licensure boards regarding the integration of touch into their practice. Laws and community standards regarding the use of touch in psychotherapy vary widely.

If your primary intervention with a client who has survived physical injuries is touch, then you absolutely need training in a system of body therapy that gives you the necessary palpation, assessment, and repair skills. Perhaps that training is part of your formal licensing process, such as physical therapy, massage therapy, or chiropractic care, but other modalities can offer helpful skills as well. Ortho-Bionomy, Feldenkrais, Body-Mind Centering, Biodynamic Craniosacral Therapy, Clinical Acupressure, or Zero Balancing are just a few examples.

If you are using touch as an adjunct to other therapeutic interventions, you don't necessarily need detailed anatomy and palpation skills. You do need to know about using touch appropriately, and you must develop an understanding of its implications for a therapeutic, healing relationship. Similarly, if you are primarily a physical care provider or an acupuncturist, you need to maintain appropriate boundaries within your scope of practice and not engage in psychotherapeutic interventions as you integrate this material. When thinking about your scope of practice, consider these queries:

- What are the primary dynamics of your client's symptoms: physical, emotional, developmental, psychological, relational, or a blend of these?
- Does your scope of practice allow you to work appropriately within the primary areas of disruption for the client? That is, if the client's primary symptoms are psychological, your scope of practice needs to include the legal and ethical right to work psychologically with that client—otherwise you should make a referral to another professional who has the appropriate scope of practice for the client's needs.

- Could your scope of practice include some of the elements of needed care for the client with supervision or in partnership with other providers? How will you and your client determine the boundaries of appropriate scope of practice?
- Physical care providers: Can you access your client's symptoms through the body—or will other forms of intervention, such as psychotherapy or spiritual direction be needed? Can your client's symptoms and responses be adequately discussed using body therapy language rather than psychotherapeutic language?
- Mental health providers: Can you access your client's symptoms appropriately within the context of a psychotherapeutic relationship—or will other forms of intervention be needed that may be outside of your scope (such as physical care for an injury or physical disorder)? Can the client's symptoms and responses be adequately discussed using psychotherapeutic, somatic language, or is the language of physical repair needed?

ORIENTATION FOR VARIOUS CLINICAL DISCIPLINES

Somatic Psychotherapists

The successful practice of body-oriented psychotherapy relies in part on the practitioner's skill in understanding a client's somatic communications. Psychotherapists rely on their senses to understand a client's inner experience: they listen not just to their words, but also for the absence of certain words—and they certainly pay attention to the client's affect, cadence, posture, and gestures. But sometimes a client's communication of their experience occurs mainly through subtle changes in their tissues, requiring a certain type of "listening with the hands" to comprehend. When a clinician's practice setting allows touch, this can become another means of understanding the inner reality of clients.

Exploring the model of the Five Elements will add yet another dimension to a mental health provider's understanding and practice of various body-oriented frameworks that have revolutionized mental health care in the past fifteen to twenty years, such as the use of "felt sense" described by Eugene Gendlin,[14] and the integration of body-oriented therapies such as the Hakomi method,[15] Somatic Experiencing,[16] Sensorimotor Psychotherapy,[17] and Eye Movement Desensitization and Recovery (EMDR).[18]

Acupuncturists

Acupuncturists who are unfamiliar with trauma physiology may inadvertently mis-attune, overtreat, or exacerbate a patient's symptoms. The treatment of trauma survivors often will not follow the example of case studies in acupuncture textbooks, which are often described with uniform, predictable, and consistently positive outcomes. These clients do not have the same physiology as other clients. Traumatic stress gives rise to unpredictable and unusual physiology and clinical outcomes that are often not accounted for in acupuncture training programs, in spite of their common presence in acupuncture clinics.

Trauma survivors may exhibit paradoxical dynamics with acupuncture needles. If the vector of a client's *qi* is moving out of the zone of resiliency toward greater sympathetic arousal, an acupuncturist risks stimulating hyperarousal and creating excessive pain with needling unless there is a shift toward regulation and less bracing before offering a needle.

If the vector of her *qi* is moving out of the zone of resiliency toward parasympathetic collapse, placing a needle will be ineffective without a shift toward regulation and more tone before needling. *Qi* travels with embodied awareness. It is less present in the survivor who experienced freeze or dissociation as a management strategy. Her *qi* is not present enough for a needle to have impact.

In either case, the client may not return for more treatment—the needles in the first session were either too painful and caused increased turmoil and activation, or they were completely ineffective. It may be necessary to use your presence, language, demeanor, or touch to help initiate movement toward regulation before a survivor can tolerate or make use of the beneficial effect of an acupuncture point.

Non-needling techniques, such as those presented in this book, using the Five Element correspondences as a guide, can support the return of a survivor's embodied awareness and his *qi*—and build enough regulation in his tissues—to give acupuncture needles more access to the energy body and make acupuncture treatment more tolerable and more effective in restoring overall regulation.

This approach can also help acupuncturists gather diagnostic information and develop treatment plans. The deactivation of braced traumatic stress often releases as a shimmer or wave on a meridian pathway. Supporting this movement with a needle, moxa, or acupressure can be a helpful way to support its deeper release. As the layers of a client's inner experience emerge out of his tissues, subtle and nuanced meaning, images, or sensations that illuminate the role of AAM organ systems or functions often emerge and can inform acupuncture treatment planning.

Physical Care Providers

Physical care providers who are skilled in supporting tissue and autonomic nervous system regulation are critical for the health and wellness of trauma survivors. Many survivors have highly developed coping strategies that can cloud a practitioner's awareness of her client's history and life experiences. Current research tells us that when traumatic experiences include physical injury, there is a greater probability of developing a traumatic stress response.[19]

The injury these survivors experienced, together with the stress associated with it, can create neuro-inflammatory changes in the central nervous system that may impact the somatic nervous system (which carries nerve impulses between the central nervous system and the skeletal muscles, skin, and sensory organs) as well as the autonomic nervous system. These central nervous system disturbances disrupt calcium signaling, impacting not only physical pain but also cognition and psychology—and contribute to the multi-symptom spectrum of the trauma spectrum response. Some symptoms may emerge immediately, while others—such as depression and anxiety—may intensify with the passage of time, as the impact of inflammation on neural structures takes its toll alongside stressors in family, work, or community life arising out of increasingly dysfunctional responses in the survivor.

These dynamics underlie the complex and multi-symptom illness that arises for survivors of severe physical injury. Physical care providers will benefit from exploring how traumatic stress can cause a patient to present or respond in unpredictable or confusing ways. Many clinicians—and many of our clients—will not have made the connection between their physical symptoms and the impact their life experiences are having on their physiology. This model may help physical care providers reconsider their approach to treatment.

If you are a physical care provider who thinks of your work as primarily helping people relax or increase their range of motion, *The Tao of Trauma* will expand possibilities in your treatment room. Beyond physical repair or relaxation, physical care providers can also

- support greater embodiment, enhanced somatic mindfulness, and the creation of a relaxed but alert state;
- recognize activation and collapse in the client's presence, affect, and tissues;
- help restore tone in collapsed tissues and soften tone in braced tissues;
- build coherence between body systems or tissues;
- support completion of self-protective responses;
- support integration of somatic experiences of successful survival;
- help build the client's capacity for somatic awareness and support healthy interoceptive awareness; and
- support regulation in the client's autonomic nervous system responses.

Medical Practitioners

AAM has much to offer modern Western medicine in terms of understanding symptoms, addressing complex and interrelated disorders, and supporting recovery from emotional and spiritual wounds. The landmark study of adverse childhood experiences at the Centers for Disease Control has made clear that wounds to the psyche produce physical symptoms. Current research about the relationship between motor vehicle accidents and the subsequent development of PTSD further confirm that physical experiences have much to do with psychological and emotional health.[20]

For those delivering care to patients whose physical symptoms may be as much an expression of their emotional distress as an indication of their physical health, this model adds another potential perspective to help understand patients' symptoms and expand treatment options. It will help medical practitioners

- gather diagnostic information from a different and fresh perspective;
- consider treatment options from an integrative medicine perspective;
- make appropriate referrals to integrative medicine professionals;
- enhance treatment possibilities for this client population; and
- work more effectively with highly sensitive patients and those with complex, multi-symptom presentations.

In Part Three of *The Tao of Trauma,* AAM's ancient and dynamic lens of relationship, context, and movement comes alive in our exploration of clinical applications. We integrate these concepts of Taoist philosophy with the neurophysiological platforms articulated by Stephen Porges's polyvagal theory and the steps of the self-protective response described by Peter Levine. Our goal is to build an integrative foundation, bringing together the gifts of East and West to help guide clinicians in restoring balance and regulation in their clients—and in the world we share.

Each of the five chapters of Part Three will orient readers to one of the Five Elements. They will provide information about each Element's role in the self-protective response, the organ systems that carry out those roles, and how both the generative and control cycles are reflected. Symptoms that may present when each Element is disturbed will be offered—and, most importantly, remedies to restore balance and regulation will be described.

We invite you to set aside literal thinking and Western physiology for the moment and to enter AAM's world of metaphor and imagery. Allow your mind to float around these images from nature without requiring them to make literal or linear sense. In time, we trust that you too will notice, and perhaps appreciate, how much the ancient Chinese people understood about how bodies work and how they heal from observing themselves and the natural world.

PART 3

RESTORING BALANCE AND REGULATION VIA THE FIVE ELEMENTS

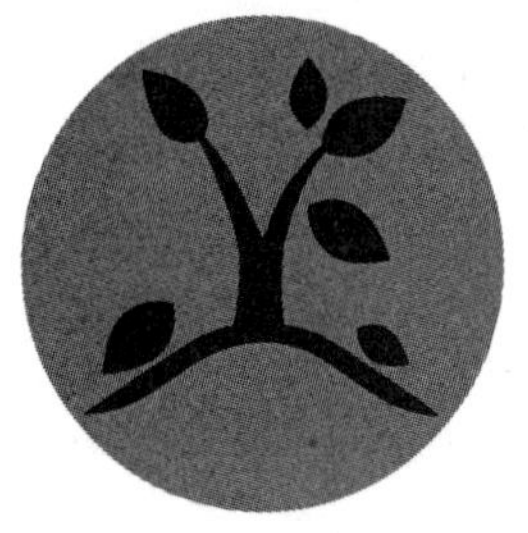

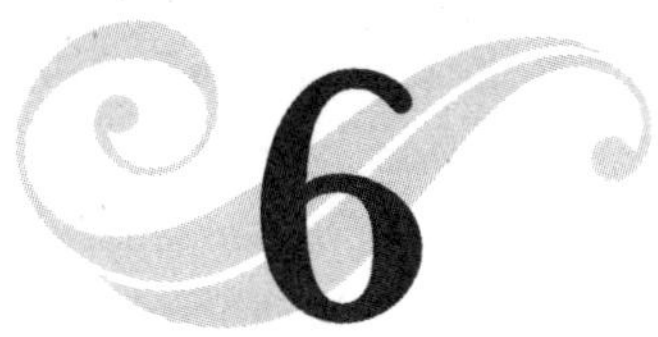

Metal and Autumn: Awaken Arousal

THE FIVE STEPS OF THE SELF-PROTECTIVE RESPONSE

1. **Arrest/Startle—Arousal Awakens Us Out of Exploratory Orienting. Metal.**
2. Defensive Orienting—Fear Signals Threat. Water.
3. Specific Self-Protective Response—Mobilization Response Initiates. Wood.
4. Completion—Successful Defense or No Threat. Restore Coherence. Fire.
5. Integration—Digest the Gristle. Harvest the Lessons. Earth.

   Cycle Returns to the Metal and Restored Capacity for Exploratory Orienting.

THE METAL ELEMENT'S season is autumn. The growing season is over, and the light is fading—there will be no new growth now. All of nature is descending into its death phase. Grief emerges as the predominate emotion of this season. The nature of grief calls us to seek spiritual answers to life's biggest questions. The clear air of autumn supports an expanded sense of connection with the heavens and our search for mystical or transcendent solutions to life's unanswerable questions.

Autumn's crisp and clear air fills every dimension of our being. We may savor the experience of feeling "inspired." Our easy breath brings with it a sense of embodied awareness. When this instinctive, open curiosity is arrested by the sense of a potential threat, it can take our breath away. If we become habituated to an unceasing sense of pending threat, we may find it difficult to inhale—to receive life and any of the gifts that are here now—or to exhale and let go of our experiences of yesterday. The predominance of grief can suppress inspiration.

Pervasive grief can leave Metal survivor types feeling shut down in a profoundly primal way. The question, "How can a loving God allow bad things to happen to good people?" can be tormenting. Our breath may be shallow, and we may experience profoundly soulful survival guilt.

When you are with your client, consider these questions to help you assess whether they may be disrupted in the arrest/startle or awakening arousal phase of the trauma response:

- *Is your client easily startled by the unexpected, such as a sound in the hallway or outside the window? Is it difficult to bring him back to an easy and full breath and present mindfulness?*
- *Does he seem to be almost suffocated by grief?*
- *Does his chest seem heavy, as if it's a struggle to inhale?*
- *Does he seem to long for a sense of inspiration that would invite a new chapter into his life?*
- *Is he able to receive a compliment or take in beauty?*
- *Can he grieve and then let go of a person or circumstance that is best left in the past?*

CORRESPONDENCES RELATING TO THE METAL ELEMENT'S ROLE IN THE SELF-PROTECTIVE RESPONSE

Element	*Metal*
Season	*Autumn*
Organ Systems	*Lung, Colon*
Emotion	*Grief, inspiration*
Role in Successful Self-Protective Response	*Restores curiosity, awakens arousal, foundation for interoceptive awareness*
Unsuccessful or Incomplete Self-Protective Response	*Hyperarousal: Anxious, jumpy, rapid breathing* *Hypoarousal: Shallow breathing, empty or "hollow" presentation, fatigued*
Engenders	*Signal for threat*
Controls	*Mobilization and orientation to threat*
Tissue	*Skin, body hair*
Virtue	*Justice*
Stores	*Qi/Energy* *Breath*
Spirit	*Po, or animal soul*
Archetypal Question	*Can I let go—allow breath to penetrate? Can I tolerate imperfection?*
Exercises to Enhance Regulation	*Awakening interoception* *Creating embodied awareness of the skin as a protective container* *Restoring regulation in the diaphragm system after traumatic stress*

ORIENTATION: THE NATURE OF THE METAL ELEMENT

Understanding the nature of the Metal Element and its role in alerting our arousal system to potential threat illuminates the role of instinct in the self-protective response and our essential animal-like nature. It gives providers a context for their efforts to help restore an embodied sense of self in clients whose traumatic stress has left them dissociated or disconnected from their bodies. It will help survivors find a fresh breath to inspire their future and support them to let go of things from their past that no longer serve life and are best left behind.

The Metal Element is associated with autumn and the dying of the vitality of the growing season. The air has left late summer's humidity behind and has become dry, light, and clear. Trees express their full beauty before their leaves make their descent. On the ground, the leaves will now rot and enrich the next growing season by bringing precious trace minerals into the soil. Falling acorns embody rest as both the first and last step of the growing season. The loss of light is tangible. Grief is in the air.[1]

While gardeners will complain about seasonal imperfections—too much or too little rain, hot spells, cold spells, or perhaps an infestation of aphids—in the grand scheme of things, the movement through the cycle of seasons is exquisite and absolutely perfect. Its essential character reflects order, regulation, and balance. The agricultural calendar provides us with an array of nourishing and wonder-filled goodness, and it guides us in a rhythm of activity and rest that provides the foundation for life. As the growing season comes to a close, we are called to honor the perfection in this intricate, paradoxical, life-giving, and magnificent cycle.

The Tao tells us that all of creation is inherently connected. The Metal Element demonstrates the depth of the Tao's wisdom on the nature of connection. Consider our acorn. It carries its connection to the oak even as it lets go and falls to the ground in the autumn. That same acorn also carries the imprint of the sun, rain, air, and soil that served its creation. In this essential act of letting go, it carries a connection with every aspect of its life. Importantly, as it lets go and falls into the void, it neither clings to what was nor anticipates what could be. The image of a small acorn, letting go without knowing whether it will give rise to an oak or simply decay and rot, has much to teach humans about letting go without regret for what was or what wasn't, without anticipation of what might be, and without any sense of attachment to the sacredness of this moment of letting go.

The Metal Element and the season of autumn support us to live in the present moment, at the fulcrum of curiosity and open exploration, without anticipation of what might be or judgment for what wasn't. In the sacred space between inhale and exhale, we live life balanced perfectly in the acorn's experience of free fall, without attachment to past or future. From this place, grief loses its power to take our breath away.

The acorn's demonstration of connection in the midst of letting go can be a reminder to us about living in the exquisite beauty of the present moment, without attachment or judgment. It can help us cope with the grief that comes when we too are called to let go and must pay the high price of loving. When life has demanded that we surrender to the loss of the tangible presence of people or experiences we treasure, our Metal also helps us remain connected to these gems. They can return to our embodied experience in a breath's moment, at our mind's mere invitation.

The Lungs are one of the two organ systems corresponding with the Metal. They serve life by receiving and dispersing the "pure *qi* of the heavens" to every dimension of our body, mind and spirit. They help us find inspiration and a fresh breath to start anew after a loss.

Every Element stores an aspect of spirit. The Metal's spirit is called the *po*, or animal soul. Our *po* gives us a sense of being animated. It inspires our most primal and instinctive nature and gives us the capacity for embodied awareness. It resides in our Lungs and travels with our breath. It brings a sensate experience of animation to every dimension of our body. It supports instinctive, reactive, physical responses, like raising a hand to protect us from an object flying at us. Spiritual practices that focus on the breath cultivate our *po*.

AAM joins many spiritual traditions that look to the breath as a tool to anchor concentration, settle the mind, and hold our universal longing for this cognitively unknowable "pure *qi* of the heavens."[2] The Chinese sometimes described the heavens as an inverted metal bowl with holes that allowed the stars to shine through.[3] This image illuminates, in a metaphoric way, the Chinese experience of the stars as sacred light, the role of the Metal Element as the conduit for this heavenly light, and an image of permeability in the lungs.

Our Colon is the other organ system associated with the Metal. It is responsible for the "drainage of the dregs." It helps us let go of regrets and move through grief and loss.[4] It supports us in the challenging task of letting go of people or experiences that are best purged—those experiences that have left us spiritually constipated, feeling polluted, blocked up, and dirty on the inside.

These two organ systems seem so dissimilar, yet they are curiously connected as pairs at opposite ends of one of life's most critical dynamics. Our Lungs help us feel inspired by life's enriching experiences, while our Colon helps us let go of experiences or people that no longer serve life—they make space available for a new chapter to begin. The Lungs receive what's new, fresh, and heavenly, and the Colon lets go of what's old, toxic, and dirty—making room for the Lungs to again receive what's pure.

Each of these organ systems requires the other for the complex dynamics of receiving and letting go to work. We can't receive without making space by letting go. Nor can we let go without inspiration to empower us to act. The Lungs and Colon are intimately connected as *yin/yang* opposite, yet connected pairs.

When our Metal is healthy, we receive inspiration from the heavens through our Lungs and let go of life's imperfections easily through our Colon. We hold life's tragedies in their broad context, and we view imperfections as part and parcel of an essentially perfect world. We connect easily with others in spite of the sure knowledge that loss and grief are part of every breath we take with loved ones. We know ourselves to be a gem and are also able to honor the gem-like nature of all others.

When our Metal is out of balance, we lose sight of our value and the treasures in others. Our difficulty letting go of experiences, people, or things prevents us from taking a fresh breath—or creating a fresh reality.

The Lung and Colon work together to support us to let go and accept the quiet and crystalline beauty of a universe that is both impeccably ordered and utterly brutal.[5] They help us find and experience a perfect world even in the midst of an imperfect life.

CONTEXT: THE ROLE OF THE METAL ELEMENT IN THE SELF-PROTECTIVE RESPONSE

The Metal Element defines life's beginning and ending via our first and last breaths. It unites the alpha and omega of life and all the movements in between—including our self-protective response. The Metal Element informs both the inception and conclusion of the 5-SPR in our interoceptive, or body-awareness, system.[6] As stated earlier, in AAM, this primal, sensation-based body-awareness system resides in the Lungs and is called the *po*.

If we are camping in the woods and hear a twig snap in the dark, we're likely to experience some sympathetic arousal—our breath may catch, and our focus will narrow as we orient our sense organs toward the sound. We are instinctively animated to respond to this embodied and sensate experience of a potential threat. We don't take time to consider whether, where, when, or how fast we should move—we respond instinctively.

Under these conditions of slight sympathetic arousal, the correspondences associated with the Metal, including our skin and body hair, our breathing and our elimination system, are awakened. Our breath catches, our felt sense of open and spacious curiosity stops, our skin may have goose bumps, the hair on our neck may stand on end, and there may be a feeling that something is "amiss" in our Colon. Our arousal systems are preparing us to act to secure our survival.

This capacity for instinctive response is the contribution of the *po*. The Lungs' function to bring the "*qi* of heaven" to the outermost regions of the body carries our sensate awareness to minute and distant locations with our breath. The vitality of our *po* provides the foundation for our capacity for an instinctive sensory response to something new in our environment—and our ability to awaken arousal to potential threats.

At the close of the 5-SPR, we experience its conclusion with an easy, effortless breath and a return to open, sensate curiosity. We are supported to reflect on our own true colors. Like the leaves that don't show their full beauty until sunlight is diminished in the autumn, our successful completion of the 5-SPR allows us to appreciate our skills and resources, as well as our unique qualities that helped us manage this experience. Our newfound resiliency supports an expansion of our sense of self-worth. We come to know and value our gem-like nature.

COMMON SYMPTOMS FOR THE METAL TYPE: THE LUNG AND COLON

If we have successfully initiated and completed each of the steps of our self-protective response, our capacity for exploratory orienting—characterized by the gentle rise and fall of the parasympathetic and sympathetic nervous systems that is mirrored in our breath—will be fully present. We will be able to notice a door closing or a loud voice in the hallway without excess activation. After slight arousal, we will easily and effortlessly return to the present moment. We can hold life's tragedies in a broader context, allowing imperfections to exist within an essentially perfect world. We take the risk of connecting with others in spite of the sure knowledge that loss and grief are the price of loving—and can take our breath away.

If the Lung's role to receive the breath and distribute it to the furthest reaches of our body is disturbed in the awaken arousal phase of the 5-SPR, our system of interoceptive awareness can be compromised. We will be challenged to accurately interpret the information that comes to us from our senses.

Our capacity for interoceptive awareness is critical for navigating life. Among other things, it tells us when we're hungry, when we need to sleep or rest, whom to trust, and when we are safe. A trauma survivor whose arousal system was repeatedly experienced as ineffective—such as an infant whose signals of hunger were not met with breast or bottle—will understandably not have a trusting or reliable relationship with the interoceptive system that sent those signals. If this is a chronic, ongoing experience, he may shut down or turn off his interoceptive awareness of hunger. The experience of life-threatening neglect was more overwhelming than the experience of hunger, so his hunger signal was turned off to avoid experiencing such unrelenting hyperarousal. As an adult, he may forget to eat or may eat without awareness of the impact his food choices have on his health. He may suffer from significant and life-challenging malnutrition, obesity, or digestive disturbance. This capacity for awareness left his body, and his capacity for receiving accurate interoceptive information is now compromised in a life-threatening way.

Interoceptive signals are provided to the brain through various sensory pathways. Research indicates that faulty evaluation of our internal state or a disconnect between our body's signal and our brain's interpretation of that signal may underlie many of the symptoms that trauma survivors experience, such as eating disorders, panic attacks, anxiety, and depression.[7] People with a history of traumatic stress have higher levels of disparity between their body-awareness signaling and their cognition, which is the foundation for their reduced interoceptive awareness.[8]

Other functions of our Metal Element and its two organ systems may also suffer in significant ways. The Lung's essential role to receive the "pure *qi* of the heavens" may be compromised. Our breath becomes shallow, we find ourselves out of breath easily, and we may feel an overall sense of weakness. We don't have the *qi* necessary to connect with others. We no longer feel inspired by beautiful things or the sacred experiences that have enriched us in the past.

The skin is the tissue associated with the Metal Element. AAM considers the skin to be a "third lung" and notes common clinical associations between, for example, asthma and eczema. Our skin is indeed a highly intelligent body system. It is our largest organ, our fundamental armor and our essential container. It also serves as a medium for the exchange of gases, nutrients, and waste. The Lungs are responsible for distributing the "pure *qi* of the heavens" just under the skin and all over the body. This helps keep the skin moist and supple so it can properly serve its function to protect us from infection or the impact of toxic chemicals. If the skin's function is compromised, we may be prone to colds or the flu and may develop dry or brittle skin. We may feel like we just don't have the necessary armor to protect ourselves from life's hard knocks. The skin also serves as a protective boundary. It differentiates inside and outside, self and nonself, "me" and "not me."

On a spiritual level, the Metal helps us know our true nature to be a gem. If our Metal is compromised, we may struggle to see our own value and lack confidence in our ability to manage life. We might look for external acknowledgment and approval to fill the depth of the hole we feel inside.

Grief may consume us, leaving us unable to create new and meaningful connections with others. It might seem virtually impossible to imagine a new reality that can replace what's been lost.

Our Colon, the "drainer of the dregs," is responsible for the final absorption of water and nourishment from our food and the elimination of waste. Disruption in these functions can manifest a sense of inner pollution that can be seen in the quality of our skin or hair, as well as the clarity of our thoughts and our underlying attitude toward life.

The most significant impact of a thwarted response in our awaken arousal phase is to our capacity for interoceptive awareness. When this function is compromised, our inner world feels less stable, and we place ourselves at greater risk of injury. Our instinctive, self-protective responses—like raising a hand to deflect a ball coming toward our head or grabbing a railing when our feet slip on a set of icy stairs—will be compromised. In fact, the successful completion of every subsequent step in the 5-SPR will be affected by disturbance here.

REMEDIES FOR RESTORING REGULATION IN THE METAL

A clinician's primary task with a Metal survivor type is to help restore the function of her *po,* or animal soul, to provide her with instinctive, embodied, sensate awareness. Stephen Porges refers to our interoception as our sixth sense and our most critical life-preserving function.[9] Without it, we are unable to evaluate and be guided by the signals that arise from our internal state in response to circumstances in our environment.

In terms of moving toward restored interoception, we suggest beginning with an approach that invites and awakens interoception using guided imagery. We will then explore how we can bring mindful touch to the skin as the associated tissue of the Metal—holding it as protective armor. Lastly, we will explore the diaphragm system—how the breath moves through the diaphragms and how they serve to contain high levels of affect after life threat.

The process of building interoceptive awareness will remain relevant in terms of restoring balance and regulation in every Element and each phase of the 5-SPR—we will circle back to this topic throughout the rest of the book, as we discuss subsequent Elements in the response cycle. The function of the *po* to bring animation to the whole body makes it foundational to restoring an interoceptive sense of embodied awareness when a survivor's system chose dissociation as its best management strategy at any point in the 5-SPR.

A Guided Exercise in Interoceptive Awareness

Our interoception is the aspect of our sensory awareness that provides information about our internal milieu, which we then use to assess not only our own state but also our experience of the external environment and the people in it. It supports us, at a gut level, to interpret safety and security, as well as danger or threat in our environment.[10] When our Heart sinks or swells, our guts tighten or let go, or our breath catches or expands, our body is informing us about our response to what is happening around us. It is guiding us to make an appropriate choice or take an appropriate action. Every tissue that has the capacity to send a signal to our brain about what our body is experiencing serves this interoceptive function.[11]

In AAM, the Metal Element, via the *po,* plays a critical role in how we sense our surroundings. Inviting a trauma survivor to explore his interoceptive awareness supports the *po* by allowing it to travel to those hidden-away creases and crevices that awareness left behind in the body's choice to manage life threat by dissociation. Providers are doing the essential work of reconnecting awareness in the body, mind, emotions and spirit when we ask questions like, "As you share that memory, what do you notice in your body?" or "I just heard your belly gurgle and wonder what's different on the inside after that release?" This creates conditions for survivors to develop a sense of knowing their internal selves. Cultivating a relationship with ourselves, based on trustworthy communication with the truth in our tissues, is an important part of trauma healing.

Many of us necessarily withdraw from our body awareness during an overwhelming experience. While this was helpful and critical for our survival in that moment, healing now requires that we reinhabit our tissues. Even if your client doesn't have the words to articulate what he senses in his body, inviting his interoceptive awareness—simply drawing his attention to those signals—will help him begin to restore the movement of his *qi*.

You may want to guide your client through this three-part exercise,[12] helping him track his sensations and titrate his arousal using the tick-tock approach, alternating attention and awareness between safety and modest arousal, as described briefly in Chapter Three and more thoroughly in Chapter Five.

Start by cultivating a sense of comfort—invite your client to explore a place where he feels most like himself:

> *See if you can remember a time when you felt most like yourself or the most like you would like to feel. Perhaps you felt seen in a deep way or loved for who you really are, or perhaps you embraced something unique about your own special nature. Just sink into this experience of feeling like your true self. Take all the time you need to simply arrive, with curiosity, in this delicious state.*

Give your client plenty of time to explore his interoceptive awareness. Invite him to notice how he actually can feel that he is in this sensate experience of "being the most like himself." What is his experience of his weight in his chair, the movement of his breath or guts, his sense of comfort or ease?

Once he is well anchored in this resource state, invite him to introduce a small but manageable challenge:

> *Now I'd like you to explore an experience of some challenge or difficulty. This could be a time where you had to struggle with yourself or your circumstances—a situation that you successfully negotiated, and perhaps one you have grown from as a result. You know that you are a better person now for having gone through this experience. Think of that occasion, and let yourself explore your state of being and state of mind.*

While it is not necessary for the client to share what the occasion was, he may wish to. The most important thing is that he notices his interoceptive experience of being in this memory of modest activation. Give him time to allow any arousal associated with this memory to rise and fall and to take in his sensate experience of the personal growth and expanded capacity that came as a result.

Next, invite your client to explore the edge of a circumstance or concern that continues to be troubling:

> *Now let's try another experience. There's no need to go into the eye of the storm—but I'd like you to bring to mind something that*

continues to bother you. Approach this concern cautiously and notice what happens as you gently bring it to mind. If you start to feel too uncomfortable, use your experience of that first place, where you felt the most like yourself, to help you manage your arousal. Let yourself explore your state of being and state of mind in this memory. Notice what's different.

Help your client track sensations that arise—his breath may tighten, his heart may race, he may feel an urge to run, kick, or punch. Encourage him to slow down and make use of the more regulated state he experienced with his first memory to manage the pace of this more difficult experience. As your client makes use of this earlier "resource state," he may notice his diaphragm relaxing, his breath deepening, his heart slowing down, or his muscles softening. You want to encourage his embodied awareness and help him stay in touch with his sensations.

You can trust that a wave of arousal will be followed by one of resolution, as long as the arousal remains within a moderate range. Use the client's experience of feeling the most like himself as an anchor for parasympathetic restoration if he appears to be moving too quickly into hyperarousal in his sympathetic system.

Lastly, bring your client back to the place where he felt the most like himself, or the most like he would like to feel:

Give yourself all the time you need to find your way back to the place where you felt the most like yourself, and sink into that experience. Notice your body awareness. Do you feel heavier—or lighter? Has something changed in your breath or your heartbeat? Is your experience of your weight in your chair different in any way?

Help your client harvest any states of greater regulation he experiences.

Client Example

Sam is a veteran of both the first Gulf War and Operation Iraqi Freedom. He uses all the bells and whistles on his smartphone to remember his appointments, medication schedule, and just about everything else his mind used to do for him before his head injury and war trauma. He suffers from chronic headaches and musculoskeletal pain, as well as debilitating anxiety and insomnia.

After a month of weekly sessions in which he was invited to cultivate his interoceptive awareness in various ways, he went to New York City for a weekend to see his daughter. While riding the subway, the car suddenly filled with too many people. For many veterans, crowds are activating, and they often cause flashbacks for Sam. In the past when he has been in situations like this, he often became violent—though with no conscious awareness of what he was doing—and later regained consciousness to find himself in jail, wearing handcuffs, with no memory of where the blood on his hands came from or how it got there. But this time—when the train came to its next stop, Sam got off. He simply got off the train.

After several sessions practicing embodied awareness, Sam was able to recognize his activation and avoid reacting instinctively. Instead, he removed himself from the activating environment. He found the space of one breath between his arousal and his instinctive response. In that precious moment, he found the values his parents had taught him as a child and the ability to make a mindful choice. He let his system settle, and when the next train came along, it wasn't so full. He knew he would be okay. He got on the train and finished his journey to meet his teenage daughter, who told him, without even hearing the story, "You're cool, Daddy. You're cool."

On that Saturday in New York City, Sam carried a new vibration into an old circumstance—and he helped himself find a new response. His daughter also benefitted, as did every rider on the train—and the NYPD. His one mindful breath allowed a different response to a familiar situation. Sam was proud of himself—for the first time in a very long time. His self-confidence expanded, and he could actually imagine himself changing and evolving into a life that felt different from the way it had been in the past.

Mindful Touch: Creating Embodied Awareness of the Skin As a Protective Container

Skin has richly sensate and strong opinions about the nature, location, quality, and kind of touch it wants. Acupuncturists penetrate the skin with needles; physical care and other medical providers touch their patients' skin in every session. This organ is our largest one and wants to be respected and heard! Being mindful about how we relate to our clients' skin is critical for all providers.

The skin provides us with critical distinctions between excitation and threat, which is important for trauma survivors. For example, our skin tells us when tickling is fun, as well as the precise moment when it becomes an experience of a loss of control or personal agency. During sexual intimacy, we can be touched in similar places with similar intensity and experience it as loving or mechanical, delicious or threatening. Our skin communicates clear distinctions between danger and delight, compassion and exploitation.

The sensory nerve endings in the skin help us pay attention to conditions and changes in the outside world. This capacity for sensate experiences of external realities lets us know when and where we can return to curious, open exploration of our world. Because of its powerful sensory abilities, and because it is often our first encounter in any circumstance with the external world, the skin can also function to store and compartmentalize traumatic experiences. It can contain a body memory of a traumatic experience. Refer to Chapter Five for more information on the role of various body tissues.

The skin can be accessed anywhere. Listen to your client's preferences about where she can safely experience touch and whether the touch should be skin to skin or over her clothing. Titrating your touch may require you, at times, to use the back of your hands, touch the back of your client's body, or the outsides rather than the insides of her limbs—thus avoiding areas that may feel more vulnerable than others.

It's important to note that skin is more sensitive over vital structures, such as major blood vessels or nerves. That means the skin is most sensitive and responsive on the "inside" surfaces of body parts, such as the crooks of knees and elbows, as well as on the most vulnerable and sensitive parts of our anatomy, such as the groin, abdomen, face, eyelids, and fingertips. More robust areas, such as the lower back, are less sensitive and deliver less sensation as a normal part of their sensory response.

When engaging a client's skin during treatment, your goals should be to

- support your client's sense of having a flexible and contiguous "container";

- help her develop an increased capacity to stay present and maintain stability even during volatile states and strong sensations;
- create a tactile interface that helps her differentiate between "me" and "not me"; and
- build coherence between her skin and other body systems or tissues.

Keep in mind, though, that we are not treating diseases of the skin. We are using the skin to explore our client's sense of having a secure and flexible boundary and to bring regulation to any states of hyperarousal or hypoarousal that may be "stored" in the skin.

We can use AAM meridian theory to help us choose the location for accessing the skin. The Lung and Colon meridians run up and down the arms from the shoulder to the forefinger and thumb. The Colon pathway runs across the deltoid muscle on the outside of the shoulder of each arm, and attention here often provides a sense of a secure boundary or container. This can be a good place to start.

As providers, we should remember that not every culture has the same relationship with touch or the same understanding of the meaning of different sensations of the skin. North American cultures, for example, utilize touch much less when compared to other cultures around the world. Many Latino and Middle Eastern cultures routinely and abundantly use touch in social interactions, so much so that it would be considered odd for there not to be touch during a conversation.[13]

In addition, some individuals may have a history of touch being used abusively or in uncomfortable and frightening ways—for control and dominance or for painful medical procedures, for instance—and so may have a different understanding of the meaning of touch than the culture at large or than that of the practitioner. It is important for any practitioner using touch to consider these potential variations and remain attentive to client education and consent when incorporating touch into any interventions and treatments. We more fully cover the various benefits and cautions of using touch in the clinical setting in Chapter Five. If the use of touch in your professional practice is unfamiliar to you, we suggest you review that chapter prior to reading the specific touch practices outlined in each of the chapters on the survivor types.

The following is a basic protocol you can use to initiate the use of touch specifically in relation to the skin:

- Educate your client on the nature of skin and why you think it would be helpful to explore the use of touch. Get his permission for touch, and come to an agreement about the amount of pressure, the location of the touch, and so forth. Titrate your touch by beginning with less sensitive parts of the body.
- Direct your attention to the client's skin. Invite his feedback, be curious, and invite his curiosity too. "One hand or two hands? Start on the right or on the left? Front or back of your hand? Which is better?"
- Bring your attention to the skin as a boundary organ and a structure that can create a sense of safe armor. Begin with your attention on the area directly under your hands. Once you and your client are settled and in relationship, let your client know that you are going to slowly expand the scope of your attention to the skin as a whole-body organ, though you won't actually be moving your hands. Invite his interoceptive awareness as you expand both the location and the scope of your attention. Hold an awareness of his skin as his most primal protective armor. Your intention will invite his awareness of his skin's experience.
- Invite your client to bring awareness to his interoceptive sense of the presence of your hand and of his skin as a container. Practice tick-tock by shifting your awareness and attention from the local area under your hand to the global experience of his skin as a boundary organ. Invite him to notice his interoceptive awareness of these shifts in your attention. If global attention on his skin is too activating for him, return your attention to the local area under your hand.
- Stay with your observation and awareness of his experience in a focused way, with an intention to not allow your attention to wander. If your mind does wander, make a mental note, "I wandered, but I'm back now." This is particularly important with a client whose interoceptive relationship with his skin has been disrupted. He will need your focused attention to help him also stay focused on the experience of touch and to provide you with needed feedback.

Client Example

Andrew is a Vietnam-era veteran, and this is his first appointment with me. "Why have I been referred to an acupuncturist?" he wants to know. "I can't have anyone sticking needles in me!"

We agree—no needles. (I never want to push needles on anyone who has to brace in order to receive them, and in fact, the use of needles is beyond the scope of this book. None of the remedies presented include the use of needles.)

I invite Andrew onto the table to see if he can find some comfort with me just using touch. He agrees. I take his hand and notice deep, dark scars covering his inner arms. I go to his feet and note how swollen they are. He says, "You haven't seen anything," and he shows me his calf, revealing skin that is swollen, pock marked, and covered in hard, knobby welts. He says, "Agent Orange. It poisoned my skin. I look like a monster."

He chooses to lie on his side. We agree that I should start my touch on the back of his forearms. I am filled with tenderness for this man and realize that probably few people touch him with kindness, comfort, or care. The anxiety he expressed when he first arrived disappears. His breath expands, his heartbeat slows, and his body softens. After a few moments, he looks up at me and says, "Let me see your hands." I show them to him. He says, "They are so soft." He gets very quiet and then softly says, "Next time, you can do needles. I trust you."

Over the course of the next three or four months, Andrew's trust in me and his healing process increased. I continued to invite his growing interoception alongside my needles and touch. His relationship with his body and his healing grew. He seemed to be increasingly substantial and less empty in his energetic presentation. He began to embrace a role for himself—he became less passive about someone else needing to "fix" him before he could enjoy life. He took a walk around the block for the first time in years—and felt great about it. He showered and shaved before coming in for an appointment. He made dinner—meat loaf and baked potatoes—for his wife. He started wearing his compression stockings and using his hearing aid.

His increased interoception supported him to embrace life more fully and to grow in his relationship with himself, his wife, and his world.

Restoring Regulation in the Diaphragm System after Traumatic Stress

The system of body diaphragms is a concept borrowed from osteopathic medicine. While the respiratory diaphragm is the only true diaphragm, it is joined in this model by additional structures that similarly serve to separate and contain sections of our body. This can be a useful conceptual framework for working with movement, brace, and collapse in the energy body of trauma survivors. We introduce it in the context of the Metal Element because the respiratory diaphragm plays a central role in the system of diaphragms and has a particular connection to the Lungs, whose job it is to distribute awareness and *qi* throughout the entire body.

The diaphragm system functions like a series of bells on a string. If one bell vibrates, they all begin to vibrate in resonance. Therefore, both braced and collapsed states in any one diaphragm are transmitted to all the others—and they influence the function of the organs and tissues contained between them. Because all the organs are held between diaphragms, you may use the diaphragm system to work with disturbances in any Element, organ system, or with any survivor type.

In this system, each diaphragm relates to its next closest diaphragm in a system of bell and bowl structures. As shown in Figure 6.1, below, the seven primary diaphragms all share this similar form:

1. **Crown:** The portion of the dura that lies below the frontal bone, occipital bone, and parietal bones. This diaphragm is contained within the dome of the top of the skull.
2. **Tentorium:** This separates the cerebellum from the occipital lobes. It is in the central part of the skull and extends from behind the eyes to the ridge at the back of the skull, near the base of the head.
3. **Cranial Base:** The portion of the dura mater that sits at the floor of the cranium. It attaches to the back of the head at the base of the skull and forms a bowl at the bottom of the head.
4. **Shoulder:** A group of structures creating a lid at the top of the chest. They include the apex of the lungs, the upper thoracic vertebrae and clavicles, and the upper border of the mediastinum. It contains the arch of the shoulder girdle.

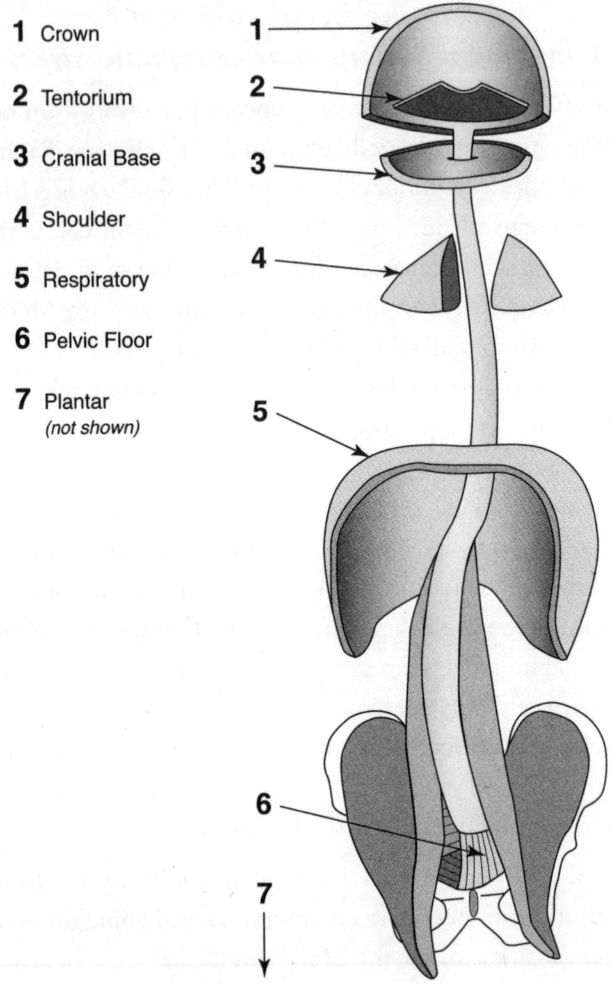

FIGURE 6.1. Primary Diaphragms

5. **Respiratory:** A muscular dome attached at the base of the rib cage, all around its circumference. It is the only *true* diaphragm. It is a complete seal, separating our body's upper chamber from the abdominal cavity, thus providing a vacuum within the chest cavity that assists drawing in and expelling air from the lungs.

6. **Pelvic Bowl:** A series of muscular bands connected to the boney structures of the pelvis that support the bladder, colon, and uterus.

They help maintain abdominal pressure, as well as continence in the urinary and anal sphincter.

7. **Plantar:** The plantar fascia is included in this theoretical framework for the sake of having a container at the bottom of the body as well as its top—creating a sense of balance in the system from head to toe. Since we are considering the diaphragm system as a full-body resonant system, we want to include the lower extremities in that resonance.[14]

The job of the diaphragms in the context of traumatic stress is to contain unbearable feelings and responses to extreme experiences of threat. In the experience of overwhelming life threat, our diaphragms help us contain what is intolerable to remember.

At the first sign of a potential threat, our respiratory diaphragm clutches, and our breath catches. If, as a small child, we were repeatedly told, "Big boys [or big girls] don't cry," we may have stored the many impulses for our tears in our respiratory diaphragm. (We tightened the diaphragm to keep us from crying, and those experiences become stored in our respiratory diaphragm's tissue memory.) It is so much better to constrict our respiratory diaphragm, stop our tears, and hold our breath than to actually experience terror—or the dissonance between our fear and the demand of our caregiver that we not cry.

Movement in the respiratory diaphragm creates the vacuum that gives rise to each inhale and exhale. Because of this unique relationship with the Lungs' function to disperse *qi*, awareness, and breath to the furthermost reaches of our body, the respiratory diaphragm is often the primary locus for work with the entire diaphragm system.

If we become habituated to holding back our tears, the resulting constriction in our respiratory diaphragm can be energetically transmitted throughout the rest of the body through the diaphragm system—via the energetic "bells on a string" metaphor. This physical strategy then becomes a surrogate for self-regulation: *I can create a sense that I'm managing it. If I clamp down and don't feel, then I won't feel scared.*

For our purposes, the diaphragms can be seen as affect and activation regulators. They help contain the out-of-control responses that can result from intense hyperarousal, which is then sometimes followed by overwhelming collapse. The primary diaphragms serve as the principal containers of affect in whole-body experiences of terror—those that reverberate through our whole body—such as being picked up and thrown by a blast or tornado or being unable to mobilize a response to repeated and compressed experiences of terror in a war zone. The most severe damage in such experiences takes place in our core organs and in our brain, and we attempt to contain the arousal in these organs with our primary diaphragms.

Infants—who are developmentally unable to mobilize a successful fight-or-flight response to what feels like life threat, such as a high fever, hypoxia at birth, a necessary surgery, or an experience of child abuse—are equally driven to use this dynamic system to contain their sense of terror. Such early experiences can affect our capacity as adults to respond to situational trauma, further compromising this dynamic system.

No matter the source of the threat to our survival, our diaphragm system serves us much like a dam holding back floodwaters, keeping us away from the damaging roar of an intolerable experience. Abject terror absolutely must be contained. The diaphragm system helps us create an inner experience that feels like everything is okay (when actually it is not). We will do anything we can to achieve a "can't feel this" state. This is why diaphragm work is critically important for survivors of life-threatening experiences—to help them relinquish some of that brace or freeze.

Depending on her constitution, a survivor's diaphragms may remain hypertonic (that is, braced and clamped down) or become hypotonic (collapsed and flaccid). Hypertonic or constricted diaphragms are more common. These survivors will present with rigid or braced expressions in their body-mind-emotions-spirit.

The hypotonic type carries greater long-term risks. There will be a lack of tone throughout—not only in her body, but also in her mind and spirit. This survivor may experience a suppressed capacity for breath, an inability to hold tone in her musculoskeletal system, or a lack of tone in her digestion, leaving her compromised in her ability to assimilate nourishment and therefore at risk of becoming malnourished.

There are significant health ramifications to the brace or collapse that may remain in our diaphragm system after physical injury or surgery. Such bracing or collapse can have a profound impact on recovery from physical injuries. If our tissues are too rigid and tight, our *qi*/energy can't flow through them. If our tissues are too collapsed, there won't be enough tone in them to carry our *qi*/energy. Our physical healing is compromised and may also manifest in anxiety, nightmares, or depression.

Both hyperarousal and hypoarousal in the diaphragms function like a barrier to sensation of life threat—like walls that muffle reverberations throughout the body—or prevent them from being felt at all. This is a brilliant and profoundly helpful survival mechanism when threats are unfolding, but it creates numerous consequences that have the potential to affect our morbidity and mortality.

Survivors use many strategies to manage the high levels of affect created by intolerable memories—isolation; addiction to alcohol, drugs, or food; or activities like work, shopping, or sex. Essentially, any behavior that contributes to brace or collapse in tissues or thoughts can function as a management strategy of one kind or another.

The diaphragm system is one way many survivors maintain what Kathy Kain and Stephen Terrell have named the "faux window of tolerance," introduced in Chapter Five.[15] By using the diaphragm system to limit the experience of the overwhelming sense of life threat, the surface waters are calmed—but at a great price. Working with the diaphragms can help you access the high levels of affect and activation that lie below your clients' management strategies.

The diaphragms are a relational system, and we need to touch them with that fact in mind. For example, as your hand and your awareness rest on the respiratory diaphragm, your client may experience a sensation in the proximal diaphragm in his shoulder or his pelvis. You may choose to move your hand and your attention to these other diaphragms in order to support a return to regulated tone in these diaphragms and in their relationship to each other.

When working with the diaphragms from a trauma perspective, titration is critical. Because the diaphragms are utilized as a braking mechanism for the fear, rage, helplessness, or other feelings related to a traumatically stressful event, their role in containing high levels of activation comes under considerable pressure. If the diaphragms fail in their job, the emotional and energetic release (like a dam breaking) can completely flood the body-mind-emotions-spirit. Think of that classic image of a driver with one foot slammed on the brake while the other is stomping on the accelerator. If the driver pulls his foot off the brake suddenly, the car will spin out of control. Our goal in working with the diaphragms is to allow shock vibration to slowly mobilize in bite-sized pieces and then disperse—something like slowly taking our foot off the brake and letting some of the energy emerge. Refer to Chapter Five for more on the concept of titration.

Because the diaphragms work together as a system, you can't simply work with a single diaphragm and invite it to fully open without initiating a significant reaction in the remaining diaphragms. Similar to gumballs in the old-fashioned gumball machine mentioned earlier, which all move when one is released, the management strategy in the whole diaphragm system will shift as we work to bring regulation to one diaphragm. As you're working with one diaphragm, look for the impact of local movement in one diaphragm on the global system of the whole body. Coherence in one area will support coherence everywhere.

The most common pattern for working with the diaphragm system is to work briefly with one diaphragm—frequently beginning with either the respiratory or shoulder diaphragms—and then move to the next closest diaphragm and do a little work there. At that point, we would assess whether or not the client's responses were sufficiently titrated, or manageable and integrated enough, to consider working with an additional diaphragm. Quite often, at the beginning of your work, working with two diaphragms is enough to initiate responses in the client that need time for integration before you would begin working with additional diaphragms. Generally, we don't work with more than three diaphragms within any single session, since we are assuming there could be strong responses to the releasing of the braking action of the constricted diaphragms. We are looking for stability in the relationship between diaphragms, manifesting with greater whole-body coherence—slow, deep breaths, breath moving through the whole body, regulated tone in the muscles, and ease throughout all body systems.

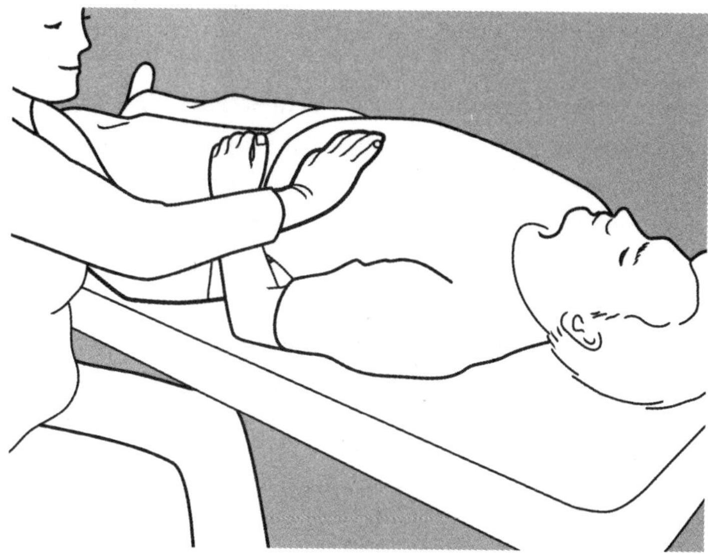

FIGURE 6.2. Touching the Respiratory Diaphragm

The diaphragm model will allow you to work with the resonant energy of the body as an integrated whole. Over time, you will develop your capacity to feel changes in the diaphragms as *qi* moves through the entire diaphragm system, gently pinging each bell in turn. Cultivate your most thoughtful observer, and invite the client's interoception to affirm or calibrate your observations. What happens when one small part of one diaphragm is able to move? What happens when breath moves into what was previously too braced or too collapsed to feel? What happens in the rest of the client's body? Look for movement in the smallest, most local aspect of your client's use of her diaphragms as a management strategy. See what happens to all the other diaphragms when she releases the bracing in just one diaphragm.

You can trust that even if you are unfamiliar with anatomy and physiology, an approximate placement of your hands with your full attention and intention on your client can access and wake up the brace or collapse that is stored in her diaphragms. You will come to know and understand anatomy and physiology more and more as you work with the diaphragms. Your client's interoceptive system especially wants to know that you are present and safe. Invite her to "micromanage" the placement of your hands—this will teach you something about her physiology and will create another opportunity for her to cultivate interoception. Conceptually, we want to move what is held strongly in the interior of the body to the periphery and finally out of the body. But to do this, we must prepare the periphery for this energetic work.

In addition to the primary diaphragms already discussed, there are hundreds of secondary diaphragms. Every location in the body where we find a space structured like a bell or a bowl—the eye sockets, mouth, and joints—can be addressed and utilized within this context. If these secondary diaphragms are not open when the primary diaphragms move, the periphery can feel painful and explosive. The shock absorber that should soften their mobilization response is not in full service. We will explore working with the secondary diaphragms in the context of repairing the self-protective response, in Chapter Eight.

As you observe your client, ask yourself: *Where is the higher charge—at the core or the periphery?* Start with the diaphragms that contain the lower charge, more balanced tone, and greatest movement of breath. If the primary diaphragms are managing a higher charge at the core of the body, begin by working with the secondary diaphragms in the joints to release the exterior. If the secondary diaphragms are managing a higher charge at the periphery, work with stabilizing the primary diaphragms first, then move to the periphery.

A person holding a braced response—a high sympathetic charge—in their diaphragms will appear tight and wiry. They may be jumpy and have a need to run or move in order to manage their arousal. In contrast, a person experiencing a collapse or freeze response in their diaphragms will appear soft or lacking in tone to the point of feeling "mushy" in their torso. They will have little motivation or desire to move, preferring to be a "couch potato." Many survivors will have mixed patterns—aspects of both brace and collapse, working with the diaphragms can help them restore overall regulation. Attending to either state with your touch and your attention can help it transform—restoring tone and more regulated function.

The diaphragm model allows you to begin work at a relatively safer distance, away from an area of the body that holds a strong affect. Once you have cleared the diaphragms with a lower charge, those with a higher charge will be more approachable as areas to continue the work. When working with the primary diaphragms, we would most commonly begin work with either the shoulder or respiratory diaphragms. Releasing brace or collapse in the respiratory diaphragm may then be carried to the pelvic diaphragm. While the pelvic diaphragm is often much too reactive a place to begin, particularly for sexual trauma survivors, dysregulation in this diaphragm may be accessible via movement emanating from a more regulated respiratory diaphragm. Similarly, clearing brace or collapse in the shoulder diaphragm may encourage the cranial diaphragms to open, while these diaphragms would be much too sensitive to work with directly if there is a history of traumatic brain injury.

It's best to only work with one, two, or—at a maximum—three diaphragms in a session, rarely more. When a diaphragm moves, it will speak to the neighboring diaphragms through a naturally resonating vibrational system. This can create an impulse for each diaphragm to come into more regulation with its neighbor—or it can cause the diaphragms to tighten, out of chronic fear of allowing the terror they contain to be released and experienced. A certain amount of tension in each diaphragm may be necessary early on for the client to feel safe enough to let go and allow vibration and movement throughout the diaphragms.

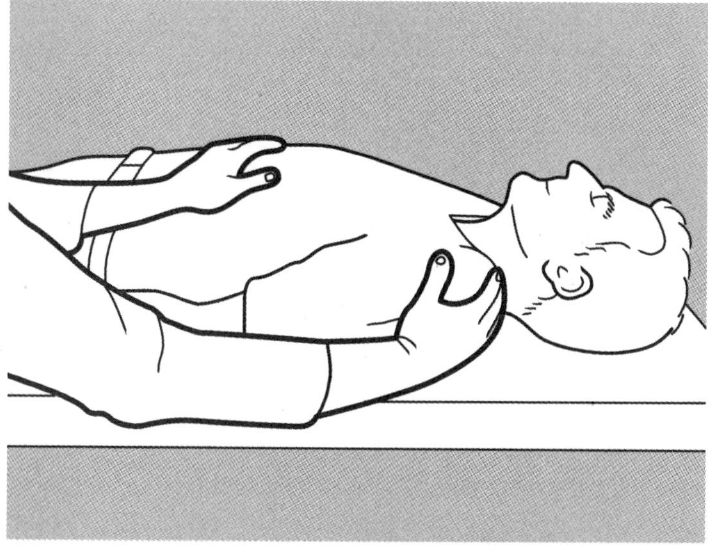

FIGURE 6.3. Touching the Shoulder Diaphragm and Respiratory Diaphragms Together

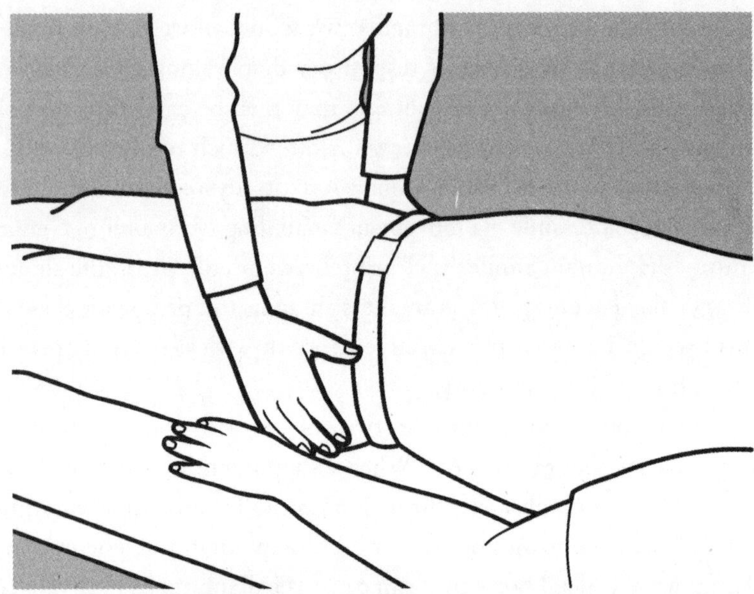

FIGURE 6.4. Touching the Pelvic Diaphragm

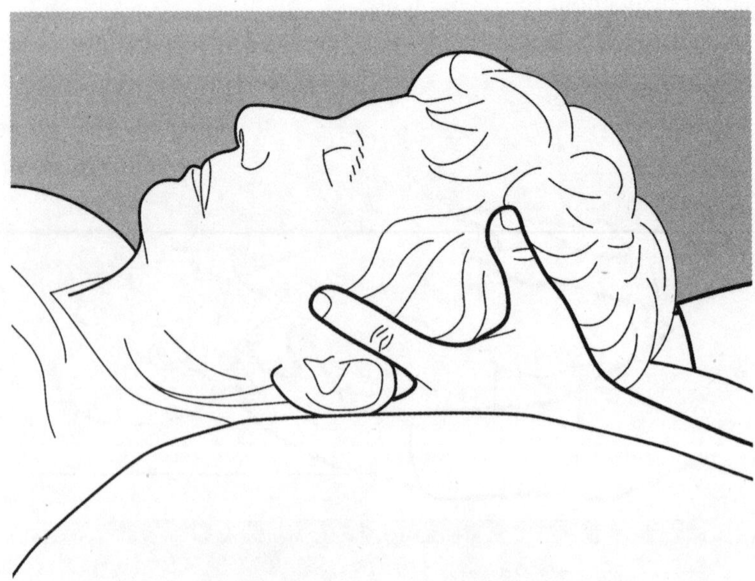

FIGURE 6.5. Touching the Cranial Diaphragms

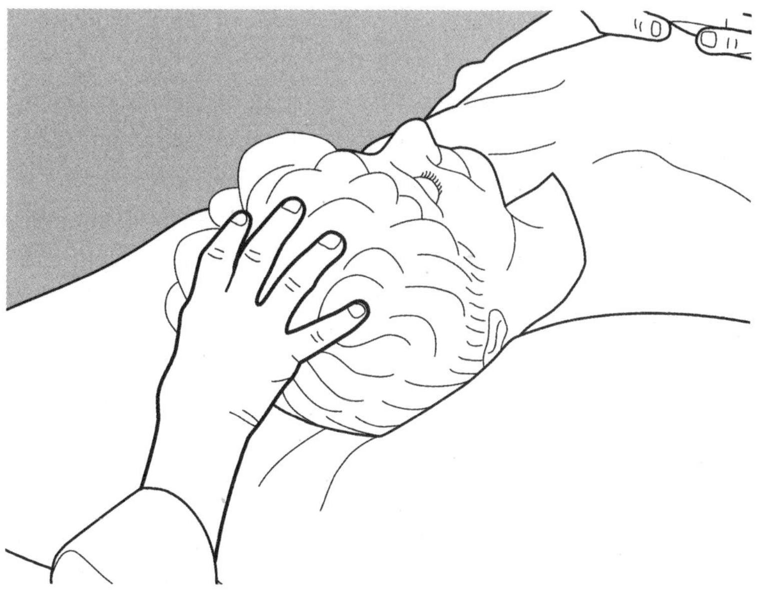

FIGURE 6.6. Touching the Crown Diaphragm

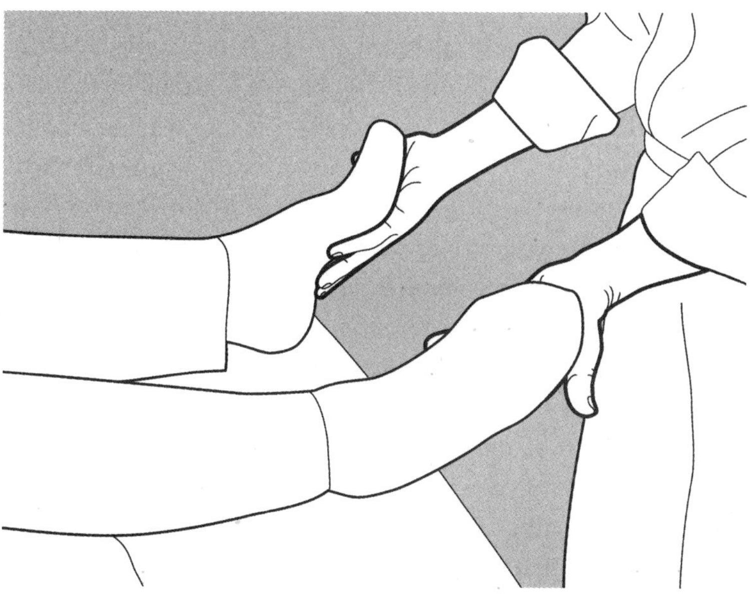

FIGURE 6.7. Touching the Plantar Diaphragm

The experience of hyperarousal, helplessness, or terror stored in a client's diaphragm system may return as the diaphragms begin to move. The survival energy that was clamped down long ago is held in his tissues as an interrupted survival effort—it needs mobilization and completion. The circumstances that gave rise to his terror are not here and now, but it may feel that they are, and he may respond by shutting down his mobilization response yet again, perhaps even more forcefully. Coaching your client on the importance of allowing an incomplete response to come to fruition and bring the threat response cycle to a healthy conclusion in order to achieve integration and recognition of a successful survival effort may be critical to help him let go and trust this process.

Dismantling the management strategy of constricted diaphragms may be frightening. Remember, it arose out of a sense of futility from a self-protective response that could not fully mobilize long ago. When we invite that energy to mobilize again, it will activate a direct connection to the historic event that required it to shut down in the first place. The halting of a mobilization response in the past was the product of strategic body-wisdom. There is no shame in making good use of a freeze response.

When working with the diaphragms, the energy that comes forward may feel to the client like it is going to kill her, but she is actually reexperiencing the great effort she made to fight for her life. She may need to mobilize an action—run, push, or stomp—to complete what was unavailable to her in the past. To ensure safety for the client, it is usually best to have her imagine performing these actions, rather than physically executing them. Especially with clients who have severe symptoms or physical injuries related to traumatic events, it is important to ensure that they don't make any sudden or extreme movements that could make their symptoms worse or reinjure them.

You may need to be quite directive in your coaching, since these diaphragm responses occurred under the influence of a survival effort and thus will tend to be automatic: "This is where you don't freeze. It wasn't safe for your muscles to kick that mugger way back then—but now you can experience your power and capacity to defend yourself. No need to stop yourself. Keep breathing." Help them notice how it feels when they don't stop their mobilization response. "This is the state we have been trying to create. This is how you can win. Let this energy come forward. This is your life force. This is you being alive."

Use language like: "Let it come down through your legs; open your pelvis; open your shoulders; be like grass in a lake, kelp in the ocean, a willow in the wind—let it move and flow." Help clients learn how to get out of the way of these sensations so they can develop a new relationship with how they experience energy and life force moving in their system.

New symptoms may show up as the old management strategy is dismantled. For example, clients may develop a skin rash as dysregulation in the interior moves to the exterior. They may develop ankle instability as the hip and knee diaphragms become less braced and as movement through the leg shifts toward greater organization. Helping patients understand the benefit of these responses can be critical in encouraging them to allow the completion of survival responses and the return to equilibrium. Our intention in working with the diaphragms is for the system to gain greater capacity for survival response. As balance and tone return to the diaphragms, a sense of spaciousness will emerge. High charge in a larger container will feel like less. Your client's capacity to manage life will expand with this growing sense of spaciousness.

You may also choose to use diaphragm work with a patient who does not have a high level of activation in this system. This can be a lovely way to finish off a session and bring a whole-body sense of integration and coherence.

Always work with the diaphragms as a system. Open a little here, then go there, and come back again. We are looking for stability in the dynamic relationship between diaphragms, manifesting with greater whole-body coherence—slow, deep breaths with breath moving through the whole body, a lack of bracing in the musculoskeletal system, and ease in both you and your client.

Client Example

Maria had been experiencing chronic pain in most of her joints, including her pelvis and shoulders, for three years. After many different tests and examinations, clinicians could identify no specific reason for the pain, yet it was severe enough that Maria could no longer work. I gently asked Maria what had been happening in the months or year prior to the onset of her pain, and she revealed she had witnessed a robbery at her local convenience store about six months before she first began developing pain. She was in the store at the time and hid in the back during the robbery, but she heard the confrontation between the store clerk and the two men robbing the store. She also heard the gunshot that badly wounded the store clerk. Even though she could see the clerk needed help, she was unable to move until after the police and ambulance arrived, and another customer had been the one to place the call to 911.

As Maria described the event, I noticed she was nearly rigid with fear and hardly breathing. I invited her to the table and asked if I could gently support her breathing by making physical contact with her ribcage. Slowly, as her breath returned, Maria began to weep. With great, gasping breaths, she talked about how frightened she had been and how horrible she felt about not being able to help the clerk. I gently coached her to let her breath move, to let her shoulders move with her breath, but to also take it slowly and not try to do too much this first time.

In each session over the next few weeks, Maria allowed more and more movement and breath to return. She felt within herself the compassion she had not only for the store clerk but also for herself, as she came to understand that her frozen state was a natural survival response to her overwhelming fear. Together, we gently explored how each joint could breathe, allowing small movements to release and open each of these diaphragms. Her pain then slowly receded as movement returned.

SOCIAL IMPLICATIONS FOR RESTORING REGULATION IN THE METAL ELEMENT

The successful completion of our survival response—whether in the direct experience of threat, or years later, using approaches such as those described here—places us in a better position to mount a successful survival response in the future. Our Metal Element's capacity to notice and alert our system to a potential risk arises out of a successful completion of previous calls to arousal.

When we are able to complete this response, our Colon can fully break down and eliminate any waste that remains. We are no longer influenced or "constipated" by a previous experience of danger. Our Lungs are able to receive an easy and fresh breath. Our *po* has returned to full function. We are open and curious about our environment; we can experience beauty and receive inspiration from the gifts and challenges in our past. Our interoception is fully available and provides us with clear and unencumbered information to inform our decisions and actions.

The social implications of living in this state are significant. We are supported in our curiosity, rather than alarmed or threatened by new neighbors or unfamiliar circumstances. We are able to find a single breath to help us notice our response, rather than instinctively reacting to these primal states of contraction and fear. We are better able to respect those we might have previously perceived as "other." This is the foundation for developing greater understanding and a more respectful culture in our homes, neighborhoods, workplaces, and beyond.

In the context of the Five Element system, the Metal engenders the signaling center for threat in the Water, and controls the mobilization response in the Wood. Arousal is designed to be slight in the Metal. It should signal the Wood via the control cycle to orient to and investigate whether a mobilization response is called for. Only if the assessment of risk is high will the Water receive the message to initiate a full-bore threat response and power mobilization of fight or flight in the Wood.

Regulation in the Metal mediates signaling in the Water and tempers mobilization in the Wood. If the Metal's task of discernment of threat becomes unreliable due to an incomplete threat response, then a lack of curiosity, a lack of respect for differences, and impulsive or reactive responses to unfamiliar people or circumstances are more likely to arise.

CONCLUSION

The Lungs receive inspiration from the heavens and disperse it to each and every distant location in our whole body. Their spirit, called the *po*, or animal soul, is the basis for our sense of being animated. It is the foundation for our sensory awareness and interoceptive capacity. The *po* awakens in us the awareness that something is amiss. If danger seems likely, it sends this message to the Water Element, which then signals to the whole body-mind-spirit that a threat is imminent and a mobilization response is in order.

The Metal and Water Elements share a special connection. Caring for Metal is one way to care for Water. AAM teaches that "Metal creates Water," and we often find Water flowing down the sides of mountains made of rocks containing metal. Rocks (and the metallic elements they contain) create natural cisterns and containers for water. A healthy arousal system in the Metal Element will similarly create a clear and powerful signal for threat in the Water Element. We will explore this signaling center for response to threat next.

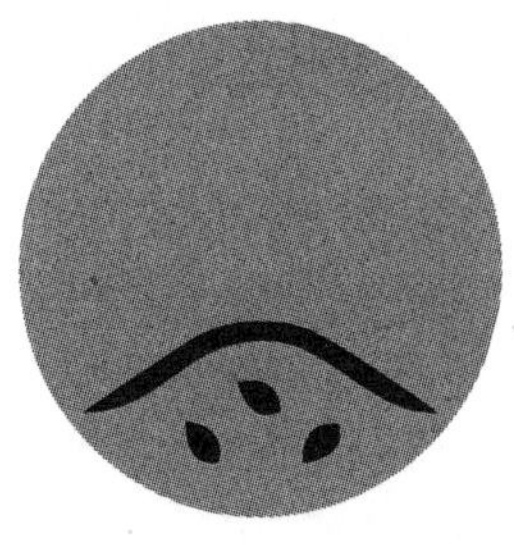

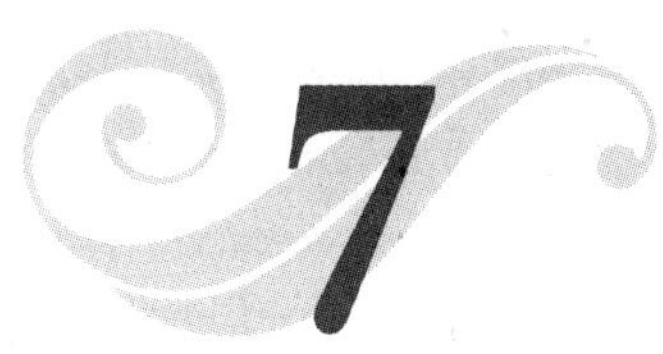

Water and Winter: Signal Threat

THE FIVE STEPS OF THE SELF-PROTECTIVE RESPONSE

1. Arrest/Startle—Arousal Awakens Us Out of Exploratory Orienting. Metal.
2. **Defensive Orienting—Fear Signals Threat. Water.**
3. Specific Self-Protective Response—Mobilization Response Initiates. Wood.
4. Completion—Successful Defense or No Threat. Restore Coherence. Fire.
5. Integration—Digest the Gristle. Harvest the Lessons. Earth.

   Cycle Returns to the Metal and Restored Capacity for Exploratory Orienting.

THE WATER ELEMENT'S season is winter. It is the darkest time of the year. Life grows cold and still. Trees stand bare before this season's harshness. Nature rests, animals hibernate, and we too want to sleep more. We contract socially and energetically. Winter is the most internal, contemplative time of the year. Wisdom grows in the depth of its quiet stillness.

When disturbed by a sense of life threat, our quiet contemplation is transformed into its opposite—consuming fear. We may find ourselves constantly scanning our environment with jumpy eyes and anxious attention. Fear can be so consuming as to make it difficult to feel a sense of safety, even when we're not under threat. Unable to sink deeply and comfortably into ourselves, we can't sleep for fear of what may come in the night. We feel collapsed, frozen, and untrusting. Alternatively, our capacity to discern danger may become unreliable. We can't utilize fear productively to guide us toward safe activities or people and instead put ourselves in risky situations. We may crave high-adrenalin experiences to help us simply feel alive.

When you are with your client, consider these questions to help you assess the ongoing impact of an incomplete response in the defensive orienting or "signaling threat" phase of the 5-SPR.

- *How is his fear-signaling system? Does he seem to know when he is safe? When he is unsafe?*
- *Does he need high-risk "adrenalin junkie" activities to help him feel alive?*
- *Does fear consume his view of the world? Does he know, in his deepest self, that he has survived?*
- *How is his essential vitality? Does he seem either exhausted and depleted or jumpy and anxious?*
- *How permeable are his boundaries? Does he know where you and others begin and end?*
- *Is he aging prematurely? Is he losing his hearing or teeth, developing brittle bones, going grey or bald at an unexpectedly early age?*

CORRESPONDENCES RELATING TO THE WATER ELEMENT'S ROLE IN THE SELF-PROTECTIVE RESPONSE

Element	*Water*
Season	*Winter*
Organ systems	*Kidney, Bladder*
Emotion	*Wisdom, fear*
Role in Successful Self-Protective Response	*Signaling center, power to fuel the mobilization response*
Unsuccessful or Incomplete Self-Protective Response	*Hyperarousal: Panic, agitation, hypervigilance* *Hypoarousal: Collapse, contraction, phobias*
Engenders	*Power for mobilization*
Controls	*Cardiac coherence*
Tissues	*Bones, brain, spinal chord*
Virtue	*Wisdom*
Stores	*Genetic potential, or jing*
Spirit	*Willpower, or zhi*
Archetypal Questions	*Do I have enough crops stored away? Do I have enough fuel? Can I survive this cold winter?*
Exercises to Enhance Regulation	*Building a felt sense of safety* *Repairing boundary ruptures* *Building capacity in the kidney/adrenal system* *Restoring regulation in the fear and terror centers of the brain stem* *Supporting bone flexibility and resilience*

ORIENTATION: THE NATURE OF THE WATER ELEMENT

Understanding the nature of the Water Element and its role as the signaling center for threat will deepen your skills as a clinician and help to normalize the experience of survivors. Understanding Water's impact on morbidity and mortality, its role in epigenetics and ancestral trauma, and the social implications of restoring its regulation will expand the context of clinical interventions and the meaning these interventions may have for survivors.

Water is the foundation of life. Humans—and all living beings—can't survive without it. The Water Element is emblematic of the mystery in the depths of the ocean, the quiet of a still pond, the movement of a mountain stream, the inexorably slow and steady power of a glacier, and the fierce power of a tsunami.[1]

Water manifests with immense power, like Niagara Falls, and with extraordinary stillness, like a frozen lake. Water is soft, yet it chisels valleys through mountains with its persistent and continuous nature. The oceans' tides, waves, and even its salinity are mirrored in our deepest cellular rhythms. Water is ubiquitous, but without a container, it has no shape and consumes everything in its path.

Fear is the emotion associated with the Water Element. Note the resonance between these images of water's expression in nature and how fear manifests in human beings:

- The power of a tsunami is mirrored in the petite woman who is suddenly able to lift a car off her trapped child or the firefighter who charges into a burning building to save its occupants. Fear is formidable, demanding, and commanding.
- Water's ubiquitous nature is emblematic of the trauma survivor whose fear borders on paranoia and consumes his world outlook. Like water, fear seeps into every crevice of his mind, consumes his attention, and feels impossible to contain.
- The act of freezing when overwhelmed by fear is echoed in the surface of a frozen pond. Freeze is a physiologically brilliant and lifesaving solution at certain critical times—it protects our heart from

the damage of prolonged tachycardia (rapid heartbeat), when our system is overwhelmed by an experience of life threat.

- The quiet of a still pond echoes our capacity to experience a deeply contemplative and meditative state *when we feel safe*. Our Water energy will sink, settle, and quiet in the absence of threat.
- Like the slow but relentless movement of a glacier, our Water Element provides the capacity to persevere on a day-to-day basis while growing up in poverty or enduring a long military deployment as an adult. It is the source of wisdom for the sage who has survived many challenges in a long life.

Fear has its most commanding presence in the wintertime. Winter brings forward ancient and archetypal questions that live as metaphors in our unconscious: *Do I have enough crops stored away? Do I have enough fuel? Can I survive the cold?* Winter is the darkest, coldest, most challenging season. There is little movement or activity, life is quiet, and our vitality is held deeply.

The two organ systems associated with the Water Element are the Kidneys and the Bladder. The drive to survive danger is embedded in our Kidneys. This drive to survive is held in the very essence of our being. After all, we don't *choose* to escape threats, we react instinctively with our innate will to survive. This compulsion and the willpower behind it—called the *zhi*—are the spiritual expression of the Kidneys.

The depth of Water is reflected in our bones, the densest tissue in the body. Our bones, together with the brain and spinal cord, are the Water Element's corresponding tissues. The brain referred to in AAM is specifically the brain stem, where our primal, instinctive, and largely fear-inspired responses are managed. It is distinguished from the mind—which is associated with the function of the Heart and refers more specifically to the frontal cortex.

AAM's understanding of Kidney function includes the protection of our most fundamental vitality. The Kidneys store a special substance, called *jing*, which is created in the union of sperm and egg at our conception. *Jing* governs our essential vitality, our genetic potential, the health of our bones, and our capacity for mental focus and concentration. It governs the pace of our physiological development—when we walk, talk, and reach puberty; as well as when we go grey or bald, lose our hearing or our teeth, or develop brittle bones. *Jing* plays a major role in our morbidity and mortality. We are born with a finite amount of *jing* and expend it throughout our lifetime. Once it is fully depleted, our life comes to its natural end.

CONTEXT: THE ROLE OF THE WATER ELEMENT IN THE SELF-PROTECTIVE RESPONSE

That inner squirrel of ours just heard a twig snap. Our sensory systems have discerned possible risk and alerted our sympathetic nervous system to rise slightly and alert our orientation system. The task of discerning risk belongs to the Metal Element. When it discerns a high level of risk, it sends that message to the Water Element via our Kidneys, and their close companions, the adrenal glands, which together create the signal for threat.[2]

Both Western medicine and AAM recognize the critical role of the Kidney/adrenal system in signaling threat. In Western terms, the adrenal gland secretes adrenaline and cortisol, the chemical messengers that provide the signal to initiate a whole-body survival response. Adrenaline causes extra calcium to enter our heart and skeletal muscles, which increases the strength of muscle contractions, relaxes the lungs to allow deeper breaths, and triggers the emotional responses associated with fear in the brain. Cortisol causes an increase in glucose levels to fuel our muscles and temporarily inhibit the systems of the body that we don't immediately need—such as digestion, the growth and repair of tissues, and immune function.

The powerful message of these stress hormones sends a message of alarm across the control cycle to our Heart Protector. As mammals, unless previously extinguished, we will first use our social engagement system—governed by our Heart Protector —to attempt a relational response to low-level threat. However, if our Heart Protector is unable to resolve this sense of threat in the context of relationship, or the threat is significant enough that it can't be dealt with by social means, this vibration of fear will penetrate the Heart. The Heart will then call into action every body system and every physiological function designed to protect and defend. Every ounce of *qi* we have available is deployed to save our life. The message of imminent life threat is sent to the entire kingdom of the body as an all-encompassing vibration, carried in the blood by the Heart's pulse. Transmission is immediate and comprehensive. The whole body moves into high arousal, with a fast and pounding heartbeat as its central feature.

In particular, the Water Element will be instructed by our Heart to provide the necessary power to mount a full-on fight-or-flight response, crafted by our Wood Element. This chapter explores the Water Element's role in signaling threat and providing the power that fuels mobilization; it also outlines what happens when that signaling function is disrupted, and it provides strategies for restoring regulation so that in the future, this important system can effectively recognize safety as well as danger.

COMMON SYMPTOMS FOR THE WATER TYPE: THE KIDNEYS AND BLADDER

The massive *qi* harnessed by the Kidneys in the presence of life threat, and the breadth of its influence, give rise to diverse symptoms, as well as many avenues for restoring its regulation. The Kidney's critical role as the signaling center for life threat makes it an important organ to work with in virtually all survivor types. AAM speaks to the significant and complex role of the Kidneys in our overall health and vitality by recognizing it as *the root of all yin and all yang*. The Kidneys are understood to be the origin and foundation for both the *yin* and the *yang* of all other body organs. Their *yin* aspect is responsible for birth, growth, and reproduction, while their *yang* aspect is the source of energy for all physiological processes.[3]

Because of its crucial and powerful role in our physiology, the impact of chronic, unremitting fear on the Kidneys is profound. Such fear creates chronic stress chemistry, which wreaks havoc on the physical body and profoundly impacts our mind and emotions.[4] This constant signaling of danger can become consuming. Water survivor types may appear to be over- or under-adrenalized—either unable to sit still or, conversely, unable to initiate movement.

There is an intimate relationship between the Kidneys and the Heart in AAM trauma physiology. Those whose self-protective response was thwarted in the signal threat phase have difficulty discerning both safety and danger, because the signaling center in the Kidneys sends the wrong messages to the Heart. The Kidneys may signal danger when there is none or may fail to signal danger when life threat is imminent. This intimate role between the Kidneys and the Heart can give rise to cardiac symptoms that are actually rooted in our Kidneys. Blood pressure and the strength of our heart's contractions are particularly impacted by kidney function.

For Water types, fear can dominate interpersonal relationships. We may have too much fear—we don't connect with or trust anyone. Alternatively, we don't use our fear effectively and are frequently hurt when we place ourselves in risky situations with untrustworthy people.

When stuck in this phase of the trauma cycle, the body makes use of cortisol and adrenalin in distorted ways, impacting the messaging of our endocrine system and, by extension, virtually every body function. When functioning well, these stress hormones rise to help us meet a challenge and then return to equilibrium when we know we are safe. In trauma survivors, the message "it's over" that is signaled by a reduction in cortisol levels is disturbed—and so the stress response doesn't return to its baseline.[5]

Our *jing*, or our core vitality—which is stored in our Kidneys—is particularly vulnerable to traumatic stress. It can be prematurely depleted by too much exercise or hard work, too many births for women, or exposure to repeated and overwhelming fear. Traumatic stress can consume our *jing*, which is why we look for early signs of aging in this survivor type—weak bones or teeth, loss of hearing, or early greying of hair are signs of its depletion. Caring for people's Kidneys protects their *jing* and, by extension, their life expectancy and essential vitality.

The bones are the tissue associated with the Water Element. They are highly vulnerable to the loss of *jing* and can lose elasticity and resiliency as the result of injury, stress, strain, age, and trauma-induced *jing* depletion. The approaches for restoring regulation in the threat-signaling center described in this chapter will help protect and restore your client's *jing* and preserve flexibility and resilience in her bones.

The Water Element helps us feel a sense of safe boundary. Water requires a boundary—the banks of a stream, a drinking glass, a flower vase. Fear is similar; it will also leak everywhere and impact everything unless it is contained. Our boundaries can become shaken and permeable after a traumatic experience. This can manifest in many ways. We might misinterpret information from our environment or feel unable to distinguish our physical, social, or emotional "edges," which may leave us more vulnerable to future injury or boundary ruptures. We may have a tendency to collapse or, alternatively, become hypervigilant in our response to intrusion of our personal space; we might also experience an absence of boundary, leaving us open to constant overstimulation; and we could also feel a rigid and inflexible boundary, leaving us prone to isolation and numbness in our perceptions of our environment. Restoring a sense of a secure boundary supports the Water Element and its function to provide us with a felt sense of safety in the "container" of our body.

A well-regulated and healthy Water Element provides a healthy container for fear, regulates the storage and movement of fluids and *qi*/energy, and supports our overall mortality and vitality. At the level of the body, the Water Element helps keep the eyes and tissues moist. At a mental level, it keeps us from becoming so anxious that our minds can't remember what we know. At the emotional level, our Water helps uncontained fear from leaving us scared speechless. And at the spiritual level, our Water helps us find the faith that reminds us that spring will come again.

REMEDIES FOR RESTORING REGULATION IN THE WATER

If our self-protective response was thwarted in this early signaling phase, our ability to utilize fear effectively will be compromised. Unable to regulate themselves, our Kidneys will be unable either to turn off the constant signal of life threat or to turn on this life-preserving signal when needed.

Helping a survivor cultivate her ability to recognize and experience safety, rather than operating exclusively from fear, is our overarching task. We are helping our clients develop a container for their fear. Uncontained fear is as corrosive to our life force as a slow leak is to the structural integrity of a basement. Our bodies will mismanage their use of cortisol and adrenalin—causing sleep disturbances, premature aging, and metabolic disturbances, in addition to inhibiting the capacity to make good choices in distinguishing safety and danger.

Our own regulated, centered presence as providers is perhaps our most important tool in helping others reestablish their capacity to recognize safety and danger. An anxious, agitated person will begin to join and resonate with a peaceful person nearby and will become calmer. As providers, we need to provide that anchoring presence. Recognizing when we are activated and cultivating resource states that return us to greater regulation builds this groundwork of safety and is the foundation for every clinical intervention. Just like the airlines advise us, "Put your own oxygen mask on first."

In addition to your own self-care, using one or more of these kinds of resource states may be helpful when you find yourself activated in the presence of a client:

- Take a moment with nature—focusing on the tree, mountain, or sky just outside your window.
- Use a silent prayer to consciously invite the presence of an important spiritual being to be with you.
- Bring attention to and join the healing vibration your professional peers are creating down the hall and around the world.
- Invite the presence of a special person or animal—someone who has helped you feel steady and more regulated—either recently or long ago.
- Shift your attention to your feet on the ground, the rise and fall of your breath, or your heart beating rhythmically in your chest.

The remainder of this chapter explores five approaches for working with Water survivor types. We begin by focusing on ways to help create a felt sense of safety as a foundation for your work. Once your client has found an embodied experience of safety, you can choose to engage in the other approaches described, which will depend on your client's history and needs—building capacity in the Kidney/adrenal system, repairing boundary ruptures, or supporting bone flexibility and resilience. We save exploring work with the brain stem for last. It is the location of many of the structures involved in our threat-signaling system, which makes it a profoundly powerful location to work with in restoring essential regulation—but this also makes it highly volatile. We recommend setting it aside until your client has achieved a relatively stable felt sense of safety. This will allow your client to more comfortably let down any vigilance the brain stem may be holding.

Inviting a Felt Sense of Safety

When we help clients cultivate a felt sense of safety in the container of their body, we help them build their capacity to renegotiate a traumatic experience. Their capacity to protect themselves, regulate their arousal, and gain insight into their experience will expand. Without this container, it may be virtually impossible for a client to renegotiate their traumatic experience. We can help create conditions for our clients to experience a somatically mindful state of greater safety, security, and capacity to cope, but the actual building of this capacity occurs inside the client—it is not something we practitioners can force to happen.

Helping clients experience their safety will help restore the rhythmic movement between parasympathetic and sympathetic, between *yin* and *yang*, Water and Fire, Kidneys and Heart. Creating a felt sense of safety in our treatment rooms is a critical foundation for healing. Here are several suggestions for helping your client shift toward regulation and away from consuming fear:

- Invite your client to choose which chair to sit in, which end of the table he would like for his head, or the distance between your chairs. Help him notice how his choices and preferences help him embody a sense of greater safety.
- Focus your attention on the end of the client's story, asking questions like, "When did you know you were going to be okay?" or "What helped you survive?" Shifting the client's attention to this part of the story and his survival gives him an implicit experience of that survival. "There and then" is not actually "here and now."
- Invite attention to experiences of safe and trustworthy connection with others, using questions like, "Who came to help you?" or "If you could imagine the perfect person there to help—it could be your fairy godmother, a person from your past, a movie star, superhero, or an imaginary friend—who would it be?" With questions like these,

you help restore lost pieces of safe attachment and the inherent healing available in social engagement.

- Let your inquiries orient toward healing. Instead of saying, "Tell me about your headaches," ask, "What helps your headaches feel better?" or "Is there a time you can remember feeling less anxious? Where were you and what were you doing?"

Client Example

Peter, an army chaplain, tells me he had been unable to speak for several months after his tour in Iraq. "That's kind of tough on a preacher," he says. "I didn't know how I was going to live my life."

I ask him, "When did you know you were home safe?" He looks at me thoughtfully. It is one of those "light bulb turning on" moments. He slowly tells me his story:

"They airlifted me to Landstuhl, Germany. My physical injuries healed fairly quickly, but I couldn't speak. One day, I went for a walk out among the trees. It looked like home in northern Wisconsin. I started talking to God. When I could talk to God, I knew I was eventually going to be okay, even though it took awhile before my speech came back."

We don't know how or why Peter had been scared speechless. But in this single, brief interchange with me, he recognized the experience of safety and his reconnection to his faith that helped him know he would be okay. He harvested an experience of safety that became the anchor for his healing. He rediscovered the dual resource of his home and his faith, shifted his orientation to safety instead of fear, and everything changed. As he remembered this reconnection and recognition that he would recover, he straightened up, appeared more solid, substantial, and settled.

Building Capacity in the Kidney/Adrenal System

A clinician's greatest service to all trauma survivors, and especially Water survivor types, is to help them build capacity in their Kidney/adrenal system to support the Kidneys to better distinguish safety from threat and to communicate these messages more accurately to the Heart. This approach to working directly with the Kidney/adrenal system will be useful for almost all clients who experienced disruption anywhere in the 5-SPR.

The braced, drawn-up, and contracted physical appearance that communicates fear is mirrored in the Kidney/adrenal system, which also becomes braced and contracted. In this state, the system releases more adrenalin and other stress chemicals that constantly communicate a message of life threat. This physiology can only support fear or terror, anger or rage, intense arousal or profound collapse. The body can become stuck in this state, signaling ubiquitous fear and constant threat.

The Kidney/adrenal "hold" is an opportunity to practice "seeing" inside the body using your hand, your mind's eye, and your intention. It requires a quiet, focused, and receptive mind. The kidneys are nestled under the respiratory diaphragm. Their color is a deep burgundy red, with a smooth, slick texture. A single adrenal gland rests atop each kidney. In the case of the Kidney/adrenal hold, clients can either lie face up on a treatment table or sit in a comfortable chair. Depending on your client's knowledge, you may need to educate her about the important role these structures play in the stress response and how supportive contact with these systems may be helpful. You will be working with each Kidney/adrenal gland in turn, and for most clients, it doesn't matter which side you begin on, but simply asking the client's preference, as noted below, will also support her growing embodiment and connection with her somatic self. For general information and guidance on mindful touch, please see our discussion in Chapter Five.

Here are specific strategies for applying touch to the Kidney/adrenal system:

1. As you prepare to bring your touch here, check in with your client, standing on one side and then the other, and ask, "Which side feels more comfortable for receiving touch?" Start with the side he chooses.
2. Then bring your attention to your own Kidney/adrenal system. You may want to look at anatomy books to help you visualize this space in the body. Imagine making gentle contact with your own Kidneys and adrenal glands or simply bring your attention to this area with your embodied awareness. This internal focus will help quiet and focus your mind.

3. Shift your attention now to your client's Kidney/adrenal system. It may take some time to experiment with the best way for you to connect with these structures inside your clients. Practicing this technique can be a helpful way to deepen the experience of connection between the two of you.
4. Notice your client's response as you share this subtle shift in your attention. Does his breathing slow? Do you see him relax? Does he close his eyes and turn his attention inward? Or does he hold his breath, brace, or withdraw from you? In the latter case, you may need to wait awhile before making actual physical contact. You might want to talk with him about what you noticed and decide together if touch feels safe enough at this stage. It is always important to notice whether or not you feel a sense of invitation from your client for your touch. Even though you asked permission before touching, there is sometimes a difference between the client's cognitive willingness to be touched and the actual somatic response once touch is imminent. Is the invitation for touch present or absent in his tissues? Wait for this sense of open invitation to emerge before you proceed. If you're not certain, you can ask verbally if it feels okay to make contact.
5. Once you've established a sense of security around touching the area, slide your hand under the base of his rib cage, at the back, just above his waist. You should feel the boney structure of the bottom portion of the ribcage under your hand, not the soft give of the tissue of the waist itself. Imagine that you can gently direct your attention through the client's skin and rib cage to find his kidney, without any increase in physical pressure. With your mind's receptive eye, look for something a bit rounded and firm. Remember, the most important thing is for you to remain present with your contact; the physical accuracy is less critical. The intention in your contact is to provide your client with a sense of supportive and calming connection, so if you are in the general area of the kidney, the touch is likely to be effective. If you are uncertain about whether or not your contact feels supportive and is serving his sense of safe connection, simply ask, "Do I need to adjust my hand up or down, in or out? How's the pressure?" Let him direct your contact. Feel free to experiment

together with what feels best. Eventually, with practice, you will develop a better sense of when you have arrived at the right spot and greater confidence about how to notice the Kidney/adrenal system using this placement of your attention. If you focus on staying present within yourself and offering connection to your client with your contact, you are doing what's most effective.

When the Kidney relaxes, you may feel this as a gentle "settling" into your hand, as if the Kidney is finding you and letting its weight down into your contact. It is moving out of its previous braced, clutched state. You may feel a sense of the blood pulsing, gently vibrating against your hand. If this pulse initially feels choppy and fast, you may then feel it slow, elongate, and smooth out. You may feel an increase in warmth or notice the client's breath moving more fully through the surrounding tissues. You may also feel your own body relax. There are so many different ways we may notice the responses in our clients; it will likely take some time to discover what the most effective methods are for you. Again, the most important thing you are offering is your focused and quiet attention on the Kidney/adrenal gland. Cradle it as if it were a newborn infant.

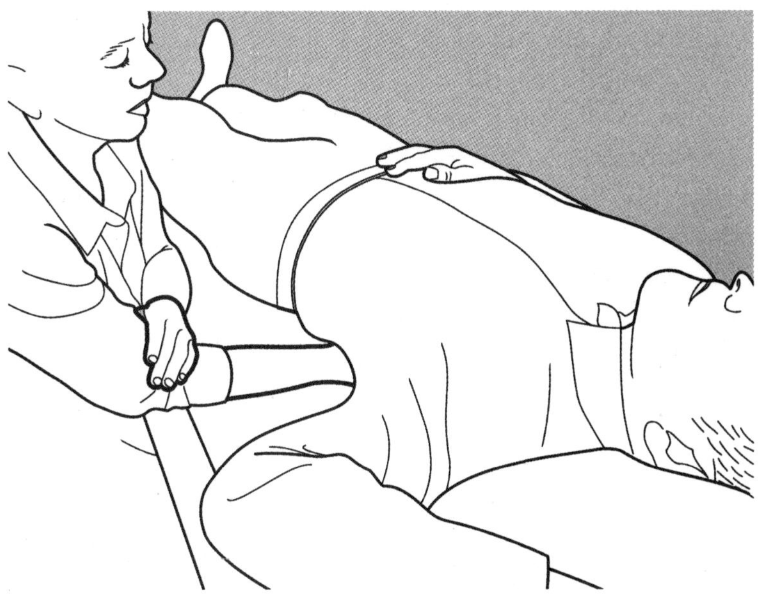

FIGURE 7.1. Kidney/Adrenal Hold, Lying on a Table

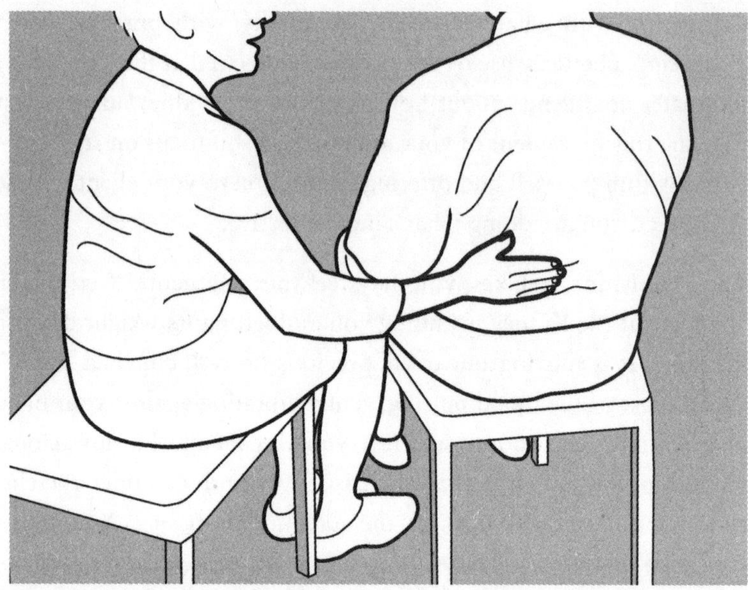

FIGURE 7.2.—Kidney/Adrenal Hold, Sitting in a Chair

During this process, you are waiting for your client's Kidney—and thus her whole system—to settle. She can't force this settling to occur. More often than not, your client will experience your contact as delicious and welcome support. Her Kidney no longer has to do it all by itself. Here, finally, is the literal support she so desperately needs and wants. She will likely experience her whole system releasing its bracing and coming alive out of immobilization and freeze.

You may also find that different clients have different preferences for how contact happens—either both sides contacted at the same time (slide your arm under her body so your palm will be on the far side and the soft, fleshy part of your forearm on the near side) or one side contacted first and then the other, shifting sides after you have been on one side for a period of time.

Help the client notice what happens as her Kidney settles, softens, and drops. Look for movement toward parasympathetic restoration and a sense of greater capacity in her system. Here are a few things you may say to help her embody her experience:

- "From the outside, I feel a pulsing in your kidney that wasn't there when I first made contact. I wonder—what are you noticing?"

- "As you took that deep breath, what did you notice in the rest of your body?"
- "That was a nice gurgle in your belly—and from the outside, your body appears softer. I wonder—what does that feel like on the inside?"

As the Kidney softens and relaxes, blood will move through it more readily, allowing you to feel your client's pulse in your hand. As the tissues that support the kidney also relax, the diaphragm itself may soften from its previous braced state, allowing a deeper breath to emerge. With increased parasympathetic restoration, any latent freeze or shutdown of peristalsis in the guts will wake up and move, often causing burps, gurgles, or flatulence. All of these are good signs of returning regulation, but you may need to reassure your client: "We are not at a formal event. I celebrate any movement in your guts as a sign of restoration of your system's vitality. I don't want you to brace against any movements in your guts."

It's important to note that dropping into a more relaxed state can feel "wrong" to a client who has been braced and activated for a long time. He may not have felt this state of relaxation in years and may not feel safe enough to relinquish his vigilance. He may have come to associate vigilance as the equivalent of (or a substitute for) safety. Letting go and relaxing could be mistaken for lack of preparedness, and it could feel overwhelmingly precarious. If you sense this reaction, slow down—you may need to remove your hand and help your client find a more settled state to pair with this arousal. Spending more time on the approaches described in the section "Inviting a Felt Sense of Safety" earlier in this chapter may be helpful.

Near the end of a session focused on the Kidney/adrenal system, you might want to offer your client some homework to help integrate any shifts that have taken place. A pair of warmed yoga eye pillows or warmed washcloths folded in quarters and placed under his kidneys as he falls asleep at night may be a welcome suggestion.

Client Example

Chuck is in his early twenties. He grew up in a military family that moved frequently. Both his parents worked in demanding positions within the military and were largely unavailable to him. He joined the army straight out of high school. Being overseas in a combat zone had been terrifying for him. He had attempted suicide once. He was chronically anxious and highly vigilant. He couldn't stop thinking about all the terrible things that could happen to him. Once home again, he spent hours each day checking and rechecking the locks on his doors and windows. In an early session with me, he told me, with racing, anxious eyes, "There is so much inside me. If you pricked me, I would explode."

Over the next several months, I used the Kidney/adrenal hold alongside acupuncture treatment. In one memorable session, as I held Chuck's Kidney, he told me, "I feel like water droplets coming together instead of being separate and apart. I'm finding myself. Like my whole entity is working as one—instead of being so scattered on the inside."

In a later session, while I continued to support Chuck's Kidney/adrenal system, he said, "I feel like I have the confidence and faith in myself that can help me heal. When I feel warm inside like this, my brain relaxes. I'm ready to open up the passageway to my heart, link my mind to my heart, end the battle inside me, and let my heart and my mind speak together. I think I can find safety by staying in my heart instead of running to anger or withdrawal."

The boyish, scared look on Chuck's face had transformed into a more mature, more manly, and more chiseled look. Shortly after, he began vocational training to become a cook, got his driver's license, and was ready to move out of his parents' home and into an apartment of his own.

Repairing Boundary Ruptures

Knowing where we begin and end, and where we are in relation to other objects, either moving or stationary, is critical for cultivating kinesthetic awareness of our physical state and place. Knowing how and where we set our own social and emotional boundaries lets us reach out for relationship while also maintaining clarity about what is—and isn't—okay in this dimension of life. We become more able to navigate our interpersonal world with ease and safety. This type of healthy boundary awareness supports our ability to make instinctive, protective responses in situations that would otherwise leave us more vulnerable to accidents or injuries. Thankfully, we can help survivors heal breaches to this most primal sense of their own container.

The techniques outlined below will help bring awareness to your client's interoception of a safe boundary, as well as any ruptures to her sense of a safe container. It is important to guide her through this experience slowly, gently touching into the edge of any experience of arousal. Use the tick-tock method, alternating attention and awareness between safety and modest arousal, as described in depth in Chapter Five.

Begin by anchoring your client's experience in a felt sense of safety, using the methods described earlier in this chapter. Then, using one of the approaches outlined below, invite her to become aware of a sense of having a boundary. You want to find the edge where her sense of safety gives way to modest arousal. Note that we want to find this edge without drastically going past it. Allow time for her arousal to rise and then time for regulation to return. You can trust that if you keep your tick-tock inside a titrated range, restoration will naturally follow arousal. The law of *yin* and *yang* confirms that prediction.

However, if the client's arousal is excessive, collapse will quickly follow—as hyperarousal is connected as a paired opposite to freeze and collapse. Titration is critical in all our work. Play tick-tock again, slowing down your investigation of her arousal to a more manageable level. Anchor each tick-tock in your client's felt sense of safety, and work the edges of her arousal pattern at a gentle, inch-by-inch pace. Working the rise and fall of this dynamic wave of arousal and safety will expand your client's zone of resiliency and her capacity to recognize safety, as well as threat.

Here are a few approaches for working to restore healthy boundaries with your client. You may develop others that better match your practice setting and client population:

- Invite your client to notice her felt sense of safety as you vary the distance between your chairs to move closer or further away from her. Find the sweet spot of comfortable distance and location, and then consciously challenge that boundary—ever so slightly—by shifting your location and then returning to the sweet spot. Invite your client's curiosity as you explore these subtle changes in your position. If she notices arousal in her body but says, "It's okay, I can take it," then stop. Return to the sweet spot, allow some time to pass and see if regulation comes on board. We don't want to violate her body's wisdom of what is a safe and comfortable boundary.

- Invite your client to notice his personal boundary when you walk toward him from across the room, inviting him to tell you when to stop. Practice tick-tock, bringing awareness to the wave of slight arousal and giving time for the restoration of regulation. You can also try approaching from the left or right side, or with him facing you, turning to the side, or facing the wall. If appropriate, you might experiment with a blindfold or invite him to close his eyes. Invite curiosity. Invite playfulness.
- Give your client a ball of string and invite her to make a circle that represents her boundary. Help her explore her felt sense of safety while placing yourself at various points on her circle and bringing awareness to any hyperarousal or hypoarousal that emerges, again playing tick-tock with her experience. Invite her to make adjustments to the string to fine-tune her felt sense of a secure and safe personal boundary.
- At home, your client can bring her own sensate attention to her skin as a safe container. She can experiment in the shower by changing the temperature or force of the water and noticing her felt sense of those changes. She can take time to apply an aromatic and soothing oil to honor her body's boundary and the protection that comes with this awareness.

Client Example

Sally was in a massive car accident as a young teen and underwent multiple surgeries that saved her life but left her with a primary strategy of dissociation as her way of managing this experience. Throughout young adulthood, she coped by opting out and seeking escape—using street drugs and alcohol and subsisting on marginal employment in an alternative community. Sally is now married and has a young adult son. She is successful at work but remains troubled in her marriage, finding her husband distant and unavailable.

When she came to see me, she complained about her husband and the lack of intimacy in their relationship. When I asked what helps her cope, she answered, "Well, I tell myself that I can't do anything about how unavailable he is, and I should forget about it—you know, just accept the things I cannot change. That helps a lot."

Except it didn't seem this strategy was helping a lot, or that accepting her husband's unavailability was a desirable choice for her or a healing one for their marriage. The management strategy she used—that of disconnection—had helped her manage her arousal state for many years, but it was no longer helping her achieve a satisfying life. She had learned long ago that she could create distance from the experience of her accident and the many surgeries—and this was how she now approached all forms of intimacy, which, naturally, only fostered distance. Her marriage now spanned a great expanse of mutual unavailability. The thick boundary she developed to protect her from a fear-filled inner reality, which had been useful once upon a time, now left her wanting more out of life.

We used the tick-tock method to explore her personal boundary system. As she lay on the table, relaxed and with her eyes closed, I stood next to her feet and then walked toward her head incrementally. Sally was amazed to observe her arousal with only the slightest micro-movements I made toward her. Her experiences of vulnerability and fear, tenderness and longing emerged. We allowed them to rise and then gave time and space for safety and regulation to return.

When she returned to see me a month later, she reported that she and her husband were listening together to the audiobook Wired for Love, *by Stan Tatkin,*[6] *going on evening walks to debrief their day, and greeting each other with a hug they held until they experienced the other relaxing in their arms. They needed to titrate the hug—it was quite activating to their capacity for connection—so sometimes they simply held each other's hands until they were able to relax together.*

Inviting awareness of Sally's boundary and offering her opportunities to experience her arousal, sandwiched between thick slices of safety, helped her cultivate the possibility of safety in relationship and a more embodied sense of wholeness. It allowed both her and her husband to begin to connect with each other in more meaningful ways.

Supporting Bone Flexibility and Resilience with Mindful Touch

The bones are the tissue corresponding to the Water Element. Though they might seem quite static, bones are, in fact, living tissue. When healthy, they are relatively solid, but they should also possess some flexibility and responsiveness to movement. We rely on our bones for a sense of our inner strength and for external protection. Our long bones provide stability in our limbs, while our cranium, ribs, and spine provide protection for soft organs like our brain, heart, lungs, and viscera.

Our long bones serve as "spacers" between our muscles. They keep our muscles elongated and give them something to push or pull against to create movement. Our stability requires dynamic tension and relaxation, with muscles and tendons pulling against bones. This relationship between the different parts of the musculoskeletal system makes it possible for us to stand up, move through the world, and know where we are in space. It allows us to exert an antigravity effort and remain upright. Working with the bones from this conceptual framework is particularly important for survivors of trauma associated with physical injury, such as motor vehicle accidents or other high-velocity injuries. These survivors may have experienced dramatic changes in their entire musculoskeletal system.

While each bone is part of the larger skeletal system, each one also exists as a clearly delineated and defined local unit. Bones are our densest tissue and have the capacity to hold very dense and intense vibrations. For some trauma survivors, this quality of density and intensity may be associated with an experience of terror. But for others, the inner structure held in our bones may provide a sense of deep self-connection and grounded stability.

The bones can be used as an anchor for high-arousal states that emerge when working with other tissues. Their unique feature of having a clearly delineated beginning and ending—an inherently segmented and titrated structure—can help contain the high arousal that may emerge when working with tissues that have an inherently whole body, global, or un-titrated nature—such as the skin or connective tissue. When working with high activation in more global tissues, you may shift your hand placement to a location where the bone is close to the body's surface—placing your fingers on your client's wrist, elbow, or ankle. This can provide quick access to a more titrated form of contact and attention. Or you may simply shift your attention deeper into your client's body, down to their bones, which can have the same effect of containing and anchoring arousal. Allow your client's arousal to settle using the skeletal structure, and then tick-tock back to the outside edge of her arousal, returning attention to the bone as needed for an experience of safe anchor.

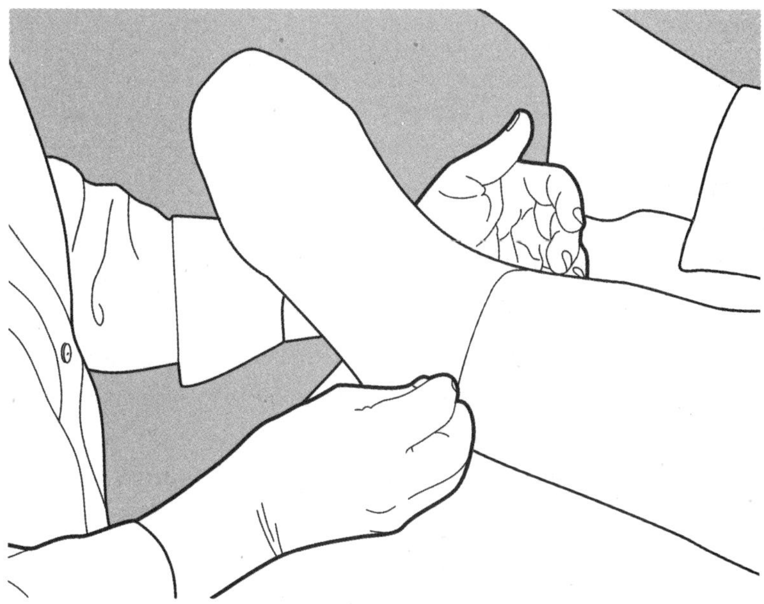

FIGURE 7.3. Touching the Bones

Client Example

Michelle had been seriously injured in a car accident a few years before she first came to see me. She had also experienced a difficult childhood, having been a witness to a lot of violence between her parents. As she told me a little about her history, she said she always felt she had to walk on eggshells at home to avoid causing explosive arguments between her mom and dad. As an adult, she was withdrawn and lacked confidence. Since her car accident, she began to experience stiffness in her legs, and—although she was only in her early fifties—had been diagnosed with advanced osteoporosis.

We began our work with the Kidney/adrenal hold. Fairly quickly, we progressed to working with Michelle's bones, particularly those in her legs, because she said she felt deep, aching sensations in her bones when I held her Kidney. Each time I made contact with her bones, she experienced waves of terror that flowed up from her legs and caused her breath to catch. Together, we waited for each wave to pass, so she could settle again. Each time, she felt a sense of greater strength flowing inside as the terror subsided.

Eventually, she began to experience a sense of power that she had never known before. She developed the sense of her legs standing strong underneath her—and the sense that she could stand her ground when she felt challenged at work. Her legs felt more flexible, vital, and substantial—and decidedly less achy.

Restoring Regulation in the Fear/Terror Centers in the Brain Stem

Both AAM and Western medicine recognize the brain stem as the site of our vigilance system. Helping people replace fear or terror with neutral curiosity requires balance and regulation in this tissue.

In AAM, the Bladder meridian, which is the Kidney's partner in the Water Element, runs alongside the brain stem and spinal chord. It plays a critical role in creating a leak-proof container for our fear and our energy—as well as our urine. If we are overwhelmed by fear, our Bladder's function as a container will also be overwhelmed and fear will spill out and consume our worldview. How many times have you heard, "I was so scared I nearly wet my pants"?

Similarly, Western medicine locates the physiological structures for signaling threat and managing responses to fear in the brain stem and midbrain:

- The reticular activating system regulates our transition from sleep to wakefulness. It interprets information about potential threats and signals us to become alert when necessary.[7]
- Both the dorsal and ventral branches of the vagus, or tenth cranial nerve, emerge from the brain stem. Discussed more fully in Chapters One and Two, it is the longest nerve in the autonomic nervous system, and it provides parasympathetic regulation to the heart, lungs, and organs of digestion.

- The hippocampus helps us process sensation-based memories. If the smell of sugar cookies in the oven transports you to your grandmother's kitchen, it is your hippocampus that has linked this smell to that memory. Similarly, if you are a Vietnam-era veteran and the sound of a helicopter overhead causes you to dive behind a parked car, it is your hippocampus that linked that sound to that memory.
- The amygdala helps us answer the question, "Is it a stick or a snake?" Often called the "smoke signal for threat," the amygdala is our primary sensory apparatus for interpreting potential threat.[8]

Similar to the Kidney/adrenal work described earlier, we can also build capacity in the signaling center for threat when we work with the brain stem. However, since your attention to the brain stem goes directly to the part of body that manages the signaling of life threat, your client may feel particularly challenged by your hand's invitation to relax her vigilance, especially when compared to similar requests with her Kidney/adrenal system. She may have linked constriction and hypervigilance in this area with her sense of safety and security. For this reason, your hand's gentle invitation to relax and settle may be interpreted by her physiology as a request to turn off her safety radar, which may—ironically—increase her sense of activation and fear. Thus, the predictability of parasympathetic restoration is less assured with brain stem work than it is with the Kidney/adrenal work.

We can not emphasize this enough: titration is critically important for all brain stem work, and it may require you to work in other parts of the client's body, such as the Kidney/adrenal system, for quite some time before moving on to work with the brain stem.

You will likely find it helpful to stabilize your client by using the other techniques discussed in this chapter—cultivating a felt sense of safety, repairing boundary ruptures, building capacity in the Kidney/adrenal system, and supporting bone flexibility and resilience—before turning your attention to the brain stem. Working directly with the brain stem must wait until your client has developed reliable and embodied experiences of successfully moving out of the terror/fear state. She needs the ability to feel safe with you seated behind her, outside of her field of vision, before you can do this work.

Indeed, Water survivor types with dysregulation in the brain stem structures may subconsciously feel this refrain quite viscerally: *I will die if I let down my brain stem.* It is difficult for them to let go of that inner reality without feeling absolutely overwhelming terror.

This is particularly true for survivors of traumatic brain injuries, for whom the traumatizing event was itself a brain injury. There is a powerful connection between brain injuries and traumatic stress responses. When we invite the brain to move and settle, we risk triggering a threat response. The client must first physiologically learn that letting down her guard does not equal a lack of safety, which reaches far beyond her preliminary intellectual acceptance of her state. Once this is achieved in the physiology, working with the brain stem can be helpful rather than terrifying.

Brain stem work is most easily done using a treatment table, with your client lying on her back. Invite her to choose which end of the table she would like to place her head, and then proceed accordingly:

- Slowly move toward her head, keeping your hands at your sides, to help titrate any arousal that may be provoked by your movement toward her brain stem. Ask her to notice how it feels to have you coming toward her in this way. Allow any arousal to peak and settle before going forward.
- Place your hands on the table on either side of her head, palms down. Again, ask her to notice how she perceives your hands. When she answers, does she do so in a *please touch me* voice or a *stay away for now* voice? Allow any arousal to peak and relax. If arousal remains high, put off this work until she is more regulated.
- Bring your attention inside yourself, focusing on the area where the spinal cord emerges from the base of your skull.
- Bring your attention to this same space in your client.
- Notice your client's response, and look for a sense of invitation for your touch—is it present or absent? If you are unclear from her body's signal, ask when she is ready.
- Bring your fingers to the base of her skull. Direct your attention just inside the skull, around her brain stem, with no increase whatsoever in physical pressure. Imagine that you could gently curl your fingers

up inside the base of the skull and lightly cup the lowest part of the brain.

- For this work, the neck must also feel supported. You can either gently place your fingers so they extend down under the neck while you focus on the brain stem, or you can use one hand to support the neck while the other remains in contact with the base of the skull/brain stem area.
- Pay attention to your client. A wide range of experiences is possible, from deep relaxation to fear. You need to be prepared to adjust or mindfully withdraw your contact if the client becomes too aroused in response to this work.
- Assess the felt sense of safety for your client, including verbally checking in to see if she feels okay with the contact and whatever may be emerging in her experience.
- Use the tick-tock method to invite a shift in her awareness between her felt sense of safety and support to the edge of any arousal that appears and back again. Go slowly.

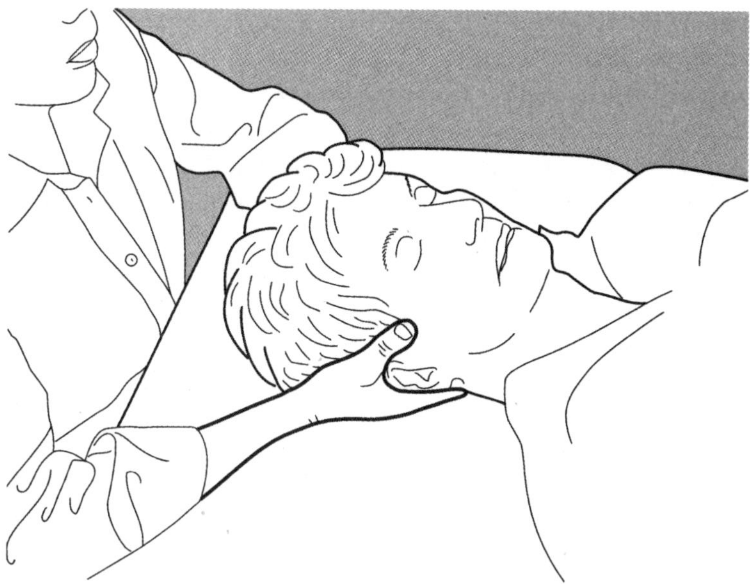

FIGURE 7.4. Touching the Brain Stem

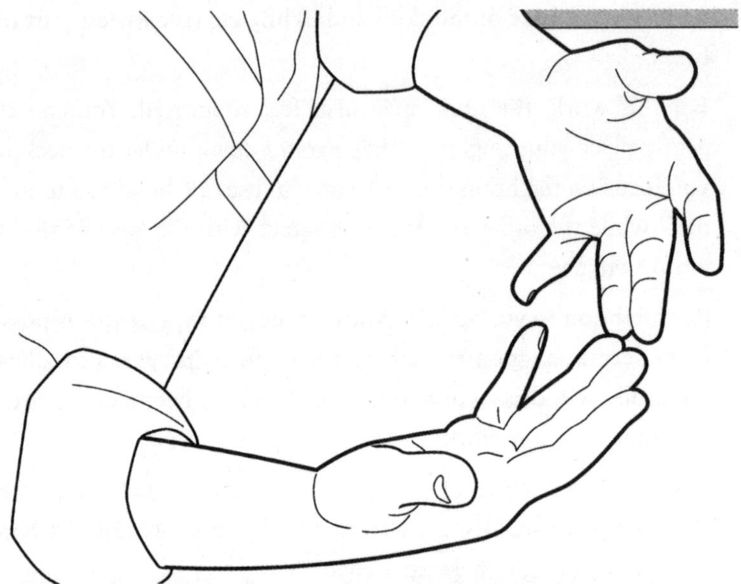

FIGURE 7.5. Position of the Fingers When Touching the Brain Stem

Client Example

Rachel was consumed by a state of constant vigilance. Simply leaving the house each morning felt like an act of bravery. Her fundamental truth was that the world is a dangerous place, and so she felt she needed to always remain prepared for possible danger to emerge. There was never a time when she simply walked down the street and enjoyed the day, never a time when she felt at ease and safe in her own home, never a time when she fully trusted any person. It was always true that danger was present, even if she hadn't yet located it. This experience of constant threat had been present for her, to some degree, even before her military service in Iraq. But since returning home to San Francisco, it had nearly taken over her life.

Rachel's arousal level was so high that we spent our first series of treatments simply holding her Kidney/adrenal system and letting her notice her response to contact, to the room, to her own breathing. After a few weeks of this, she began to experience at least some settling in her vigilance while on the treatment table. We then turned our attention to her brain stem, and she allowed me to make contact with the base of her skull, slowly bringing attention to her brain stem. Initially, she felt such a jolt of fear that she literally jumped up off the table. Together, we walked quickly up and down the hallway outside the office, letting her physiology complete the urge for flight that had been initiated by her self-protective response.

Once she was ready to lie back on the table, we slowed down and used the tick-tock method to help her notice her brain stem only in the smallest possible "doses" of attention. This still produced surges of fear, but not so much that she felt compelled to act. After a few rounds of working in this way, we returned to Kidney/adrenal work for the remainder of the session. Slowly, over many weeks, Rachel was finally able to feel herself—for a few moments at a time—letting down out of her vigilance even when we had turned our attention to her brain stem. Her breath deepened, and her inner awareness expanded. "I'm not sure I've ever actually felt this before," Rachel told me. "Is this what feeling safe feels like?" We spent the next few months expanding and exploring her increasing capacity for noticing safety.

SOCIAL IMPLICATIONS FOR RESTORING REGULATION IN THE WATER ELEMENT

The nature of the Water Element is as deep as the ocean. Disturbance in its role as the signaling center for threat is equally deep. It impacts the health and welfare, morbidity, mortality, and potentially the epigenetics of all survivor types, and, by extension, it has a profound affect on public health and community life.

When our Kidney/adrenal system signals the structures in our brain stem that life threat is imminent, our frontal cortex is relegated to the backseat. We won't have easy access to more relational, thoughtful, and nuanced responses to something new in our environment. This quality of fear tends to be contagious, influencing not just our personal experience but also the experience of everyone around us.

In the presence of overwhelming fear, decisions tend to be impulsive, reactive, primal, and geared toward lifesaving. We won't pause and consider thoughtfully an answer to the question, "Is that a snake or a rope?" We live our lives convinced that we are moments away from immediate danger. The neurological platform for fear, anchored in the brain stem, moves rapidly and becomes utterly consuming, while the neurological platform that supports relationships and executive function, rooted in our frontal cortex, becomes subverted or repressed by this powerful fear response.

In this state, we are unable to consider questions of meaning, long-term implications, or matters of the Heart. We simply react in order to "kill the snake," which can have unfortunate social implications if that "snake" turns out to be a rope (or a relationship or an opportunity for growth). When fear is consuming, our task as healers is to help people and their communities remain in the dynamic and relational tension of social discourse, to move between fear and thoughtfulness, between the lower structures of the brain stem and the frontal cortex.

Traumatic stress too often results in a loss of trust in other people or a sense of disconnection from our own true nature. But when the Kidney and the Heart—the brain stem and the prefrontal cortex—are in healthy and dynamic relationship, uncertain futures and unknown people feel less threatening, and decisions can be more thoughtfully considered for the good of community life and our children's children. Better, more positive and lasting outcomes can be put in place to enable more peaceful and productive living.

An individual, community, or nation whose signaling center for threat is stuck in the "on" position will have a different response to perceived threat than an individual, community, or nation that feels safe, valued, and respected by peers. Because of the fundamental relationship between interoceptive awareness of safety and healthy outcomes, the work of healers to restore balance and regulation in trauma survivors ripples outward and can impact interactions between individuals, communities, and nations in critically important ways.

Of particular concern in our study of trauma physiology is the impact of ongoing and high levels of stress chemistry on morbidity and mortality in survivors. According to information in the National Death Index[9] and the adverse childhood experiences study[10] at the Centers for Disease Control, survivors of severe prenatal and perinatal trauma died nearly twenty years earlier than a paired sample of people who did not experience childhood trauma. One explanation lies in the strong correlation between early trauma and the use of coping substances, such as nicotine, street drugs, and alcohol.

Looking more deeply, there are also strong correlations between early trauma and heart disease, cancer, chronic lung disease, skeletal fractures, and liver disease, as well as major mental illness and suicidality.[11] Virtually every public health concern has roots in the dysregulation of the autonomic nervous system by trauma.

AAM's understanding of the impact of traumatic stress on *jing,* introduced earlier in this chapter, can bring an additional dimension of understanding to the impact of traumatic stress on morbidity and mortality of survivors, as well as to the intergenerational impact traumatic stress and the study of epigenetics.

Early medical writings from both Eastern and Western medicine suggest that they saw disease arising from a lack of food and shelter; the presence of pathogens, such as bacteria or viruses; or accident and injury. Today, chronic illness is less likely to arise exclusively from infectious disease or a lack of food or shelter. Instead, stress chemistry is more often implicated in chronic noninfectious illnesses, as well as the vitality and function of our immune system.[12]

Jing determines the growth and development of children, the sexual maturation and reproductive capacity of adults, and our overall constitutional vitality. At birth, we are full of potential, possessing great vitality. Our skin is fresh and soft, our hair is shiny, and our hearing acute. As we age, we "consume" our *jing,* and this vitality diminishes. Our hair turns grey, our teeth fall out, our libido decreases, and we become hard of hearing. These are all functions regulated, informed by, and in resonance with the Kidneys and the Water Element.

Experiences that are likely to consume our *jing* prematurely include overexercise, overwork, giving birth to too many children (for women), and *being exposed to overwhelming fear.*[13] Traumatic stress necessarily includes overwhelming fear as its signal, and such experiences significantly tax our *jing.* Caring for our clients' Kidneys and helping them find their way to a sense of safety is critically important to protecting their *jing* and, by extension, their life expectancy and essential vitality.

Restoring regulation in the signaling center for threat and thereby building a protective container around a survivor's *jing* is worth exploring as a means of reversing the overwhelming impact of traumatic stress on life expectancy.

An exploration of the impact of traumatic stress on survivors would not be complete without a brief exploration of the science of epigenetics. Epigenetics explores the impact of external circumstances—such as exposure to toxic chemicals or traumatic stress—on genetic expression and function.

Recent research has demonstrated that traumatic stress can cause modifications that turn on or turn off the expression of genes.[14] War and natural disasters, as well as physical and emotional abuse, leave marks on families that can be traced through generational lines. Trauma-induced epigenetic changes can influence as many as *three* subsequent generations.[15]

Children born to mothers pregnant at the time of the Dutch famine in 1944 and 1945 were understandably smaller than normal. Interestingly, these children also experienced higher rates of schizophrenia, anxiety, diabetes, cardiovascular disease, and obesity in adulthood—after the war and its food shortages were long over. Even more striking is the hypothesis that epigenetic changes in women affected by the famine are the basis for significantly lower birth weights in their grandchildren, who were not exposed to famine.[16]

These children and grandchildren became more susceptible to genetic changes that left them at higher risk of cardiac, pulmonary, and autoimmune diseases. These descendants also experience higher rates of addiction and suicide, as well as mental health disorders. Such epigenetic changes can last a lifetime.[17] AAM's understanding of *jing* is one way to understand the impact of traumatic stress on the epigenetic expression of trauma survivors. Their *jing* has been disturbed by traumatic stress, and this permeates not only the survivor's immediate physiology, but likely also that of their descendants.

Epigenetics helps us more clearly understand that traumatic stress that impacts large groups of people simultaneously—such as those living in a war zone, or those exposed to a natural disaster, widespread starvation, or the 9/11 attacks[18]—can result in broad and long-lasting imprints on the biology (as well as the world outlook and culture) of whole regions or nations.

The dynamic interaction between traumatic stress and epigenetics and AAM and *jing* provides a deeper understanding of the imprint of pervasive, culturally embedded, and multigenerational oppression on health disparities in African Americans,[19] Native Americans,[20] and other communities of color, and in clusters of symptoms found in second- and third-generation Holocaust survivors.[21]

Curiously, the epigenetic impact from traumatic stress in previous generations leaves some children and grandchildren more vulnerable to physical and psychological insults while others become more resilient. Epigenetics conveys that human beings are, at the same time, both predestined and highly malleable creatures. It offers some promise that the negative effects of trauma can also be reversed or remedied with treatment anchored in regulation and capacity-building around states of fear. Even though offspring of survivors may be somewhat more genetically vulnerable, they also may be able to shift their genetic expression in ways that can transform or reverse the impact of a previous generation's experience.[22]

It follows that building resiliency in the Kidney/adrenal system may be one way to significantly impact the epigenetic impact of transgenerational transmission of traumatic stress.

CONCLUSION

Overwhelming fear is the signal for life threat. Fear alerts the Kidney/adrenal system to initiate appropriate signaling in the brain to mount a whole-body response to threat. Because of the Kidney's fundamental role as the body's signaling center, almost every survivor will benefit from a reboot of this organ.

The Water Element's relationship via the control cycle with the Fire Element illuminates the fundamental relationship between the Kidneys and the Heart in traumatic stress. This relationship is expressed through the Five Element correspondences as the relationship between the brain stem and the frontal cortex, the dorsal vagus and the ventral vagus, and between primal fear and thoughtful relationship.

The Kidneys are a potent reservoir of *qi*/energy. They function like a battery pack of *qi*. They provide the power for robust mobilization of the fight-or-flight response, governed by the Wood Element explored in the next chapter.

The Water and the Wood Elements share a special connection. Caring for Water is one way to care for Wood, as AAM teaches us that Water feeds Wood. Just as watering a plant helps it grow, healthy water in the right amount is vital for healthy wood. A healthy signaling of threat in the Water will give rise to a clear and powerful fight-or-flight response in the Wood.

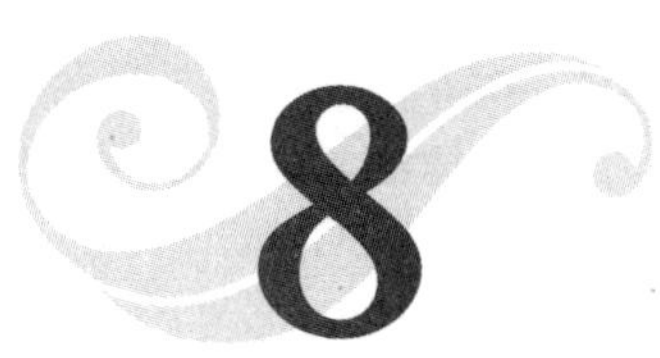

Wood and Spring: Mobilize a Response

THE FIVE STEPS OF THE SELF-PROTECTIVE RESPONSE

1. Arrest/Startle—Arousal Awakens Us Out of Exploratory Orienting. Metal.
2. Defensive Orienting—Fear Signals Threat. Water.
3. **Specific Self-Protective Response—Mobilization Response Initiates. Wood.**
4. Completion—Successful Defense or No Threat. Restoring Coherence. Fire.
5. Integration—Digest the Gristle. Harvest the Lessons. Earth.

   Cycle Returns to the Metal and Restored Capacity for Exploratory Orienting.

THE WOOD ELEMENT'S job is to protect and defend. It is always on and carries tremendous power to organize and manifest a fight-or-flight response when we or those we care about feel threatened. If our impulse to protect others and defend ourselves is thwarted or unavailable, this quality of benevolent power becomes similarly impeded, giving rise to anger or frustration.[1] *We may find it challenging to use our anger effectively. We could find ourselves braced—so tight, angry, and resentful that we can't use our creativity when confronted by a new threat. We may not even check to see if the door is unlocked before breaking it down. Alternatively, we may find ourselves collapsed—our anger seems absent, and we feel immobilized, anxious, and depressed. We are unable to protect ourselves or defend others. We can't find hope for our own growing season. In either manifestation, growth toward our ultimate purpose, our destiny—our personal "spring"—is compromised.*

As you are with your client, observe her with the following queries in mind. They will help inform you about the ongoing impact of a thwarted experience in the mobilize a response phase of the self-protective response.

- *Does anger frequently blind her capacity to see solutions to problems?*
- *Is it challenging for her to strategize solutions or prioritize tasks in difficult or complex situations?*
- *How well does her mobilization "thermostat" work? When she feels angry, is it commensurate with the level of threat she is navigating here and now, or is it colored by the there and then?*
- *Does she frequently feel invisible in a group?*
- *Is it challenging for her to defend herself when she feels insulted or threatened?*
- *Can she envision her future? Can she see the steps on the way to creating this image?*
- *How is her kinesthetic sense? Is she injured frequently? Does her body seem confused about where it is in space?*
- *Does she present with pain patterns that baffle her medical providers?*

CORRESPONDENCES RELATING TO THE WOOD ELEMENT'S ROLE IN THE SELF-PROTECTIVE RESPONSE

Element	*Wood*
Season	*Spring*
Organ Systems	*Liver, Gall Bladder*
Emotion	*Anger, hope*
Role in Self-Protective Response	*Mobilize a response; orient to threat; strategize, implement plan for fight or flight*
Unsuccessful or Incomplete Self-Protective Response	*Hyperarousal: Rigid impulses, thoughts, emotions and tissues; constantly mobilizing for threat with chronic and unreasonable anger and volatility, tight, painful tissues.* *Hypoarousal: Flaccid or passive impulses, thoughts, emotions, and tissues; little initiative to respond to threats; a sense of not taking up space.*
Engenders	*Cardiac coherence*
Controls	*Integration and digestion*
Tissue	*Ligaments, tendons, sinews*
Virtue	*Benevolence*
Stores	*Blood*
Spirit	*Ethereal soul, or hun*
Archetypal Question	*How do I navigate obstacles as I sprout and grow? Is there hope for my growing season?*
Exercises to Enhance Regulation	*Restoring protective and defensive responses and proprioceptive function in the secondary diaphragms* *Integrating motor and sensory function in the orientation system* *Restoring vitality in the blood*

ORIENTATION: THE NATURE OF THE WOOD ELEMENT

Understanding the nature of the Wood Element and the way in which it mirrors the power of the sympathetic nervous system can help providers and clients uncover new possibilities for their work and their lives. Restoring function in the tissues holding thwarted mobilization responses can help replace brace or collapse with strength and flexibility in the body, mind, emotions, and spirit. Providing opportunities to complete frustrated impulses to fight or flee can replace unremitting anger or anxiety with benevolent and expansive vision. These individuals will then influence their families, and communities with their experiences of success in strategizing solutions and navigating obstacles. A sense of possibility for nonviolent transformation of conflicts in families and communities emerges—and demonstrates the importance of this work to providers and their clients.

The Lunar New Year marks the arrival of spring and the Wood Element—the time when the sap in trees begins to soften and move in early February. Like all visions, dreams, and aspirations, spring's vibration begins long before it manifests in tangible form as sprouting plants. What has been held deeply within during the winter now takes shape and form. All of creation comes out of hibernation with a full tank of *qi* and dynamic vitality. Warm winds pick up. Mating season begins. We feel a spring in our step. Signs of life return. Along with the animals around us, we become more active. Spring is "a time when life is sprouting . . . the condition of the universe when life is ready to come forth, to spring up and to sprout." Winter creates spring. Water creates Wood—watering plants supports their growth. Spring arrives in punctuated bursts, with force and power. It is a time of fresh beginnings.[2]

The Wood Element is responsible for smooth movement in every dimension of the body, as well as the mind, emotions, and spirit. Its essential nature is to flow flexibly, like the swaying of willow branches, which don't break even when the winds are strong. In spring, grass demonstrates the power of the Wood Element when it grows right through concrete. Anger has a similar power and is therefore the emotion corresponding with the Wood Element. Like bark on a tree, anger serves to protect our soft inner layers from harmful external influences.[3]

An acorn can only become an oak. A fluffy dandelion seed can only become a dandelion. Every seed contains the essential plan for that plant's manifestation. Our Wood Element echoes this metaphor of strategic planning and vision for the destiny we too will manifest as our life unfolds.

The Wood's two organ systems are the Liver and the Gall Bladder. AAM texts refer to the Liver as the organ system "holding the office of General of the Armed Forces. Assessment of circumstances and conception of plans stem from it."[4] The Liver is responsible for strategic planning, long-range vision, forcefulness in executing actions, and protection of the body. In health, its strategic plans are strong and forceful—yet flexible enough to change easily as new circumstances emerge.

The Liver also plays the important role of storing and restoring blood and ensuring its smooth movement. In the metaphorical world of AAM, the blood carries the messages of the Heart to the kingdom of the body. If our Heart has had to repeatedly signal threat, without time or opportunity to come back to peaceful regulation, the blood may continue to carry this sense of alarm. The Liver's function of restoring the blood plays an important role in restoring balance and regulation to this critical messenger once an experience of life threat is over.

AAM understands the Liver to be responsible for the smooth movement of blood throughout the body during the day—nourishing and moistening the eyes, muscles, tendons, and ligaments, and ensuring the smooth flow of the menstrual cycle—all functions in the resonant field of the Wood. The blood is then said to travel back to the Liver at night, where it is restored during sleep. The Liver's function of restoring the blood can be overwhelmed by the amount of traumatic stress carried in it. Traumatic stress can create a vicious cycle—the high level of arousal in the blood disturbs sleep, and the Liver's task of restoring the blood is disrupted by the lack of rest.

The Gall Bladder works closely with the Liver. It is "responsible for what is just and exact. Determination and decision stem from it."[5] It is known as the organ system responsible for wise judgment and decision making—it helps every other organ system make decisions and navigate life on a moment-by-moment, day-to-day basis. It helps regulate all our body systems and is therefore critical in trauma physiology. Even those of us who have had our gall bladder removed continue to carry the Gall Bladder's function of wise judgment in every cell of our body. Without this function, cells would not know how to appropriately divide or take up their tasks in coordination with other cells.

The Liver makes our broad strategic plans, and the Gall Bladder carries them out, step-by-step and moment by moment. In its most balanced and healthy state, our Wood Element, via these two organ systems, helps us chart new beginnings, see our future, make good decisions, mobilize responses to threats, and flow smoothly around obstacles and through life.

The Wood Element's virtue is benevolence. Consider how trees support all life on earth by transforming carbon dioxide into oxygen through the process of photosynthesis, a gift to the life force of every living thing on the planet.

The Wood Element mirrors the sympathetic nervous system. In health, it is always on, always available to protect us. It uses good judgment in mounting creative and flexible responses appropriate to the level of threat we are experiencing. As discussed in Chapter Two, the sympathetic nervous system requires the parasympathetic nervous system to manage its arousal. Our capacity to deeply rest, quiet our mind in meditation, assimilate nourishment from food, and experience the give and take in personal relationships would all be unavailable without the ability to temper the Wood Element/sympathetic nervous system's constant protective stance.

Outside the context of threat, our Wood provides the energy for all creative, assertive, and strategic actions. It supports leaders to make decisions, artists to create, and visionaries to see possibilities. In health, the *qi*/energy of the Wood is designed to rise, take necessary action, and then fall like a wave. Once it experiences success, it returns to our zone of resiliency.

CONTEXT: THE ROLE OF THE WOOD ELEMENT IN THE SELF-PROTECTIVE RESPONSE

Our inner squirrel has heard that twig snap. A message of fear has alerted our Kidneys and their close companions, the adrenal glands. The Kidneys first direct their signal of fear to the Fire Element. If we are unable to resolve this threat via relationship and social engagement, the Heart commands every Element and every dimension of the body to respond with every ounce of *qi* they have available. Our Water Element provides the power to fuel mobilization in the Wood.

The bio-behavioral model of the 5-SPR puts the function of orienting to threat in the previous defensive orienting step, as a prelude to mobilization. AAM puts the functions of orienting to threat and strategizing a response more closely together and groups them in this mobilize-a-response step.

Our Wood Element will receive the power of the Water and use its own capacity to orient to threat and strategize how to implement a necessary fight-or-flight response. It will send all our blood and *qi* to our muscles and joints to carry out whatever actions are necessary to protect and defend us and those we care about. It mobilizes all of its mighty power to defend life.

If this particular threat happens to be bigger than our capacity to successfully respond, then this colossal force will meet a proverbial brick wall. Perhaps we were hit by the pressure wave of an improvised explosive device, leaving us unconscious, or perhaps our impulse to escape a car accident was thwarted when our legs were trapped underneath the vehicle. Unable to successfully mobilize, our body will continue spinning its wheels, trying to complete a response it cannot launch.

Our Heart is now sounding the message of life threat with every fast and pounding beat. It can maintain this level of alarm for only a short period of time without sustaining damage. At a certain point, our survival demands a halt to the mobilization, because we have no hope of success. The ventral vagus has been unsuccessful in mitigating arousal using our social-engagement system. A full-on dorsal vagal parasympathetic response, just as powerful as the Wood's mobilization, is required to stop our Heart's hyperarousal.

Part of ensuring the success of the fight-or-flight response involves the Liver sending a controlling message to the Spleen and Stomach to shut down peristalsis. Digestion, while critical for long-term health, is irrelevant when we perceive immediate life threat, when all our energy is needed in our limbs. If our attempts at active protection are thwarted or unsuccessful, we will plunge into this high-tone, dorsal vagal, parasympathetic freeze response. This protects our Heart and conserves physiological resources, helping us to survive until help arrives. Digestion continues to be inhibited in this physiological state, again as a way to conserve energy. This inhibition in the viscera is intended to be of short duration.

Note Figure 8.1 below. The jagged line overlaying the zone of resiliency (described in Chapter One) describes this dynamic in visual terms. The power of the Wood Element to harness all available resources to defend our life or the lives of others is now performing above our normal zone. We are more powerful, more focused, and stronger than ever. As the body is unable to maintain this state of arousal beyond a certain length of time, the parasympathetic system issues an equally powerful command to halt this mobilization. Our energy then falls below our normal zone. These two states are designed to be short-lived, followed by a natural return of our *qi* to the area inside our zone of resiliency. However, if our impulse to protect and defend is thwarted, we will experience the dysregulation resulting from physiology that remains stuck in a survival effort.

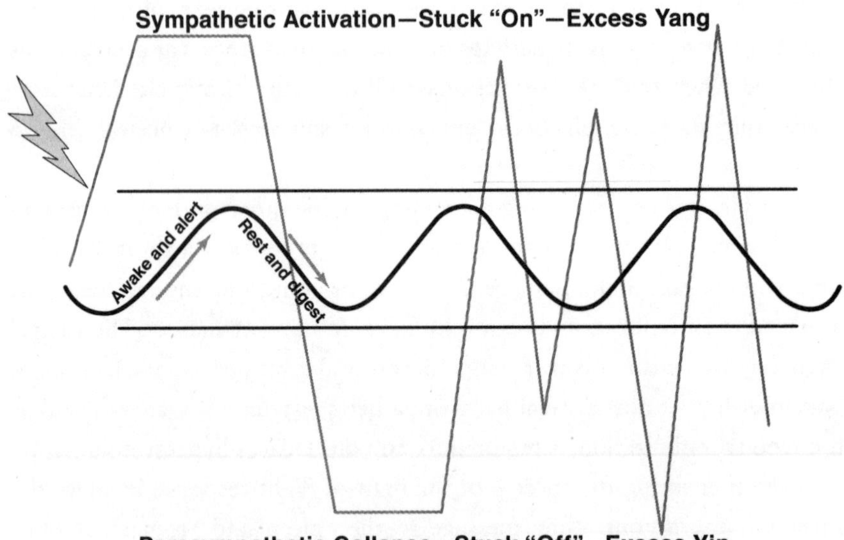

FIGURE 8.1. Zone of Resiliency with Overlay of Traumatic Stress

Imbalance in the Wood Element arises from such unsuccessful mobilization responses. Our impulse to move forward in the generative cycle, toward the Fire Element, where successful completion would be recognized, has met a formidable wall. We may find ourselves stuck in the on position, revving our engines at high throttle but never getting into gear. Alternatively, we may experience collapse and feel similarly stuck in a state of immobility. We also may find ourselves fluctuating erratically between these two states. This incomplete mobilization causes significant dysregulation in our *qi*/energy—illustrated on the far right of this image—the rapidly fluctuating rise and fall, as the gas pedal and the brake are applied simultaneously.

COMMON SYMPTOMS FOR THE WOOD TYPE: THE LIVER AND GALL BLADDER

Symptoms in the Wood Element arise from an imbalance in these dynamics of sympathetic arousal and parasympathetic inhibition that remain in our tissues—even after the moment has passed. We may be stuck in either high arousal or collapse, or we may rapidly cycle between arousal and collapse. In the most challenging version of this imbalance, the gas pedal and the brake are pressed equally to the floor, causing us to alternate between arousal and collapse—a highly tenuous physiological state. If what was thwarted was a fight response, rage may consume us. Or if what was thwarted was a flight response, anxiety will dominate.

When disturbed, the Wood's function of ensuring the smooth movement of *qi* leaves Wood survivor types particularly vulnerable to symptoms of hyperarousal manifesting as stagnant *qi*. We will feel braced and constricted in every dimension of our being. Our body becomes so rigid and tight that our *qi*/energy can't easily move through us.

On a physical level, stagnant *qi* gives rise to pain patterns, including headaches and musculoskeletal or menstrual pain, and it can cause *qi* or blood to accumulate and congeal in cysts or tumors. In this state, our emotions may feel explosive. Rather than anger or frustration rising and falling smoothly, it bursts out in pushy or unnecessarily oppositional ways. On a mental or cognitive level, stagnant *qi* makes it challenging to think through step-by-step solutions to problems, resulting in frustration or difficulty navigating new situations. And on a spiritual level, it makes it hard to see new possibilities or find hope for our future.

Designed to be brief, this state of hyperarousal puts us at risk of habituation to the message from the Liver to the Spleen/Stomach to shut down digestion. Liver *qi* is now chronically invading our Spleen/Stomach across the control cycle. This constant overpowering of the Spleen/Stomach can cause digestive disturbances like irritable bowel syndrome, the inability to metabolize particular nutrients, or weight gain in the middle, arising from the Spleen's inability to transform food into *qi* and blood, instead causing it to stagnate as excess weight. Metabolic syndrome, in which hypertension, high cholesterol, obesity, and high blood sugar converge, is an extreme manifestation of this Wood/Earth dynamic. We will explore the impact of the Liver over-controlling the Spleen/Stomach in greater detail in Chapter Ten.

In addition to an imbalance that arises from hyperarousal, our body, mind, emotions, and spirit may also manifest imbalances that arise from collapse, or hypoarousal. Unable to safely maintain the higher level of arousal, we have collapsed into a dorsal vagal dominant (parasympathetic) freeze state. Our DV is over-controlling our SNS. We feel flaccid and limp in every dimension of our being. We lack the capacity to defend ourselves when we feel insulted or threatened, our emotions are flat and lack animation, and we feel physically weak and have little zest for life. There is insufficient tone in our body tissues to carry our *qi*/energy. Our *qi* is predominantly operating below our zone of resiliency.

The sense organ corresponding to the Wood Element is the eyes. They are critical in our efforts to successfully orient ourselves to threat so we can defend ourselves. Wood survivor types may find their eyes are easily distracted, jumping around and unable to rest or focus. They may also be dry, red, and irritated.

Our capacity to orient to threat involves all our sensory systems, not just our eyes, of course. While the eyes are the sense organ associated with the Wood Element, the entire function of orienting to threat also belongs to the Wood. If our orienting system was disturbed in this mobilize a response step, it will manifest in one of two ways.

In the first, we may be hyperalert to threats that appear similar to one we experienced long ago. If we were sideswiped on the right side of our car, for example, all of our focus may be drawn now to our right side, because that's where bad things happen. We have "over-coupled" our awareness of threat with our right side, and we are so focused on the right that we don't see the baseball careening toward the left side of our head. When we have over-coupled our experience, we are less able to assess our current circumstances and are more likely to be injured.

Alternatively, we avoid the stimulus of looking toward the potential threat. The accident happened on the right side of the car, so we don't look that way. We keep our attention to the left, becoming hypo-alert to things on our right, and we find ourselves unaware of the small child learning to ride a bike who is tottering toward us on the right. We have "under-coupled" our awareness of threat on our right side, and so we experience repeated accidents on that side. In both under- and over-coupling, we are more likely to be injured in the future, because we are no longer processing information about our environment in the present moment—and in a balanced way.

In each of these examples, our over- or under-coupling involved not only our vision but also our kinesthetic sense. All of our senses work together to help us navigate the obstacle course of life. Restoring regulation in any one sensory system will influence the function in all the others. Later in this chapter, we will introduce a hearing exercise designed to restore our orienting system. The dynamics of over- and under-coupling can manifest in any of our senses. In terms of our auditory system, sirens screaming or the whop-whop-whop sound of helicopters overhead may bring us immediately back to a previous life threat. In such cases, we have over-coupled sounds from the past to a sense of threat in the present. On the other hand, some sounds may be too frightening to ever hear again, so we turn off our capacity to hear them at all, so it is no longer available to us as a signal of a change in our environment.

The same or similar dynamics of over- and under-coupling can also apply with smells, tastes, or textures. When dinner burns, we are consumed by memories of a house fire we survived as a child; when we taste crab—even though it's perfectly fresh—we become nauseous, as we did when we experienced food poisoning after eating crab years ago. Sometimes we don't recognize our association between a particular sense and an event in the past; we just know that we have an immediate reaction to it. For example, all we might know is that we don't like the texture of crisp cotton sheets—we haven't realized that they take us back to scary nights in the dark at our grandmother's house, where the beds were always made with starched sheets.

In Wood survivor types, the tissues and the senses corresponding to the Wood Element—our eyes, ligaments, tendons, and blood—will be particularly affected by these coupling dynamics. Each of these tissues can become stuck in a state of brace or collapse (dry and brittle or weak and flaccid) if they were not allowed to fluidly complete their role in mobilizing our response. This can have a profound affect on our ability to accurately orient to future threats and successfully mobilize appropriate responses.

If an active defensive response is thwarted or overwhelmed—such as when our arms brace against the steering wheel or our foot futilely attempts to brake our out-of-control car during an accident—the thwarted activation may be stored in the joints in our limbs: our hands, wrists, elbows, ankles, knees, or hips.

Our joint structures—including tendons, ligaments, synovial fluid, and the space within the joint capsule itself—act as shock absorbers between our bones and provide stability and organization for the movement of our limbs. These joint structures manage how tight or loose the joint needs to be to perform its various functions, as well as the amount of space needed within the joint to support the flexibility and power it needs to properly respond. These functions can be severely compromised when high states of arousal are thwarted, with nowhere to go—such as when our hands were braced against the steering wheel in a car accident. These dynamics are often significant players in chronic pain patterns.

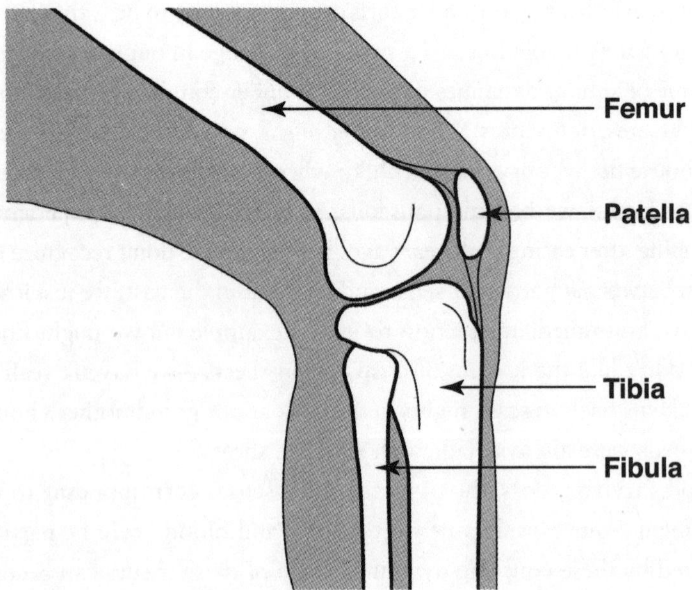

FIGURE 8.2. Secondary Diaphragm in Joint

Physical injuries sustained during such thwarted defensive responses can stun or destroy our proprioceptive receptors—these specialized nerves lie primarily along muscle fibers and in the tendons that connect muscles to bones. Proprioceptive receptors provide information to our brain about where our body is in space and how it is moving. They also contribute to the structure of secondary diaphragms and inform our muscle tone, body image, control of effort, and relationship with gravity. The main proprioceptive beds reside in the ankles, pelvis, and upper neck.

High-impact injuries can severely impact our tendons and ligaments—and thus the proprioceptive receptors that reside within them. Injuries to these receptors can compromise our kinesthetic sense—our awareness of movement and acceleration of our body while in motion; our proprioceptive sense—our awareness of the relationship between different parts of our body, and the strength of effort we are employing; and particularly in head injuries, our vestibular function—which supports our balance and spatial orientation. We may trip or fall frequently. We may not know exactly where our body is in relationship to this curb or that table—and so we run into things.

Damage to these proprioceptive receptors compromises our capacity to orient to our environment and strategize responses to safety and danger. We may experience dizziness, loss of balance, nausea, poor depth perception, motion sickness, or headaches. We can be easily disoriented. The relationship between our torso and limbs becomes confusing, and physical responses are challenging to organize. Head injuries resulting in brain or cranial nerve damage can leave us particularly vulnerable to "Proprioceptive Disinformation Syndrome," in which the brain gives incorrect commands to muscles and joints, putting us at risk of re-injury. The bottom line is: we are more vulnerable to future threats.

As noted above, the Wood Element corresponds not only to the eyes, ligaments, and tendons but also to the blood. In AAM, blood helps maintain flexibility in our tendons and ligaments, supporting the function of the joints to move, twist, and hold stability—and thus our capacity to both orient to threat and mobilize defensive responses.

Understanding the Liver's contribution to AAM blood physiology and function is central to our study of the traumatic stress response. If we sense a tiger outside our tent, our Heart communicates alarm to the kingdom of the body via the blood, with a fast and irregular pulse. Threat is communicated to every cell with each heartbeat. Transmission is immediate and comprehensive. The whole body is called into high arousal. We will further explore the role of the Heart in communicating threat in Chapter Nine.

While the Heart's communication via the blood is central to the management of the threat response, the Liver supports the blood in critical ways. First, AAM classical literature tells us that the Liver is responsible for the smooth movement of blood. It oversees the blood's movement through the body all day, nourishing, moistening, and supporting the function of our eyes, muscles, tendons, and ligaments, as well as the smooth flow of the menstrual cycle. These tissues all correspond to the Wood Element and rely on the blood to keep them flexible and strong. If this function of smooth movement is disturbed, the stagnation that results will cause "congealed," or stagnant blood, characterized by fixed and stabbing pain. In extreme cases, this disturbance in the blood can lead to the formation of dense cysts. The menstrual cycle may be impacted, with large clots, painful menses, or fibroids in the uterine wall.

Important in the context of trauma physiology, AAM understands that the blood travels back to the Liver at night, where it is stored and "restored" while we sleep. This function of restoring the blood can become overwhelmed if the blood is carrying high levels of dysregulation rooted in traumatic stress, or if the function of the Liver is compromised by previous experiences of thwarted mobilization. The blood's function to nourish and moisten our body, as well as our mind, emotions, and spirit, will be compromised.

The spirit of the Liver, called the *hun* (or ethereal soul), is said to "rest" in the blood. The *hun* is associated with our ability to see our destiny, manifest our life plan, experience spiritual insights, and have a vision for our future. If our blood is disturbed or deficient, as occurs in cases of severe blood loss, malnourishment, or Liver *qi* disturbance, it will not provide an adequate resting place for our *hun*. This leaves our *hun* unable to rest at night, manifesting with insomnia, disturbing and vivid dreams or nightmares, or sleepwalking. We find ourselves caught in a vicious cycle: We are unable to sleep; therefore, our blood is not restored. Lack of restoration of our blood, in turn, leaves us unable to sleep. Without a healthy *hun,* we may feel dreamy, unfocused, and confused; we lack a sense of direction or purpose, or we feel separated from our body.[6]

The emotion associated with the Wood Element is anger. When our Wood is out of balance, we can become "blinded" by anger, further illuminating the correspondence of the eyes with the Wood Element. On the mental/emotional plane, we can't see hope for the future of our growing season; we are either depressed and immobilized, or we can't find our way around obstacles, finding ourselves tight, angry, and resentful as we break through every obstacle we encounter. We later regret the unnecessary fights, road rage, or broken dishes that resulted from our overwhelming and impulsive anger. Our growth toward our ultimate purpose, our destiny, is compromised.

REMEDIES FOR RESTORING REGULATION IN THE WOOD

Wood survivor types may benefit from work that focuses on building capacity in the Water Element, as described in the previous chapter, before providers move to more directly attending to the tissues and functions of Wood. The wisdom of AAM teaches us that a deficiency of Water will deprive a plant of its appropriate flexibility and strength. A tree will be brittle and easily break, or a plant will lack appropriate turgidity and become too flaccid. Because Water creates Wood, stability in the Water Element feeds the Wood Element.

In terms of the 5-SPR, if our Water Element has not nourished our Wood properly, our self-protective response can also be dry and brittle—and we will be more vulnerable to disruption as we orient to threat.

The approaches we describe below are all geared toward restoring capacity in the tissues and functions related to the Wood Element and its role to orient and strategize responses to threat and to mobilize actions to defend and protect us. Restoring regulation in these defensive functions involves helping our clients complete their as-yet-incomplete mobilization response.

Restoring Protective/Defensive Responses in the Secondary Diaphragms

The first step of the self-protective response calls on our Metal Element, using the interoceptive capacity of the spirit of the Lung, the *po*, to bring awareness to something amiss in our environment. The Metal Element sends a message across the control cycle to the Wood Element to initiate orienting to a potential threat. Our body assumes a predictive reflexive startle posture. We turn our body and all our senses toward the potential threat, duck our head, crouch to prepare our muscles and joints to respond, and begin to strategize our survival. This posture is a precursor to our fight-or-flight response.

If our mobilization was thwarted as we assumed this posture, a state of hyperarousal or hypoarousal may be contained, managed, and hidden from view in our diaphragm system—as described by the faux window in Chapters Five and Six.

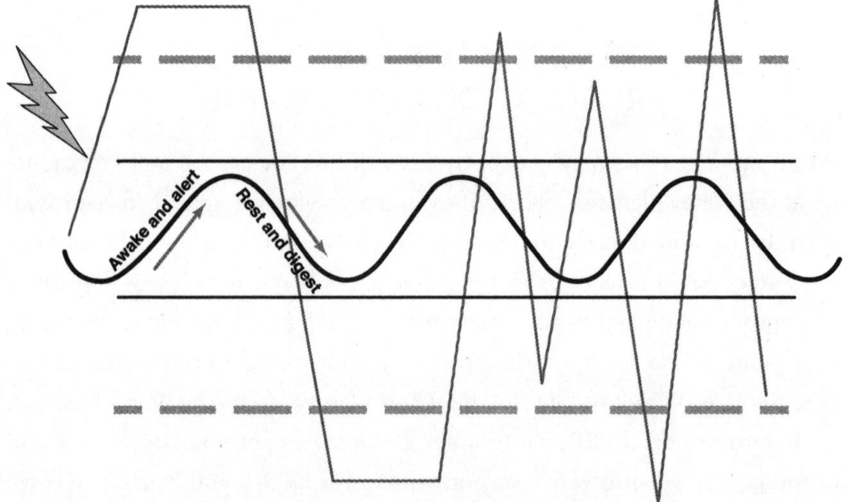

FIGURE 8.3. Faux Window of Tolerance

Of note, the Wood's Gall Bladder meridian traverses all of the primary diaphragms, as well as the secondary diaphragms in the hips, knees, ankles, and feet that support this reflexive startle posture. Together with the Liver, the Gall Bladder supports our orientation to threat, governs the tendons and ligaments that provide the structure of our joints, and brings energy to our proprioceptive function.

As discussed in Chapter Six, the diaphragm system includes both the primary diaphragms in the torso and cranium and the secondary diaphragms any place within the body where a bell or bowl structure is present, primarily in the joints. Working with the joints in the context of the system of secondary diaphragms can help move dysregulation, caused by a thwarted defensive response, out to the periphery of the body to be released.

Titration, discussed in depth in Chapter Five, is critical when working with either the primary or the secondary diaphragms. In the context of trauma physiology, the diaphragms help us manage extreme states of arousal. In the car analogy used previously, if we take our foot off either the brake or the gas too quickly, the car will spin out of control. We must instead take a little pressure off the gas and then a little off the brake, alternately, to regain control of the car. In the context of diaphragm work, as you note a change in one diaphragm, you will see it influence another. Moving between them, in a relational context will serve this principle of titration.

The clinical challenge is to engage the mobilization response, work with it in bite-sized portions, and help it find completion in a manageable, titrated way. It is as easy to overwhelm a client as it is to fail to access the activation contained in the diaphragms when working with arousal inside the faux window.

Releasing the full magnitude of our client's mobilization response all at one time can provoke overwhelming, consuming rage. Many people will feel shame in the presence of the enormity of this rage and will go into an even deeper freeze state. Their high level of arousal required an equally strong brake to temper it. This deep freeze then gives rise to greater dysregulation instead of greater regulation—and has the potential to jeopardize the relationship between client and provider.

There is also risk in being too cautious and never accessing the thwarted response that remains contained and hidden away in our client's diaphragm system. He may be using highly developed, finely tuned, difficult-to-access, and *unconscious* management strategies to contain his hyperarousal. Providers who lack the skills to access the power of the hyperarousal contained in the diaphragm system will never be successful in thawing the freeze response that is paired with it in their clients.

If your client struggles in a general way with self-regulation and then experiences a thwarted defensive response—such as his hand braced against the steering wheel in an automobile accident—releasing the high level of activation stored in his elbow or wrist can overwhelm rather than encourage the repair of his orienting and defensive response. In this case, as a practitioner, you may choose to spend several sessions working with the Kidney/adrenal hold in order to establish an anchor of safety and support his capacity for self-regulation as a foundation to later support repairs to his Wood's orienting and defensive system. Establishing an experience of a resourceful anchor will help titrate the arousal that may be contained in the diaphragm system.

When you and your client are ready, choose the distal joint in a limb that is either functionally impaired or in chronic pain after an earlier accident or injury. Begin by mindfully holding an ankle or wrist—or a finger or toe joint. Circle the joint with one or both hands and look for the sensation of a wave coming through your client's experience and into your hands, as if the joint is breathing. Depending on your client's history and constitution, this may take several minutes or several sessions. It has the potential to wake up the diaphragms in the knee or hip, elbow or shoulder—or the primary diaphragms in the torso—through the naturally resonant system of bells and bowls of the diaphragms.

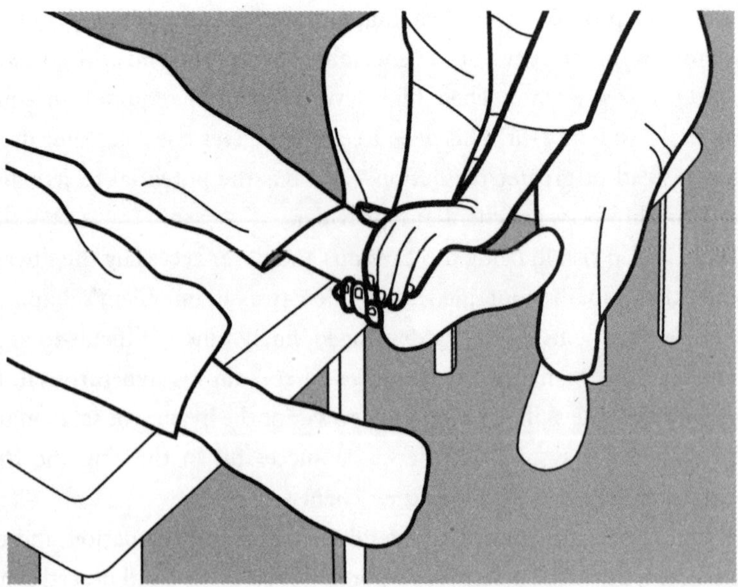

FIGURE 8.4. Touching the Ankle Joint

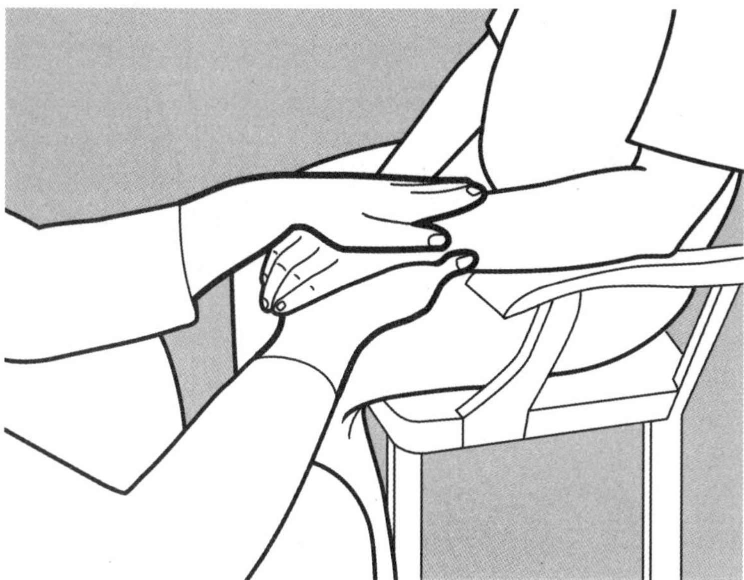

FIGURE 8.5. Touching the Wrist Joint

In order to find deeper healing, clients may need to experience and complete the action that was thwarted long ago—the impulse to run, push, or stomp may need physical expression in order to move hyperarousal contained in a secondary diaphragm out of the body. It is important to do this only in controlled ways to avoid further injury or over-activation of the mobilization responses. You may choose to work only in the imaginal world, having the client imagine she is making the movement rather than having her physically perform it. If there is sufficient regulation on board, it may be safe to have the client physically express the completion of the action—always staying at safe levels of speed and forcefulness of effort.

As with the primary diaphragms, when working with the secondary diaphragms, you will be supporting the movement of the bound energy of thwarted survival responses out of the diaphragms, while also attending to an increase of coherence. In the joints, coherence tends to manifest as an increasingly balanced and rhythmic movement of the breath through each joint in turn. It can feel as if the joint itself is breathing, that a wave of breath is moving along the arm or leg and gently moving the next joint in turn.

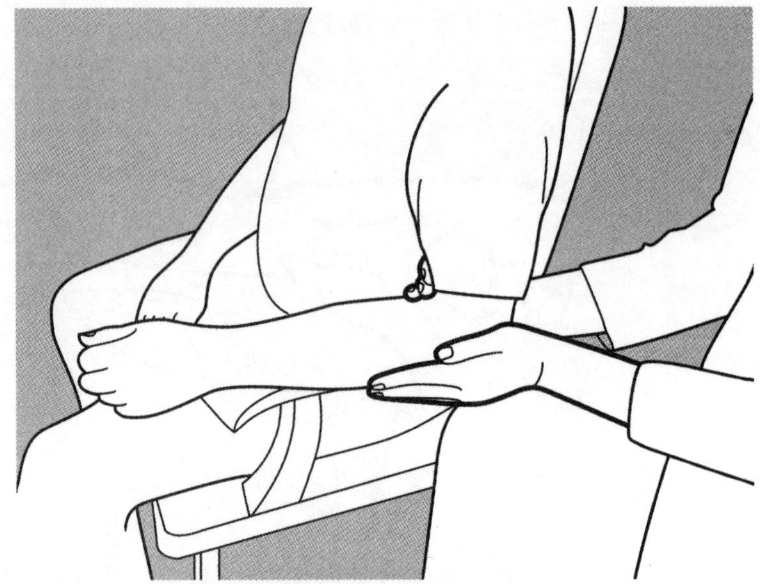

FIGURE 8.6. Touching the Elbow Joint

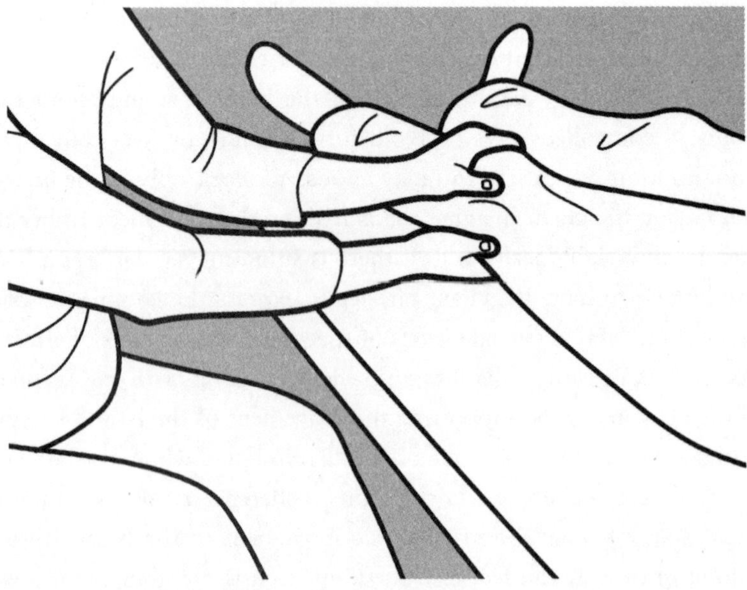

FIGURE 8.7. Touching the Knee Joint

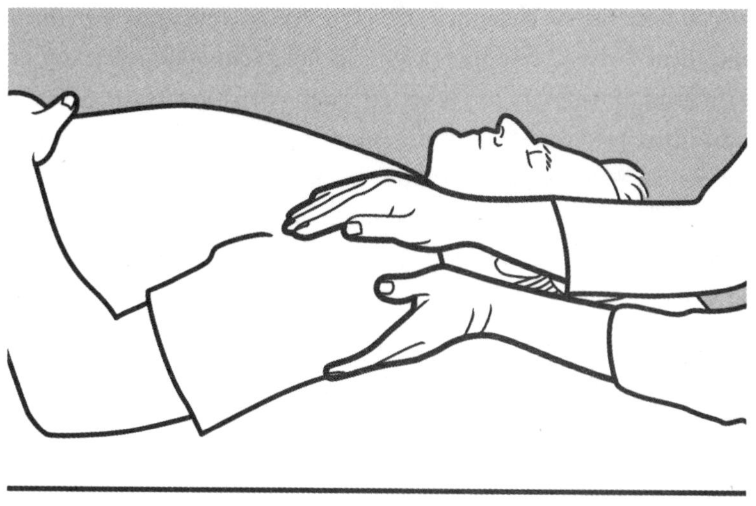

FIGURE 8.8. Touching the Shoulder Joint

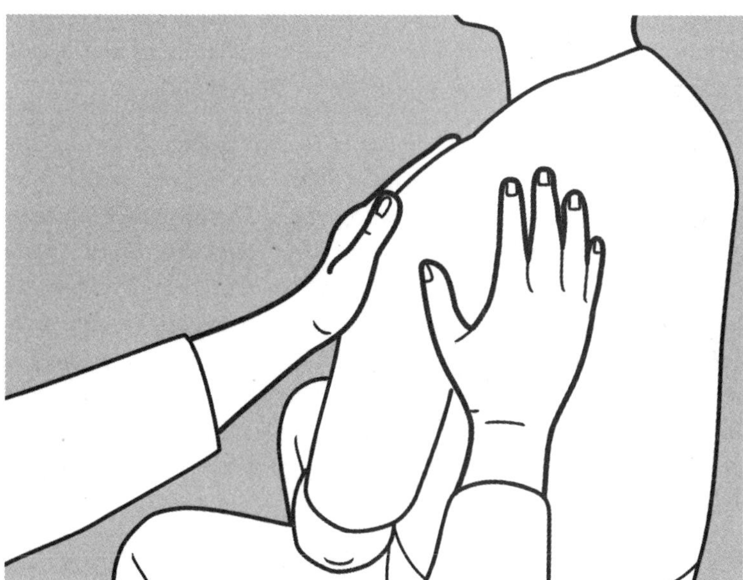

FIGURE 8.9. Touching the Shoulder Joint, Seated

As you notice these changes in the peripheral diaphragms, you can monitor the client's overall response to your contact. Does he tighten up or "go away" when I move his joint? What's the nature of the weight of his limb in my hand? Is it braced and lifted off? Is it too light, airy, or lacking presence? Has he withdrawn his presence from his joint—does it feel less alive and responsive? What is my response to this contact? Am I feeling more coherence within myself? Is coherence propagating—in myself, his breath, his joints? Coherence grows coherence. Coherence propagates itself. Look for it.

Building coherence in the secondary diaphragms is the foundation for bringing regulation to the muscle system, which we will explore in Chapter Ten. The sinews, muscles, and bones all work in an integrated fashion. Restoring regulation in any one aspect of the musculoskeletal system brings regulation to all aspects.

Client Example

Dewayne is eight years old. He was born with a congenitally malfunctioning kidney. His doctors put off surgery as long as they could and finally decided his kidney needed to be removed. While it was the right decision for Dewayne's long-term health, recovery from surgery was tough. A month later, he remained anxious and unable to sleep at night, which affected his entire household.

One of the functions of anesthesia is to immobilize us during surgery. Our limbs are often restricted from moving by straps so we don't risk injury while the surgeon operates. This approach is meant to ensure the safety of patients and physicians, but there can be repercussions from this immobilization that require some attention. It is not uncommon for surgery patients to experience thwarted mobilization responses as a side effect of surgery. From a survival perspective, our body doesn't know the difference between a scalpel and sharp claws, yet we are necessarily physically and pharmaceutically prevented or thwarted from fighting or fleeing during a surgical procedure.

As I worked with Dewayne's peripheral diaphragms in his ankles, he was filled with an impulse to run. In spite of all the reports of his exhaustion and sleeplessness, he really wanted to run—and run fast! He climbed off the table, and together we (slowly) ran in place. I directed him to run toward a safe place. In his case, this was his grandmother's kitchen, where cookies were baking. (On occasions where a client experiences a flight impulse, it is preferable to have them run to a safe place rather than run away from a dangerous place.)

That night, Dewayne slept through the night for the first time since his surgery, and he continued to sleep well over the coming weeks. The pain at his surgical site fell dramatically. His whole family was also able to sleep better—and manage the emotional drain of this critical time in their family with more ease.

Integrating Motor and Sensory Function in the Orientation System

The eyes are the Wood Element's sense organ. The Wood helps us see what is tangible, as well as what is intangible. It helps us envision our future, see new possibilities, and visualize in our dreams what we can't see with our eyes. Combined with our senses of hearing, smell, taste, and kinesthesia, they support the Wood's function to orient to our surroundings, assess threats, and strategically plan successful mobilization responses.

Just as an unusually warm or dry winter will influence the number of blossoms that will set on the fruit trees the following spring, if the function of our Water Element to provide us with a sense of a safe and secure boundary (which we explored in Chapter Seven) was ruptured during a traumatic experience, our Wood Element's function to accurately orient to threat and strategize solutions can be compromised. We will be either hyper- or hypo-aware of the region of our boundary where we experienced that rupture. Our eyes, the sense organ corresponding with the Wood Element, will be particularly compromised when we need to orient to another threat.

This is another example of how the Water Element feeds the Wood Element. Stability in the various functions of the Water Element will be a critical foundation for moving into and repairing the motor and sensory functions that belong to the Wood. In particular, it may be quite important to first repair any ruptures in your client's capacity for a safe and secure boundary before proceeding with repairs to their motor and sensory functions.

Eye placement in predatory animals is different than that in prey animals. Predators need to see long distances, across a wide range, to seek out prey. Their eye placement is necessarily oriented in the front of the face, with round pupils. Cats, coyotes, owls, and humans all have predator eye placement.

Prey animals, on the other hand, need to see up close and in all directions in order to optimize their ability to perceive threats. Their eyes are particularly attuned to movement. Prey eye placement is necessarily on the sides of the head, giving them highly tuned peripheral vision. Rabbits, squirrels, and mice all exhibit this type of eye structure and function.[7]

Human beings are sometimes predators and at other times are prey. We need to have the capacity to support success in both roles. Our eyes are positioned at the front of our faces, allowing us to scan across large areas and distances, like a predator. Our neck allows us to move our sense organs around to locate and interpret threats and to facilitate exploration and navigation of safety. It is our neck that helps us function when we find ourselves in the position of prey. It helps us aim our senses to discern potential threats when circumstances require it. Neck function is critical when we feel threatened. Clients who have been preyed upon may feel safer and less activated when care providers keep their bodies still and avoid placing themselves in the client's peripheral vision. Clients will want to see the care provider with their central vision.

If, for example, a heavy book were dropped behind you, your reflexive startle response, explored in the previous section, would cause you to simultaneously turn your head and orient to the sound's origin and to duck by collapsing your neck. The tension inherent in the opposing movements of twisting and ducking often explains the constriction and neck pain we find so often in trauma survivors. If we become habituated to this neck constriction, or if our self-protective response was thwarted as we attempted to locate a threat, traumatic stress may be stored in the tissues and structures that support and stabilize the neck. We will be less able to move our sense organs fluidly and interpret our surroundings accurately. Our safety will be compromised.

If our physiological capacity to orient to threats is compromised, we won't be able to gather information from our environment or orient to and complete a successful threat response. We can't feel safe if we can't orient to our environment, we will therefore remain in hyperarousal and will be unable to regulate ourselves.

One exercise that gently challenges our orientation system and integrates motor function in the neck with the auditory aspect of our orientation system involves beanbags, bandannas, and a quiet space. As you establish the context for this exercise, it is important to be clear that there is no shame in being unable to orient to a sound—just as in an eye exam, there is no shame in being unable to read the smallest line in the chart. This is a method we use to assess and repair over- or under-coupling in the sensory system's orientation function, which may remain if a survivor's response was thwarted in this orienting phase. We are exploring the client's capacity for auditory orientation and for coherence between her hearing and the functions of her neck.

It is common for trauma survivors to feel wrong or broken because their physiology has been so impacted by their experience. This is why it's important that you do your best to help the client anchor herself in a state of curiosity, rather than competition, a need for perfection, or holding judgment about her success.

You will need two sets of three or four beanbags, each set a different color, but identical in weight and size. Give one set of beanbags to your client, while you retain the other. Check in to be sure that your client feels comfortable having her eyes covered by a bandanna to remove vision from her orientation function (she can simply close her eyes if the bandanna idea is too activating).

Explain that the two of you will be standing about six to eight feet away from each other. You will toss a beanbag onto the floor near her (in front of her, on either side, or behind her), and invite her to notice where she hears the bag fall. When she hears one of yours fall, she will then toss her beanbag, trying to match the location of yours. This exercise explores coherence between her neck and her hearing, and it assesses disruption in the auditory aspect of her orienting system.

If her beanbag lands close to yours, this is an expression of coherence in her auditory orientation system. Throw your next beanbag to a new place near her. You are looking for gaps in her capacity to hear a signal in her environment. If her beanbag lands at some distance from yours, throw your next beanbag to land *between* your previous beanbag and her response to it. Repairing her orienting system comes alongside this evaluation. You are creating conditions for her to experience success with the gentlest of demands on her auditory system. This will support her body to organically restore this function. If her next beanbag lands closer to yours, this is an indication that she has integrated improved function in her capacity to orient to sounds in her environment. You will likely note that hyperarousal in her sympathetic system has calmed in the presence of this success.

However, if her next beanbag is yet further away, it is best to stop this exercise. You don't want to ask for what she can't do, make demands she can't meet, or overstimulate her system. You won't be able to fix her auditory orientation by overwhelming it or provoking shame. Use the tick-tock model to help bring her back to a more regulated state. She may benefit from some Kidney/adrenal work or other resource-building activities that are meaningful to her. Come back to this work during a future session, when she is ready, and go slowly with it.

Client Example

Marina, a nurse, had been experiencing chronic headaches and neck pain after an injury at work two years before. She had entered a storage room to collect some items from a shelf at the end of her shift, and as she turned to go back out the door, she heard an odd sound. Just as she began to turn to see what it was, a heavy box toppled from a top shelf and hit her on the top of the head. At the time, it seemed she had not been seriously injured, but over the next two weeks, she noticed she was jumpy at work, and she began to experience headaches. After three months, she was barely able to turn her head, and the headaches were occurring at least three times per week.

We began our session with the beanbag work discussed above. With the first toss of the bean bag, behind and to Marina's right, she felt her neck "lock"—she was trying to turn her head both to the right and the left at the same time, and she couldn't figure out where the bean bag was. At the same time, she was shaking and perspiring, feeling mysteriously frightened and disoriented. We took a few minutes to help Marina settle and to bring her breathing back to normal.

We then began again. This time I suggested she keep her eyes open so she could see clearly where the beanbag landed, and this time I tossed it almost directly in front of her, so she could see it as it landed. We repeated this with another couple of tosses, and then returned to her closing her eyes, since her neck was no longer reacting so strongly to the process of noticing where the beanbags landed. Slowly, we worked our way back around to the same position as the first toss. Each time Marina became activated, we took time for her to settle. On the final toss, Marina was able to hear the beanbag land and tossed her own beanbag almost on top of it.

As we were still standing, a few feet apart, after her successful final toss, I asked her to imagine the moment she heard the noise in the storage space. As she did, she turned her head to the right, and—without even noticing she had done it—stepped forward. Turning back to me with a wide grin, she said, "If I'd just known what I was hearing, I could have gotten out of the way!" We practiced a few more times—she imagined hearing the noise and experimented with ways she could have avoided the falling box. Her body had the opportunity to experience successfully orienting to the falling box and mobilizing a successful response, completing the thwarted step in her 5-SPR.

Even after that single session, Marina's headaches and neck pain were significantly improved. After another six sessions, she was free of pain.

Restoring Vitality in the Liver Blood

Attending to the blood in the Liver with mindful touch can help restore balance and regulation and relieve the blood from the message of alarm it's been carrying. Working with the blood can help restore its capacity to nourish and moisten the body, mind, emotions, and spirit—and provide a place for the *hun* to rest. This work allows providers the opportunity to practice "seeing" with their own *hun* what may be tangibly invisible to their fingers.

You may wish to refer to Chapter Five for more detailed information about mindful touch. For now, here are specific strategies for applying touch to restore function to the blood in the Liver:

1. Refer to the section of this chapter called "Common Symptoms for the Wood Type: The Liver and Gall Bladder." Share with your client the importance of the Liver, its role in blood physiology, and why it could be helpful for him to receive this attention with touch. Get explicit permission for this type of contact.
2. Sit on your client's right side. He can be seated in a chair or lying on his back on a table.
3. To help quiet and focus your mind, bring your attention to your own Liver. It is a large organ, lying under your right ribcage. Your respiratory diaphragm is above it, and your right kidney is behind and slightly below.
4. Bring your attention to your client's Liver, without physically touching him. This can deepen the experience of connection between the two of you.
5. Notice your client's response; note any sense of invitation for your touch—is it present or absent? Wait for a sense of invitation to emerge.
6. If there is an invitation to touch, place your hand gently over the middle of his right rib cage. Direct your intention through his skin and rib cage to "see" his Liver with your hand. With your mind's eye, look for something dense and large. At first, it may feel quite dry, but in time, you may feel a pulse moving through his Liver, and you may sense it becoming more juicy and taking up more space. You are looking for a sense of smooth movement or "filling in" of his Liver.
7. Using the skills for enhancing interoception explored in Chapter Six, ask questions like, "As you notice your Liver softening and expanding, what do you notice in the rest of you?" Help your client embody any sense of fullness, juiciness, or smooth movement he experiences in his Liver. Help him note any sense of greater regulation in his whole system when his Liver feels more full, juicy, or smooth.

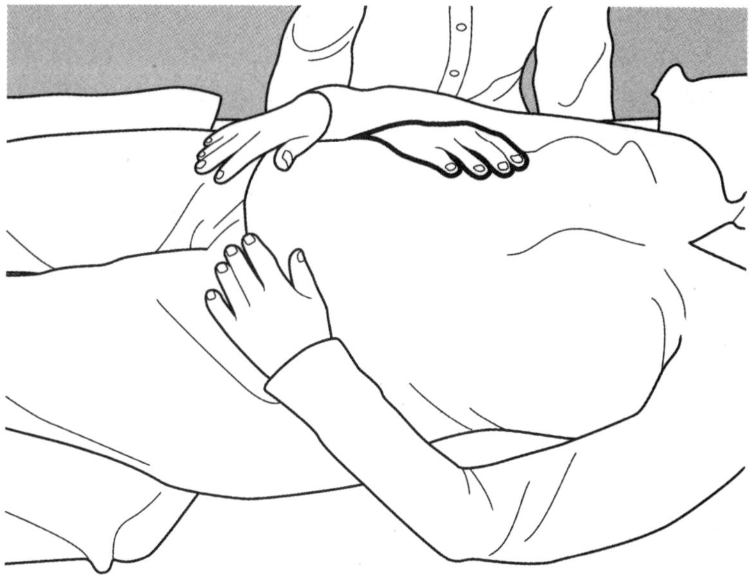

FIGURE 8.10. Touching the Liver Blood

Client Example

Sue is in her early twenties. She did well in high school but never went to college and could not figure out "what she wanted to be when she grew up." She now lives with her parents and works as a clerk in a department store. She has always been somewhat timid and indecisive.

Sue was born with a cleft foot, which required two surgeries before she was three years old. During the second surgery, she was given too much anesthesia and nearly died. She now has trouble drifting off to sleep and can remain awake well into the night. When she does sleep, she is often troubled by frightening dreams.

I spent several sessions helping to quiet Sue's sense of anxiety by using the Kidney/adrenal hold before coming to focus on her Liver blood. Once she was ready for this work, I rested my hand on her right ribcage and directed my attention to her Liver and the blood it contained. After a few moments, I began to feel a gentle pulsing. It felt like a balloon slowly being filled with warm water. It gradually began to feel more substantial, kind of soft and squishy. Sue looked up at me with wide eyes and said, "Instead of feeling like a flat, empty envelope, my liver feels full and round and vital. I've never felt this way." In a subsequent session, she said, "It feels like some major artery in my liver just opened up and is filling my legs. In fact, all my vessels feel like solid tubes with bright red blood flowing through them now."

Sue began sleeping through the night on a regular basis. Always good at math, she enrolled in a computer science program at the local community college and began making plans to move out of her parents' house and into an apartment with a friend from high school.

SOCIAL IMPLICATIONS FOR RESTORING REGULATION IN THE WOOD ELEMENT

Restoring regulation to the sympathetic nervous system in trauma survivors can have a profound social impact. People who have experienced thwarted impulses to protect others or defend themselves can have significant blocks in their physiology—as well as their mind, emotions, and spirit. Our inability to complete an impulse to protect or defend is a powerful and profound impulse that remains behind in every aspect of our being. Conscious—or even unconscious—experiences from there and then consume our responses in the here and now. Our capacity to accurately orient and appropriately respond to a sense of threat has become distorted.

The goal of our work is to help clients complete what was disrupted so they can move on to the next phase and eventually complete the entire self-protective response. Healthy functioning is rooted in an experience of successful survival.

If, for example, an attacker overwhelmed us as we first noticed him on the street and began orienting to his approach, our mobilization response was unsuccessful, and we collapsed into a freeze state. The thief took our wallet and left us with a state of hyperarousal in our muscles and joints buried beneath our experience of collapse. While we surely feel grateful to have survived, we also have a need to feel powerful and capable of defending ourselves, instead of collapsed and frozen. We need to complete the punch that was blocked by this thief.

Similarly, and perhaps of even greater significance, if we descended into a freeze state repeatedly as a small child or infant, we may be particularly vulnerable to the overwhelming rage that remains hidden away under what became, way back then, a chronic freeze state. It risks leaking out as domestic or community violence.

We may have felt threatened by high fever, a difficult birth, prenatal drug or alcohol abuse, mental illness or violence in our homes, or by living in a war zone. We didn't have the developmental capacity or social context to support us in initiating or completing a mobilization response, so our only choice was to freeze in order to quiet the overwhelmingly high arousal in our Heart.

In the context of developmental trauma such as this, we are at significant risk of this collapsed state becoming chronic. We didn't have an opportunity to experience a successful completion of our impulse to survive. Our sympathetic nervous system was initially turned on, but it was developmentally impossible to fight or flee before we could walk, run, or make a fist, and so, needing to protect our Heart from hyperarousal, we collapsed into a freeze state—perhaps over and over again.

These kinds of experiences can leave our mobilization thermostat dysregulated. We may have a rigid bearing, with high levels of impulsive anger. Our need to get that bully on the playground or to respond appropriately to even mild disagreements with friends or coworkers is influenced by our historic inability to respond to threats we experienced as an infant or small child. We may dream of showing *them* our true power—but end up choosing the wrong time, the wrong person, and the wrong level of response. Our strategy for responding to perceived threat goes from zero to sixty before we have a chance to think. This largely unconscious impulse to complete a defensive response that occurred before we even had language to describe it may be an important underlying factor of mass violence in our schools and communities.

Conversely, we may appear completely passive, with others constantly taking advantage of us. However, the potential for murderous rage remains underneath our collapsed appearance. This is the backstory in the newspaper article that reports friends or coworkers of a perpetrator of mass violence saying, "he always was so quiet and kept to himself."

Providers may be called to work directly with the Wood Element, using some of the approaches introduced in this chapter. As we discussed in Chapter Six, we may also support a Wood survivor type through work with the Metal Element, which serves as a controlling influence over the Wood. Cultivating an inherent sense of respect for those who are somehow "different," which is a quality engendered by Metal, can help mitigate simmering mistrust or anger. Acknowledging the positive aspect of someone's anger, by saying, for example, "I am moved by witnessing how deeply you care for your child's well-being," can mitigate the somewhat misplaced rage a client may feel toward his child's teacher or principal.

As we discussed both in this chapter and in Chapter Seven, AAM also teaches us that the Water nourishes the Wood. Helping survivors build capacity in their Water Element to recognize safety—as well as danger—will provide more accurate threat signaling for the Wood. Replacing fear or anxiety with wisdom and peace in the Water Element will restore flexibility in the Wood. Anger will soften, and survivors will be less influenced by the thwarted experiences from the past, and their Wood Element's essential function to support creativity, planning, and decision making will return.

Thwarted mobilization responses are an important aspect of understanding the complex dynamics of violence in our homes and on our streets. The most important contribution to conflict resolution providers can make is to provide conditions that allow our clients' thwarted mobilization responses to complete in a titrated, paced, and safe manner. Survivors need the opportunity to access the impulses hidden beneath their unsuccessful mobilization—and allow them to complete. On an emotional level, this impulse will present as anger, frustration, or rage. It will remain until a survivor experiences the full success of his thwarted response, allowing it to disperse out of his system.

Once this happens, survivors will be able to see new possibilities for themselves, their families, and our communities, instead of feeling blinded by rage—our ability to creatively respond, instead of instinctively react, to life's challenges returns. Our Wood Element can return to its inherently benevolent nature.

CONCLUSION

The Wood Element feeds the Fire Element. A successful mobilization response will send a clear message of success to the Fire, which will communicate this message with a regulated, coherent vibration in the pulse. Our next chapter will explore the impact of the message of life threat on all matters of the Heart.

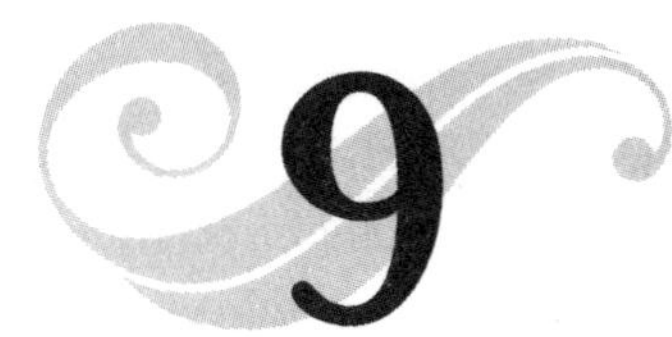

Fire and Summer: Restore Coherence

THE FIVE STEPS OF THE SELF-PROTECTIVE RESPONSE

1. Arrest/Startle—Arousal Awakens Us Out of Exploratory Orienting. Metal.
2. Defensive Orienting—Fear Signals Threat. Water.
3. Specific Self-Protective Response—Mobilization Response Initiates. Wood.
4. **Completion—Successful Defense or No Threat. Restore Coherence. Fire.**
5. Integration—Digest the Gristle. Harvest the Lessons. Earth.

   Cycle Returns to the Metal and Restored Capacity for Exploratory Orienting.

THE FIRE ELEMENT'S season is summer. Our Fire oversees all "matters of the Heart" and embodies joy and peace, tranquility and propriety in the center of our being.

When our Heart is penetrated by a commanding message of life threat, every organ system is called to arousal. If we are repeatedly called into this response, we can become habituated to a sense of constant threat and may have trouble realizing that the threat is over and that we have survived. We can feel anxious and uncentered and struggle with our cognition, focus, or memory. We may not sleep well—our mind can't rest peacefully at night. Our eyes, as well as our emotions, may be flat, and we may feel profoundly sad. Social interactions leave us feeling inhibited and awkward. We struggle to feel vulnerable and safe in relationships. Alternatively, disembodied joy or hysteria may overwhelm our capacity for meaningful presence and connection. We may have a sense of heightened sexual expression—but this expression lacks intimacy, connection, or engagement.

As you are with your client, observe him with these questions in mind. This will help inform you about the extent to which your client knows that the threat is over—and that he has restored coherence in his Heart and his whole system.

- *Does your client engage easily with you and others? Does he have relationships with people or with animals that are loving and supportive?*
- *Is there sparkle or twinkle in his eyes? Does his face shine?*
- *Are his social interactions appropriate to his age and culture?*
- *Is his memory clear and his mental focus sharp? Is he often forgetful?*
- *Can his mind rest at night? Does he fall asleep easily and remain asleep through the night?*
- *Can he find joy? Or does he seem heavyhearted?*
- *Does he find passion and pleasure, intimacy, and connection in his sexual expression?*

CORRESPONDENCES RELATING TO THE FIRE ELEMENT'S ROLE IN THE SELF-PROTECTIVE RESPONSE

Element	*Fire*
Season	*Summer*
Organ Systems	*Heart, Small Intestine, Heart Protector, Triple Heater*
Emotion	*Joy, panic*
Role in Successful Self-Protective Response	*Restore coherence*
Unsuccessful or Incomplete Self-Protective Response	*Hyperarousal: Panic attacks, mania, dark humor, insomnia, racing thoughts.* *Hypoarousal: Dissociation, flat eyes and emotions, hard to connect, poor memory and focus.*
Engenders	*Digestion and harvesting*
Controls	*Sensate curiosity*
Tissue	*Vessels*
Virtue	*Propriety*
Stores	*Spirit or mind*
Spirit	*Consciousness, presence*
Archetypal Question	*How do I find the one great Heart that beats in all Hearts?* *Can I find love and joy with other beings?*
Remedies to Enhance Regulation	*Restoring interoception in the gates of the Heart Protector*

ORIENTATION: THE NATURE OF THE FIRE ELEMENT

Understanding the nature and function of the Fire Element in the self-protective response is central to working with trauma survivors. Our Heart is the primary organ system of our Fire Element—and our entire body. It oversees our essential regulation. Its job in the 5-SPR is first to command every system of the body to fully participate in a response to life threat and then to signal a return to coherence and equanimity when we have successfully completed that response.

Knowing in our Heart of hearts that we have survived restores system-wide regulation, bringing peace and equanimity to our body, mind, emotions, and spirit. Taoist medical scholars acknowledged the resonant connection between the Heart and the mind in their calligraphy—the character for the Heart is identical to the one for the mind. This articulates a truth that is easily embraced today—a disturbance in our Heart affects our mind, and a disturbance in our mind affects our Heart.

If we are a Fire survivor type, we are more likely to have been interrupted during the completion, or restore coherence, phase of the 5-SPR. Unable to recognize our survival, our Heart—and each of our organ systems—remains poised in response to a message of life threat. We will struggle to integrate an embodied experience of our successful survival, leaving every organ system on high alert. We may struggle to trust our instincts and our abilities. We constantly feel we got it wrong. This pervasive sense of failure is the hallmark of interruption in this particular phase of the 5-SPR.

On the other hand, when our Fire Element is balanced and healthy, we experience joy and readily find peace. Our Heart's steady and quiet rhythm communicates a coherent beat that brings regulation to every organ system. We experience openhearted relationships with others and feel compassion for those who suffer. We enjoy our sexual expression and find pleasure in life. We feel peaceful when our heart is peaceful.

Summer, the season of the Fire Element, emerges out of spring and the Wood Element. AAM's declaration that Wood creates Fire is both literal and metaphoric. Adding more wood to a fire creates more flames and heat. This declaration also tells us metaphorically that summer's fruit emerges out of spring's flowers—spring's cool, windy, and rainy nature gives rise to summer's long, warm, and bright days. Similarly, a successful mobilization response, governed by the Wood Element, will naturally give rise to a message of completion and equanimity in the Heart, governed by the Fire. The sun reaches its zenith in the summer. We spend more time outside and thus engage more with others. The bright sun seems to inspire joy and more playful interactions. "All things in creation flourish and grow."[1]

The sun is nature's expression of the Fire Element. Like our Heart, the sun is central to life. Every living thing—animal and plant—relies on it for survival. It provides a coherent rhythm to our days and nights, and its light and warmth sustains everything we rely on for life. A bright summer sun is emblematic of our need for coherent regulation and rhythm in our being, as well as the warmth, compassion, and vitality we find in loving connections with others.

In the AAM framework, the Fire Element contains twice as many organ systems as the other Elements—four versus two. This speaks to the complexity of matters of the Heart that are understood in every culture!

In AAM, the Heart is paired with the Small Intestine, both of which together relate to the expansiveness of the mind—they call us to higher consciousness and relationship with all of humanity, and all of life. The Pericardium (also called the *Heart Protector* or the *Circulation/Sex organ system*) and its partner, the Triple Heater (also called the *Triple Burner* or *Triple Energizer*), relate to our connections with other individuals, allowing us to take joy and pleasure in our relationships, especially our most vulnerable, intimate, or sexual expressions.

The Heart—or, in AAM, the Supreme Controller—is described as holding "the office of Lord and Sovereign" in classical AAM texts. "The radiance of the spirits stem from it."[2] Our Heart is responsible for ensuring system-wide coherence and regulation. It is responsible for our sense of self-awareness and inner connection, and for our capacity for mental cognition and focus. In health, its essential nature is joy, contentment, propriety, and order.

Just as the results of Western medicine's research on the electromagnetic field of the Heart points to the impact of cardiac coherence on whole-body function, AAM will say that the welfare of the entire body depends on the Heart. A coherent electromagnetic field in our Heart influences our brain waves and the brain waves of others up to eight to fifteen feet away from us.

In terms of physical health, a regulated heartbeat provides a coherent rhythm that brings order and organization to the entire body—our central and autonomic nervous systems, as well as our neurological, pulmonary, metabolic, immune, and endocrine systems—and each and every cell.[3] Beating quietly and steadily in the background, it encourages the integrated and healthy functioning of our body, mind, emotions, and spirit—and it sends a regulating vibration to those in close proximity. Thus, when the sleeping partner of a trauma survivor is brought into greater cardiac coherence, the survivor will also experience greater regulation simply by resting next to her more regulated partner in the night.[4]

The *Yellow Emperor's Classic of Internal Medicine* is the oldest known textbook of internal medicine and still informs AAM training all over the world. It is wise in its understanding of the impact of traumatic stress on the Heart:

> *If then the sovereign radiates (virtue), those under him will be at peace. From this the nurturing of life will give longevity from generation to generation, and the empire will radiate great light.*
>
> *But if the sovereign does not radiate (virtue), the twelve charges (the twelve organ systems) will be in danger, which will cause the closing and the blocking of the ways, finally stopping communication, and the body will be seriously injured. From this the nurturing of life will sink into disaster. Everything that lives under Heaven will be threatened in its ancestral line with the greatest of dangers.*[5]

The Heart governs and stores the most etheric of all substances, the Heart's spirit, or *shen*. Mirroring the function of the ventral vagus nerve (described in Chapter Two), the Heart's *shen* is visible in the sparkle of the eyes and the shine on the face. The term *shen* is used in two ways. It is sometimes translated as "mind," and in this context it relates to consciousness, memory, keenness of thinking, and balance of emotions. It supports our short-term memory and our capacity for a sense of internal control and focused and stable thinking. *Shen* is also translated as "spirit," and as such, it encompasses the spirits associated with each of the Five Elements. The Heart's *shen* oversees and informs Water's *will power,* Wood's *ethereal soul,* Fire's *mind,* Earth's *thoughtfulness,* and Metal's *animal soul.* When traumatic stress penetrates the Heart, these spirits are all called upon—and if this alarm persists, we are thrown into system-wide chaos at the deepest level of our being.

The Heart's partner, the Small Intestine, has the job of sorting the pure from the impure. On the level of the physical body, it receives digested food, further transforms it, determines what is pure to absorb, and passes the impure to the Colon for elimination.

The larger job of the Small Intestine is to ensure that only the purest impulses reach the Heart. While food is the obvious substance requiring this kind of sorting, the Small Intestine also helps us sort the pure from the impure in other aspects of our lives. Movies and television, music and books, people and politics are great examples. Our Small Intestine helps us determine what we want to integrate of all the things we see, hear, and experience. A dysregulated Small Intestine may allow in too much of the impure or fail to absorb the right amount of the pure. For example, we may overload ourselves with too many scary movies or books or extreme and inflammatory opinion pieces in the news, and this will influence our inner balance and regulation. Similarly, without a competent sorting mechanism to retain what is true, beautiful, and life-giving, we can miss opportunities to enrich our lives and grow in new and meaningful ways.

AAM's identification of the Heart Protector and Triple Heater provide a helpful framework that is largely unacknowledged in Western physiology. In AAM classics, the Heart Protector is referred to as "the Heart's ambassador"—"from it, joy and happiness derive."[6] It gives us our capacity for intimacy, vulnerability, and engagement with others. It helps us radiate and receive the warmth and joy of connection, affection, and love. It opens the gates of the Heart for relationship and closes those gates, when necessary, for our protection. The important thing is that these gates stay lubricated, opening and closing appropriately and easily, so the Heart can love, be loved, and be protected.

The Heart Protector's partner, the Triple Heater, performs complex and helpful functions in the context of the 5-SPR. It is not an organ in the sense we are most familiar with—it is more like an energetic impulse that carries a coherent message that connects and influences all our organ systems.[7] It is referred to as "an organ with a name but no place."[8]

The Triple Heater is the first organ system to develop embryologically. It gives rise to the "three burning spaces"—a division of the torso into the chest, the area from the respiratory diaphragm to the waist, and the area from the waist to the pelvic bowl, and all the organs those three areas contain. It distributes the primal energetic imprint that we receive at conception to each meridian pathway. Its function to distribute this "original *qi*" throughout our body serves to create a whole-body message of coherence.[9] The Triple Heater is fundamentally about connection and coherence.

There are notable similarities between the Triple Heater and connective tissue. Like the Triple Heater, connective tissue is understood to be the first tissue formed embryologically. It similarly is understood to give rise to many body structures—including our bones, muscles, organs, nerves, tendons, fascia, blood, and lymph. Connective tissue is a web-like matrix that penetrates, wraps, and connects all body structures. It is embedded inside and coats the outside of each structure. It creates a container for and connects each structure with all other structures. It follows every shape, crease, and fold in our bodies. In fact, if we removed everything from our bodies except our connective tissue, we would still be completely recognizable. In *The Tao of Trauma*'s integrative sense, the Triple Heater can be thought of as the energetic function that is carried in our connective tissue.

The Triple Heater also distributes warmth throughout our system. It ensures the proper temperature for the smooth operation of each body function, as well as the appropriate and distinct degrees of warmth that will support our relationships with others in our life—our letter carrier, coworker, childhood friend, and intimate partner.[10]

The remedies described later in this chapter will engage these organ systems to bring them into greater regulation and support the healthy functioning of the ventral vagus nerve.

CONTEXT: THE ROLE OF THE FIRE ELEMENT IN THE SELF-PROTECTIVE RESPONSE

When our inner squirrel hears that twig snap, our sensory systems discern possible risk and alert our sympathetic nervous system to rise slightly and orient us to this potential threat (described in Chapter Six). A message of fear alerts our Kidneys and their close companions, the adrenal glands (described in Chapter Seven). This fear creates an initial impulse for connection with our tribe.[11]

The experience of fear in our Kidney/adrenal system reaches across the control cycle to our Heart Protector. As humans, our first instinct, unless it has been extinguished by earlier experiences, is a relational one. Our Heart Protector is the vehicle that helps us to be in relationship with and seek help from the people around us. We are social animals, and when we are in good health, our ability to engage with our tribe can make a world of difference in how we experience the impact of threat.

If our Heart Protector is able to resolve a conflict and mitigate our arousal using our capacity for connection and relationship, there will be no need for our Wood Element to mobilize a fight-or-flight response. In the language of polyvagal theory, the social engagement functions affiliated with the ventral vagus nerve have been successful in mitigating low-level arousal in our sympathetic nervous system.

For example, a coworker keeps "borrowing" pens from our desk, which becomes increasingly irritating to us. On a day when we feel well rested and poised, we raise our concern in a light-hearted and relational way that is also clear. We buy him a box of pens, tell him that we have an uncanny and perhaps silly sense of propriety about our pens, and ask him to please not take them from our desk anymore. He apologizes, buys us lunch, and we remain in collegial relationship. Our Heart has been protected from hyperarousal by our capacity to negotiate a disagreement in the context of relationship. This is the function supported by the ventral vagus nerve in the language of Western neurophysiology, or the Heart Protector in AAM.

However, if our capacity to negotiate a low-level conflict while remaining in relationship has been compromised by previous trauma, our Heart Protector will be unable to manage a conflict like this one within its function of social engagement. Instead of this light-hearted but clear resolution that allowed us to remain in relationship, we harbor anger and resentment. We may refuse to speak to our coworker, ultimately blowing up at him over an unrelated matter in a staff meeting. We not only lose relationship with him, we also develop a reputation for being volatile and unpredictable, which impairs friendship opportunities with all our coworkers.

Similarly, if we are unable to ask for or receive help from others, if our tribe is unavailable to us, or if we are responding to a towering threat—a tsunami, hurricane, or earthquake—our Heart Protector will be unable to prevent the sense of life threat from penetrating our Heart. AAM holds that nothing should actually touch the Heart, so when the Heart Protector is overwhelmed, and a message of life threat enters this sacred chamber, a tremendous, system-wide alarm is created.

If, at this stage in the self-protective response, the threat continues to mount, the Heart is catapulted into potentially life-threatening arousal in its attempt to help us respond to danger. The Heart sounds every alarm, dispatching all the fire trucks in the firehouse to tell the kingdom of the body that life threat is imminent. The message that the Heart has been penetrated is sent to the entire kingdom of the body as an all-encompassing vibration. It is carried in the blood, by the Heart's pulse.

This is essentially a physiological coup d'etat. The Heart, which supports the good, rhythmic, and coherent functioning of our whole body, has been overtaken by the crushing power of fear from the Kidney. Our entire body-mind-spirit and every organ and cell receives this alarm. Our Metal Element is commanded to provide the breath necessary to create the *qi* we need in this moment and to dump excess weight we may be carrying in our Colon by purging our digestive tract. Our Water Element is told to provide the power to fuel mobilization. Our Wood Element is ordered to strategize how to use that power, to send all blood and *qi* to our muscles and joints, and to carry out the necessary actions of fight or flight. And our Earth Element is commanded to temporarily shut down digestion and all functions of the enteric brain (often called our "belly brain") so all energy can be directed to our muscles and joints to respond to this immediate threat. Every ounce of *qi* we have available is called upon to save our life.

This is our body taking care of us. This is exactly what we want it to do when we are confronted by life threat. It only becomes a problem if, when the threat is over, the Heart is unable to signal a return to coherence and equanimity and instead continues to signal a need for this high state of arousal.

Note that the signal for threat arises from the Kidney and the Water Element, but the command to respond to that threat arises from the Heart and the Fire Element. These two organ systems function in close relationship in the 5-SPR. Building capacity in the Kidney to recognize safety will result in more accurate messaging of threat to the Heart Protector and the Heart.

The Heart oversees the functions of the frontal cortex, while the Kidneys oversee the functions of the brain's lower structures. When the Water's terror consumes us, the more thoughtful and relational functions of the frontal cortex are taken hostage. AAM would say that Water has overwhelmed Fire. Western neurophysiology would say that there is concurrent high tone in both the sympathetic and parasympathetic nervous systems. Arousal in the SNS has been turned up to its maximum, which, in turn, requires the dorsal vagal PNS to turn itself up to its maximum tone in order to apply an emergency brake to temper the extreme arousal in the SNS. This braking system will send us into a freeze response. If we become habituated to that freeze response, chaos will reign in every aspect of our body and its functions.

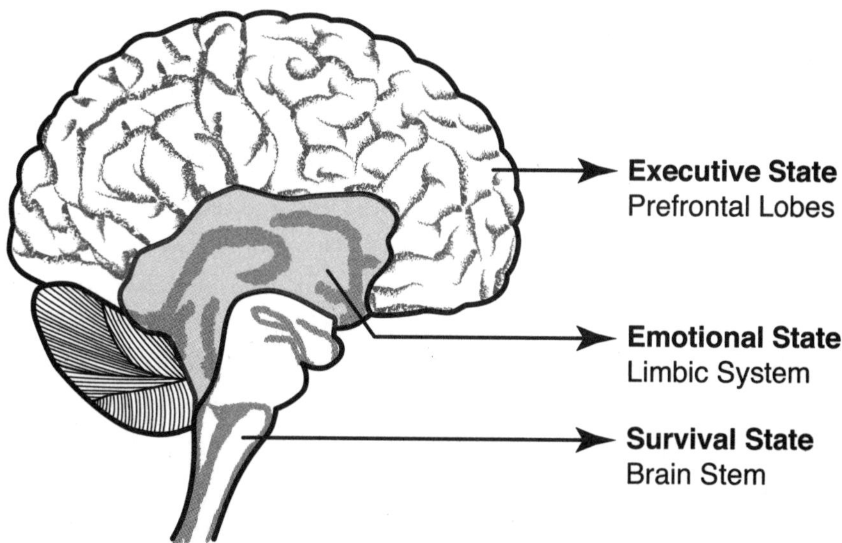

FIGURE 9.1. Brain Structures

If we are successful in our response to threat—either there was no threat (it was a rope, not a snake), or we successfully mobilized a fight-or-flight response—the Liver (known as the General of the Armed Forces) reports our success to the Heart (the Supreme Controller). We take a necessary moment to notice this: *I survived. I'm safe. It's over.* The Heart signals successful completion to the body-mind-spirit in the form of a regular heartbeat that stabilizes the kingdom of the body. Our breathing slows, and digestion returns. Balance between *yin* and *yang,* SNS and PNS, coherence and regulation is restored.

Dysregulated survival physiology can impact the Heart in two ways. We may become habituated to overusing our dorsal system and therefore respond to low-level threats as if they are life-threatening, habitually going into a freeze state. We will chronically put too strong a brake on our heart. By contrast, we may over-respond from our SNS and unnecessarily engage a mobilization response when a relational one, using the ventral vagal's PNS would be more appropriate.

COMMON SYMPTOMS FOR THE FIRE TYPE: THE HEART, HEART PROTECTOR, SMALL INTESTINE, AND TRIPLE HEATER

If we don't have time to return to equanimity, coherence, and regulation before our Heart is once again called to respond to life threat, we can become habituated to a sense of constant threat, and the functions of our ventral vagus nerve will be compromised. The relationship between our Heart and our Lungs can be profoundly affected, disturbing the important connection between our breath and our heartbeat. We may struggle to trust people and not understand nuanced meaning in facial expressions or tones of voice. Our sense of connection with our own true self—and our role in family and community—will become distorted, illusive, and confusing.

In this state, the many functions of the Fire Element—the most important of which is the regular rhythm of the heartbeat, which provides the signal upon which whole-body regulation and coherence is built—can become chaotic and asynchronous. We may become prone to panic attacks, experience impaired memory and cognition, or find it challenging to take control or command of situations that require nuanced discrimination between safety and threat. We may experience cardiac arrhythmias, hypertension, congestive heart failure, or other symptoms that require the care of a cardiologist. We may also experience a sense of general dysregulation in multiple body systems and exhibit symptoms that affect, for example, our endocrine, immune, pulmonary, or metabolic function.[12]

Significantly, it is our blood that carries the vibrations of our Heart to the furthest reaches of the body. The Heart's spirit, the *shen,* resides in the blood. If our blood is dysregulated, our *shen* will be uprooted and unable to find a home. This can cause anxiety, agitation, restlessness, forgetfulness, or an unsettled mind. We will have trouble quieting our mind for sleep and may be awakened by disturbing dreams.

In AAM, the Heart governs speech and supports heart-to-heart communication. The tongue is considered an offshoot of the Heart, and traumatic stress may manifest as stuttering or a compromised capacity to communicate with speech.

If the sorting function of the Small Intestine has been impacted by trauma, we may struggle to make distinctions of propriety. Social conventions will elude us—for instance, we may not know when and where to tell an off-color joke and end up making an inappropriate remark at a funeral. We may make errors in interpreting the nuances of facial expressions and tones of voice; we might misinterpret sounds. We can feel socially awkward and engage in inappropriate interpersonal interactions. These are ways the AAM Small Intestine organ system embodies aspects of the function of the ventral vagus nerve.

If our Heart Protector has been wounded by intimate betrayal, it will be less able to serve as a protector in subsequent relationships, and threats will more easily penetrate this vulnerable but vital space. It may misinterpret who or what should enter the Heart. Also called the *Circulation/Sex Organ System,* the Heart Protector helps us manage our most vulnerable and intimate expression. When it is compromised, we can make errors in judgment about our choice of sexual partners and sexual expression. The gates of our Heart Protector may be left wide open, causing us to experience heartbreak again and again. Or its gates may be closed tightly, making intimacy next to impossible, leading to overwhelming sadness and loneliness. Sadly, we can also become so driven to satisfy our sexual desires that we engage in violent or abusive sexual expression with unwilling or inappropriate partners.

Our Triple Heater, functioning like our connective tissue, can be disturbed by major surgery or high-velocity injury, such as an explosion or certain motor vehicle accidents. The high level of arousal that results from these sorts of injuries can be held in our connective tissue. The Triple Heater's global nature will carry these states of terror to virtually every aspect of our system. Injury to connective tissue can manifest with chronic, unremitting, and baffling pain patterns. Tissues that should fluidly glide against each other instead become dry, thickened, or sticky, causing them to abrade against each other, obstruct the flow of *qi,* and cause pain.

Connective tissue's curious function to simultaneously make relationship and create boundaries also plays an important role in the interpersonal impact of trauma on us. Especially after a breach in relationship, our psychological boundaries can become so thick or inflexible that it can become difficult for us to connect with others or navigate the dynamics and distinctions of relationship and separation in our families and communities. Working with connective tissue can support the healing of these psychological wounds in our Triple Heater. Similarly, cultivating psychologically healthy relationships will influence and instruct our connective tissue's physical function.

REMEDIES FOR RESTORING REGULATION IN THE FIRE

The Fire Element mirrors the function of the ventral vagus nerve. The remedies for dysregulation of the Fire Element described in this section all share the overarching goal of enhancing the ventral vagus's function of mitigating low-level arousal using our social-engagement system—and establishing system wide coherence.

Helping trauma survivors restore their inner regulation occurs in the context of relationship. No one can achieve deep or lasting reregulation outside the context of safe relationship, which is why it's essential that we provide our clients with the experience of attunement with our own (hopefully) more regulated nervous system. This is one reason why it is critically important to attend to our own inner regulation—it is our most important clinical tool. Cultivating our capacity for relationship is a critical and ongoing practice for all care providers.

The Fire Element's functions of relationship, connection, and coherence are deeply impacted by trauma. Profound vulnerability requires nuanced approaches to restoring the Pericardium/Heart Protector's portals of connection, the Triple Heater's infrastructure for connection, and the *shen*'s comprehensive gift of coherence and regulation.

Restoring Interoception in the Gates of the Heart Protector

Supporting the function of our Heart Protector helps restore our social-engagement system. It enhances our capacity for relationship and our ability to seek out and engage the assistance of others when we feel threatened. We are, after all, tribal animals; we are meant to live in community. The unnecessary engagement of our sympathetic nervous system can give rise to an off-putting, rigid, and argumentative style of interpersonal interaction. If we lose our capacity to resolve conflicts in the context of relationship, we will, over time, lose our place in the community. Our ability to survive is compromised if we don't have a community or if we lose our ability to seek out and welcome help when we need it.

In the context of trauma-related morbidity and mortality, a well-functioning Heart Protector protects our Heart from being penetrated by messages of low-level threat. It decreases demand for our sympathetic system to mobilize and for our dorsal vagus nerve to brake hyperarousal in our Heart. If our Heart Protector cannot keep such messages at bay, we will unnecessarily engage a mobilization response. Not only does this place a high metabolic demand on the body, it can also give rise to tragic mistakes resulting in breaches of relationship, at best, and heart-rending domestic or community violence, at worst. When our Heart Protector is working well, our whole body and its mind, emotions, and spirit are protected from the negative impact of engaging in either unnecessary sympathetic arousal or collapse.

The Heart Protector opens its gates to relationship when it is safe to do so and closes them when it is not. Ideally, these gates are easily accessed and wise in their opening and closing. The following exercise explores and cultivates the function of the Heart Protector, as well as your client's interoceptive awareness of his vulnerability and personal power.

Your client can be sitting in a chair or lying on a table. Allow him to express all his questions or thoughts about the purpose of this exercise to ensure the integrity of his consent. You don't want him to override the vulnerability inherent in your request for this touch. This is not the touch of a handshake or pat on the back. You are inviting him to explore the hinges in the gates of his Heart Protector, including their capacity to say yes and no to physical touch and connection.

Together, choose a location on your client's body where he feels it is safe for you to explore his yes and his no to your touch. It is best to choose a place that doesn't typically provoke extreme vulnerability—such as the back of his hand, the outside of his knee, the back of his forearm, or his shoulder. Touching with the back of your hand rather than your palm or fingertips may also help your client feel less vulnerable. Simply ask your client, for example, "May I touch your hand?" Encourage your client to take time and notice whether he feels a yes or no within himself, and always honor his answer. It is more important for him to respect his own interoceptive knowing than to answer yes, if a yes means that he overrides his vulnerability in order to please you. Give your client lots of time to thoughtfully explore whether his answer is yes or no—or perhaps "not yet." Invite him to notice any sense of habitual response that he becomes aware of.

If your client feels comfortable being touched, invite his continued curiosity. Explore variations to the touch—for example, the difference between when he has his eyes open or closed. Change the location of your touch from his hand to his knee, shoulder, or over his heart. Each time, be sure to ask his permission: "May I touch your 'X'?" Always honor his answer.

In health, we have capacity to say both yes and no in different circumstances and with different people. Invite your client to explore both his yes and his no. He may say yes a dozen times before a no emerges, or he may say no a dozen times before finding a yes. Give each inquiry its own time, attention, and opportunity for unique discernment.

With each answer, cultivate your client's awareness of what happens inside himself to prompt a yes or a no. Help him track these interoceptive messages. Provide an experience of safety or comfort as a resource to tick-tock with any arousal that emerges. In cultivating function in the Heart Protector, it can be especially useful to use an experience of safety that is based in a relationship, such as your presence or the imaginary presence of a safe and loving person from your client's present or past. Help him harvest the dynamics of both personal power and vulnerability that may emerge.

As waves of arousal are given time and context to find regulation, your clients' capacity to make use of their social-engagement system to manage threats will increase. Instead of going directly to a freeze response or unnecessarily initiating a mobilization response at first indication of threat, they will be better able to resolve low-level threat in the context of relationship. They will feel safer, their interpersonal relationships will be more functional, and they will likely be more able to find joy.

Client Example

Kahalia's story unfolded over several months of our work together. She suffered from almost constant anxiety, unable to sleep and almost paralyzed with fear in social situations. She was isolated, rarely going out, and attending social events only if they were required for her work or if her family pestered her to attend. She would then stay only the minimum amount of time she felt she could get away with. She felt a deep sense of shame about her inability to connect with others. She longed to be in a relationship but despaired of ever being able to meet anyone and manage the dating process.

Kahalia's father had died when she was ten years old. She had had a close relationship with him and had witnessed his death—a car hit him as they crossed a street together. Kahalia had sustained only minor physical injuries but developed severe anxiety after the accident. Her mother was devastated by the death of her husband. She became hyper-protective of her daughter, constantly monitoring Kahalia's activities and reminding her to be careful whenever she left the house.

In our initial discussions, it became apparent that Kahalia's life was ruled by fear and that she had never really had a chance to grieve and recover from her father's death. The extreme fear she experienced in the accident had overwhelmed her ability to access her feelings of loss and heartbreak.

At first, just sitting directly across from each other and looking face-to-face was activating for her. I could see her chest become tight, her breath become shallow, and her hands shake. We negotiated the distance between us, and I titrated my gaze by taking time to look away periodically. After a time, we began our work with the touch exercise described above. She agreed that the outside of her knee was a safe area to use as the starting place for the touch and that I would begin by using the back of my hand. After my seventh inquiry in this session was met with another no, I again asked her if I could touch her outside of her knee, and she hesitantly said yes. I touched her, but only briefly. We took some time together to simply allow the arousal she experienced to dissipate. A few more nos came before another yes. I then allowed my hand to stay in place slightly longer. Her arousal softened more quickly this time.

Over time, Kahalia came to a yes with my open palm on her knee. Tears came to her eyes as she remembered her father's loving touch. We sat together for an extended period of time, allowing her tears all the time they needed and giving her system time to deeply take in the love her father had had for her, and she for him.

Her whole body softened and a smile came to her face. "I was so lucky to have him as long as I did." While she continued to miss her father and struggled to negotiate her independence from her mother, she was also increasingly able to manage occasional social engagements and interactions with others. She became less anxious and experienced more vitality and self-confidence.

Using Co-Regulation to Restore or Support Self-Regulation

The function of whole-body regulation and coherence belongs to the Heart in AAM and to the ventral vagus nerve in Western neurophysiology. We are born with the hardware of our ventral vagus nerve in place, but it needs to be stimulated in our infancy and childhood for it to properly and fully function.

The ventral vagus is critical to our emotional intelligence—our social intelligence. It is developed in the context of loving and safe relationships in our infancy and childhood. Through such relationships, we develop our ability to discern the nuances of meaning in voice inflections, to look with soft eyes into someone else's, to interpret meaning in facial expressions accurately, and to develop a sense of emotional congruence with others.

At the same time that our social-engagement system is being cultivated with this co-regulatory play, our ventral vagus is also developing our ability to invisibly regulate things outside our conscious control—our immune function, breathing, heartbeat, assimilation of nutrients, and hormonal regulation.[13]

Interactions between children and their caregivers cultivate co-regulation in the infant. They bring energy to the developing ventral vagus nerve—and cultivate an infant's capacity for her own self-regulation. The sparkle in our eyes, the prosody in our voice, the songs we sing together, and the ball we toss all help build a young body's capacity for self-regulation, arising from the developing ventral vagus nerve. Our system learns—at a deep, regulatory level—exactly how to digest and assimilate nutrients by experiencing loving relationships around the dinner table.

At this early stage of life, these autonomic functions are still developing and vulnerable. If traumatic stress disrupts our ventral vagus nerve during this period, we are at particular risk for disruption to our autonomic regulation as adults. Lacking the proper stimulation to cultivate full ventral vagal functioning, traumatized infants and young children miss the acquisition of the full range of these autonomic functions, including the gentle and nuanced regulation of the cardiac, pulmonary, metabolic, and social-engagement systems.

Thankfully, providers can offer various reparative experiences to restore functions that were missed or disrupted developmentally. Playing patty-cake in a slow, deliberate, and mindful way is one example of a co-regulatory activity that can help repair and build a survivor's capacity for self-regulation. Such experiences of low-level sympathetic arousal—excitation without fear, and thus without stress chemistry—can grow the delicate and nuanced functions of the ventral vagus nerve as your client learns to play and enjoy the full range of his autonomic responses in the absence of fear.

It is important for providers to set the context when using this exercise. Playing patty-cake is not competitive, and it doesn't matter how good we are at it. It is an opportunity to cultivate co-regulation. Setting a slow pace will help you mirror each other. Make your movements simple. We want to minimize the possibility of shame that could develop from an inability to keep up with a fast pace or a complex pattern.

Sit across from each other, negotiating a distance that feels comfortable. The important thing is to be in safe relationship. It might be good to start with a tap on the knees and a tap on each other's hands, without crossing over the body's midline. The neurological demand of crossing over the midline (bringing hands together diagonally) can be challenging and can simply be too much for someone who has experienced the disruption of her brain development that can occur in the face of severe early trauma. It can also be too challenging for those who have experienced traumatic brain injury. Don't ask your client to do what she can't do. The risk of exacerbating a state of vulnerability or shame that likely already exists is much too high. She may be only able to tap her own knees while you tap yours at the same time. In this case, you can engage with your eyes and your smile while you take pleasure in sharing the rhythmic tapping.

Help your client track her sensations. Titrate your play as you experiment with different or slightly more complex movements. Waves of arousal and emerging regulation may arise. Allow time and space for these waves to come and go. Give plenty of time for arousal to resolve and for your client to harvest states of growing co-regulation with you and her own inner self-regulation.

Watch for occasions when she is ready to try crossing over the midline, which demands more complex brain integration, by tapping opposite hands or opposite knees before experimenting with more complex movement sequences. Note the impact of breaches in relationship if one of you misses the other's cue for a next movement or goes faster than a pace you can both follow.

Client Example

Yosuf spent the first two years of his life in an orphanage in Afghanistan. Although his adoptive parents were loving and excited about finally having a child to care for, they struggled with Yosuf's lack of engagement with them. Over time, they gave up trying to engage him in play and simply cared for him as best they could, loving him in whatever way he seemed able to receive. Yosuf is now in his late twenties. He tells me his parents' account of his childhood and says it matches his own memories—he felt loved by them but doesn't remember much play or playful interaction. Yosuf has always had learning challenges, as well as a tendency to feel anxious when he's trying anything new, even if it's something he's interested in.

It's likely that Yosuf's time in the orphanage meant he had limited access to normal co-regulatory experiences like snuggling and playing. His capacity to connect with others, particularly in ways that offer co-regulation, is somewhat limited. His lack of access to healthy co-regulation has also inhibited his capacity for self-regulation.

When Yosuf came to see me, we began by playing patty-cake. Yosuf was surprised when he found he couldn't do it. He couldn't simultaneously track his own movements and mine, so we sat together, each tapping our own knees and finding a rhythm we could share. In our first attempt, this is all we did. The second time, we again found our rhythm and added in a clap of our hands: three taps of the knees, then clapping our own hands together once, then another three taps on our knees. After practicing this briefly, Yosuf was interested in trying the same rhythm, clapping each other's hands. We both noticed that he was feeling a little anxious about doing this, so we took a few minutes for him to settle and decide if he really wanted to try that next step.

He'd been enjoying our game and said that he wanted to try, even though he was still nervous. We agreed on three knee taps, one hand clap, three more knee taps, and one more hand clap. We did this in slow motion so he had a chance to carefully match his movements with mine. When he was successful at our pattern, he giggled with glee and wanted to do it again. This time, I let him set the pace, and he was able to do it more quickly—and even when he made a mistake, he was able to laugh about it. We had started our journey of co-regulation together.

Restoring the Infrastructure for Connection

As noted earlier, there is no physical organ called the *Triple Heater.* Its energetic function most closely matches the structure of our connective tissue. For our purposes, we will consider the Triple Heater to carry the *qi,* the energetic impulse for connection that, through this integrative lens, is found in connective tissue. Together, the connective tissue and the Triple Heater serve as the tangible and intangible dual infrastructure that supports coherent connection within our bodies and appropriate connection in our relationships with others. When we mindfully touch the connective tissue, we also touch the energetic function of the Triple Heater.

Connective tissue can be either gel-like or solid, depending on temperature. When it is cold, it is hard and stiff, but when warmed with friction or external heat, it can be remolded and reshaped. In theory, connective tissue is universally elastic. However, we all have areas that are thickened and bound as a reflection of our life experience. Strong, habitual emotions or physical postures can cause contractions in connective tissue. Elasticity in our connective tissue influences flexibility in our emotional life.

Connective tissue is particularly vulnerable to high-velocity injuries and is almost always affected by blast injuries. It is the web that receives the impact when we fall or are thrown a distance. Our connective tissue acts as a shock absorber to dissipate that impact and is likely to be injured in the process. If it becomes rigid as a result, it can't dissipate force as easily in future experiences—even in experiences that someone with elastic and flexible connective tissue would recover from quickly.

Injury, surgery, or inflammatory responses can create scar tissue, which is a thickening and stiffening of connective tissue. In some cases, this is essential, such as the thickening in a bone after a fracture. But in other cases, the scarring can disrupt healthy functioning by limiting movement, joining things that should glide and slide separately, and binding and pulling in ways that create pain and further irritation, possibly even further inflammation.

You may choose to work with connective tissue if your client is tight or rigid and wants more flexibility or if he is slack and needs more tone. If he feels fragmented or lacks a sense of his inner connection, integrity, and wholeness, then connective tissue is a perfect tissue to work with. It inherently carries the information and experience of our connectedness.

Our challenge in working with connective tissue is the titration of arousal. Unlike bones or muscles, which have a clear beginning and end, and thus a more local nature, connective tissue is inherently global. It goes everywhere and connects everything. It is effective at carrying information through the whole body, mind, emotions, and spirit. When we facilitate greater communication within this system, it tends to spread and be shared throughout the entire body and the individual's sense of self. If the information being shared is terror, a client who struggles with self-regulation may quickly go into hyperarousal. While we ultimately do want this sense of terror to move out of the body, we don't want to awaken it in a global and consuming way, because it will terrorize the client and risk deepening his habituation to either freeze or hyperarousal. This is why we must carefully and thoughtfully choose the timing for this work and not proceed until the client has basic regulation on board.

There are several useful places for finding connective tissue. It is easiest to find in fleshy areas. You will feel its wrapping nature over large muscles, such as the biceps or triceps in the upper arm. You will feel its clear, sheet-like quality in the lower back. Your hands' "eyes" can look both superficially and deeply for it. Your touch will primarily be a still one—and you may sometimes feel called to look for elasticity and glide with gentle kneading of his tissues. Be curious about flexibility, movement, connection, and boundaries as you work. Your client will likely find it less intimate or threatening if you work with his connective tissue over his clothing.

Titration is critical when working with connective tissue. Use the tick-tock method, moving attention and awareness to the smallest and most preliminary awareness of threat—which might manifest with modest anxiety, fear, or anger—and then inviting your client to come back to a safe or comfortable state, allowing any waves of arousal that emerge to come back into regulation. Then invite his awareness back to the next incremental experience of arousal. Work slowly and for relatively short periods of time. You may choose to periodically move your hand or your attention to tissues with a more local nature, like bones or muscles. Using the Kidney/adrenal system to support regulation can be a good choice if your client goes into high arousal—such as a state of panic. (See Chapter Four for a discussion on the nature of different body tissues.)

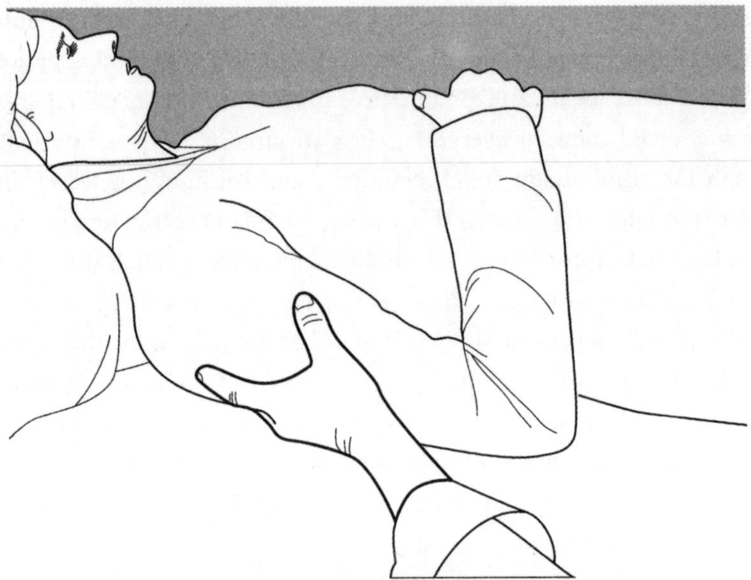

FIGURE 9.2. Touching the Connective Tissue

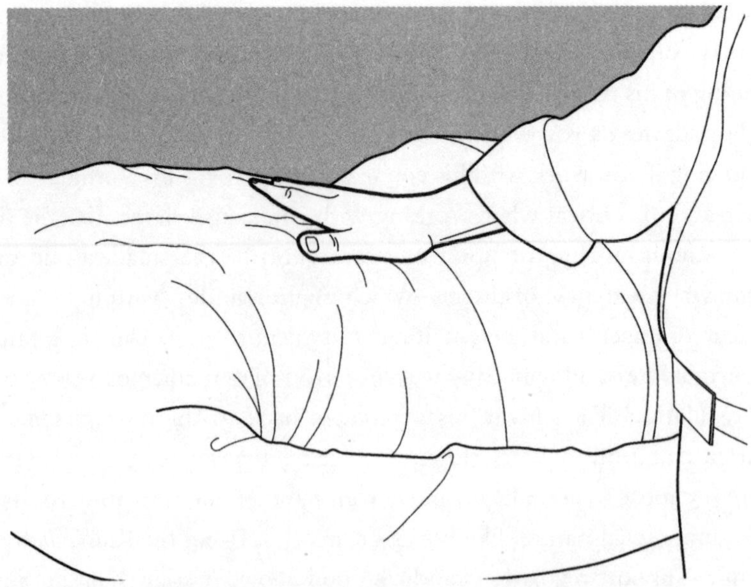

FIGURE 9.3. Touching Connective Tissue on the Back

As you move arousal out of the connective tissue, your client will increasingly experience ease in his whole system. Your goal in working with connective tissue is to replace global terror with global regulation. As the following example indicates, the result can be powerful.

Client Example

Joan is a Fire survivor type. She laughs easily and finds connection with others to be central to her healing journey. She is well liked by her colleagues and friends. Joan's physicians discovered cancer in her esophagus a year ago and surgically removed the upper half of her stomach. Her surgery was extensive and required broad exploration and incisions in related tissues—she has a scar extending from her lower abdomen up to her chest

While the surgery was necessary to save her life, it left Joan in a state of hyperarousal in both branches of her autonomic nervous system. During any surgery, our sympathetic nervous system cannot engage a fight-or-flight response to our surgeon's incision—anesthesia induces paralysis (thankfully), and straps may also help keep surgical patients immobilized while undergoing such procedures. Our organs of digestion don't like being touched, and they are particularly vulnerable to freeze after surgery. Joan's stomach as well as her small and large intestines were affected. She suffered from significant post-surgical pain, as well as impaired metabolic and digestive function.

We began by supporting her general and whole-body regulation with the boundary work described in Chapter Seven. With this work, her arousal level decreased, and she began to sleep better at night and feel less anxious during the day. She also experienced a return of peristalsis in her guts. While her digestion remained problematic, her weight stabilized, and her bowel function returned.

Once she was stabilized after surgery, she underwent chemotherapy and came to me with the common side effects of nausea and compromised assimilation of nutrients. She lost weight and experienced chronic diarrhea. Radiation treatment left scar tissue throughout her abdomen. We continued to support whole-body regulation with the Kidney/adrenal touch.

Once Joan had completed her chemotherapy and radiation, gained some of her weight back, and began eating and eliminating with more ease, we started working with her connective tissue. I placed my hand lightly on the back of her upper arm and allowed my attention to sink into the connective tissue around her triceps muscle. Before long, she began to feel her attention drawn to her viscera. Her legs began to shimmer and shake with what appeared to be a discharge of arousal.

We had no way of knowing if the discharge of this arousal was the result of the straps that prevented her from moving during the surgery or if the Stomach meridian, which runs down the legs, was carrying arousal out of her Stomach organ system. Whatever the reason, giving time for this arousal to complete and allowing her system to let go of some of its brace helped her to experience ease in her viscera. Joan's face lit up, and she said, "I feel connected inside myself in a new way. I feel whole." We gave her time to take in this important interoceptive message arising from her guts.

In a subsequent session, as our attention moved from my hand at the back of her arm to her viscera, she again began to feel the same pleasing sense of inner connection. After a few moments, she turned to look at me and said, "I feel connected to myself, but also connected to you. I'm my own person, but we're together. I feel a deep sense of safety in my connection with you."

Joan is now able to work full time again, and she enjoys going dancing with her husband and friends. She needs to eat small, frequent meals and take vitamins, but she enjoys her food and eliminates without a problem.

Restoring the Spirit of the Heart

The mediastinum is the central membrane that divides the two sides of the chest from each other. It does not actually touch the heart, but surrounds it, with a layer of fluid between it and the pericardium. Another layer of this same structure attaches to the entire surface of the respiratory diaphragm and reflects upward onto the surface of the inner walls of the chest. It has yet another layer that attaches directly to the surface of the lungs. At the back, it attaches to the fat and tissue that are directly in front of the spine, and on the front, to the inside of the sternum. All the various layers of this complex structure create a dynamic and responsive system that allows the heart to beat unimpeded while simultaneously supporting both the heart and lungs. The mediastinal structures, quite literally, protect the expansive function of the Heart as understood in AAM.

Most medical and surgical textbooks will refer to it as a completely passive and unimportant physical structure that separates the two sides of the chest cavity. In the context of the trauma spectrum response, we hold it as a physical structure that also maintains an important vibrational field around the Heart. It is this energetic function of the mediastinum that makes it an important gateway for accessing and restoring coherence to the many functions of the ventral vagus nerve in trauma survivors.

The mediastinum and its contiguous tissues in the chest can carry deep and heartfelt emotion, especially in the context of chronic relational trauma. It is particularly vulnerable after thoracic surgery, and brace or collapse in this membrane may be an aspect of the all-too-common experience of depression or anxiety after heart surgery.

The mediastinum's physiology is quite complex. It touches and can impact several different systems and their multiple functions. It supports the rhythms of the heartbeat and the breath—thus supporting the distribution of *qi* and blood. It gathers in the throat, and influences speech and strength of voice. It has profound spiritual and psychological functions.

If a client needs help unifying her Heart and mind, this membrane is a useful place to begin. We can use the mediastinum when a client is prepared to engage with herself and others with an open Heart. This type of work is precious and particularly nourishing to a wounded spirit, and it can serve as an inoculation against future traumas. It can help restore a sense of lost self.

The mediastinum can be accessed from any of its many points of connection: the sternum, the upper thoracic vertebrae, or at its connection to the respiratory diaphragm along the edge of the ribcage.

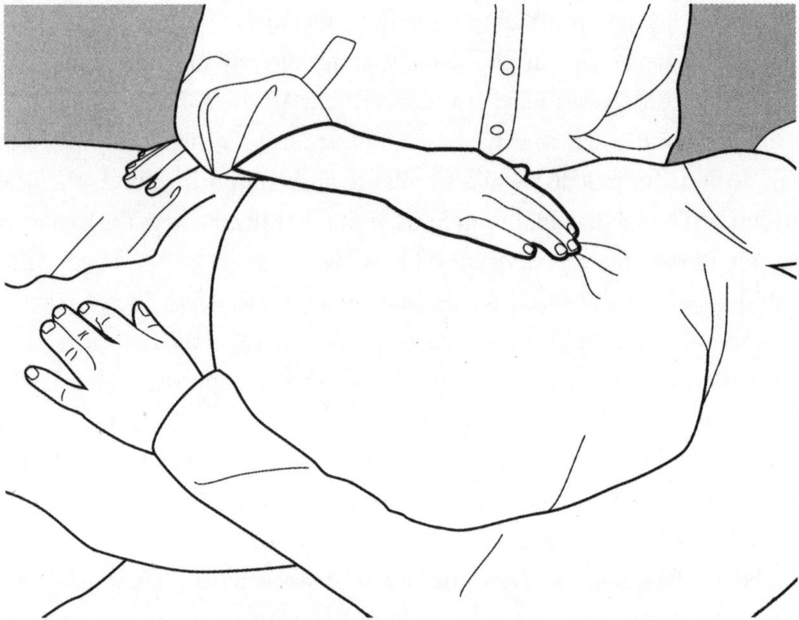

FIGURE 9.4. Touching the Mediastinum

Begin, as always, by bringing spacious attention to the equivalent structure in yourself—in this case, with awareness of your Heart space. This will help center, focus, and calm your attention. Then bring your attention to your client's Heart space before allowing your hand to organically follow your attention. Note any sense of relationship with your client that emerges. Maintain awareness of your own mediastinal structure while working with your client's. Allow your awareness to trace the anatomy of this structure in your client, noticing any areas that feel bound, tight, or missing. If touching into deep structures of the body is unfamiliar to you, you can read Chapter Five for information about using these methods.

Look for a deep sense of timelessness and a profound sense of connectedness between yourself and your client. You want to cultivate interoceptive awareness and support your client to harvest any states of greater regulation that emerge. Be in resonant relationship with your client. This may not require words at all. Engaging the mediastinum is often a deeply internal experience for your client.

Client Example

Donald had had a heart attack more than a year ago. He had been cleared by his cardiologist to return to normal activity months before his appointment with me but remained almost paralyzed by a fear that he would cause another heart attack if he exercised or otherwise raised his heart rate and blood pressure. He no longer engaged in vigorous exercise, even though he had been a lifelong athlete. He confided that he had not made love with his wife since his heart attack, and he was no longer willing to take the mountain-climbing trip they had dreamed of for three years to celebrate their anniversary.

He asked if there was something we might do that would help him overcome this deep sense of fear, which he felt as a constriction in his chest. The many scans and tests he had requested to identify this constriction had convinced his physicians that the causes were related to stress and were not physical.

We decided that I would start directly with the mediastinum, since he felt an urgency to get some relief. As Donald lay on the table, I gently placed one hand on his chest, right over his heart, and slipped the other opposite his heart, under his back. I invited him to join me in his heart space. As he did that, he experienced a wave of fear of what he might find there. I explained that we could bring our attention to his mediastinum, the structure that provided protective support for the heart. That gave him a sense of immediate relief, since he wouldn't "have to know" if his heart had been damaged.

Together we explored the sense of support he felt as we connected to his mediastinum. He slowly began to feel curious about exploring his heart more directly. He imagined that he could take a little tour, like a physician in a white coat, slowly walking around his heart. "Hmmmm," he said, "things don't actually look too bad here." I invited him to notice each area of his heart that he had felt concerned about. He noticed there was more health present than he had imagined.

Much to my surprise, he burst into tears. "My mother has been dead for twenty years, but after I had the heart attack, all I wanted was to feel her holding me and reassuring me that I would be okay. I longed for contact with her in a way I hadn't since the months after her death. As you are helping me find my heart space again, I feel like I am finding that support and reassurance that I couldn't connect with through my fear."

By the end of the session, the constriction in Donald's chest had eased completely. As he began to feel his fear lessening, he realized how far away he had gotten from his connection with his wife during the time since his heart attack. His fear had caused him to isolate himself—he was no longer letting his wife's loving attention penetrate through that cloak of isolation.

When Donald came back the next week, he reported that he had gone home and spoken with his wife about his experience of finally letting down his fear. They had agreed to reschedule their anniversary trip for a year from then—to give him time to regain his fitness and to give them time to reconnect in their relationship so it could truly be the trip they had dreamed of.

SOCIAL IMPLICATIONS FOR RESTORING REGULATION IN THE FIRE ELEMENT

The Fire Element ensures the coherent rhythm of our Heart, reinforces the executive functions of our frontal cortex, supports our capacity for connection internally and with others, and generates pleasure in our sexual expression. It mirrors the function of the ventral vagus nerve in its influence on the sparkle in our eyes, our facial muscles that express emotions, and the muscles of the ear that help us discern subtleties of meaning in speech. These functions support the depth of communication and connection necessary for healthy and loving relationships in our homes, neighborhoods, and workplaces. Interactions that emerge or fail to emerge from this regulated and peaceful center have an enormous impact on families and communities.

Recall that our Pericardium is also called our *Circulation/Sex Organ System*. This refers to its role in helping us navigate the complexities of the circulation of our sexual interest and its expression. Because of the Pericardium's close proximity to the Heart—we can easily over-couple the high arousal we experience in sexual intimacy with other experiences of high arousal that were also felt in our Heart, such as terror or life threat. If we have become habituated to go into high sympathetic arousal when our heartbeat escalates, we may have flashbacks of terror or engage an inappropriate fight response in the midst of sexual intimacy. Domestic violence can be the tragic result.

Joe is an example of this. Married and in his early twenties, he found when he returned home from Iraq that every time he became sexually aroused, he would have flashbacks of battle experiences. Sexual intimacy was problematic for him until we were able to uncouple the pounding heartbeat of his arousal and mobilization on the battlefield with the pounding heartbeat from the arousal he experienced making love with his wife. Thankfully, he did not become one of the many statistics about domestic violence in military veterans.

Traumatic stress resulting from the intimate betrayal of rape or incest can leave long-lasting imprints on this Circulation/Sex organ system. We may make errors in judgment about our choice of sexual partners and sexual expression, creating complex and hurtful dynamics in our families. We can also express our sexuality in mechanical, abusive, or even violent ways—with profoundly personal ramifications for all those involved, as well as criminal penalties that can follow people for the rest of their lives. The fabric of our communities is wounded when there is a lack of safety and respect in how sexual expression manifests. Many perpetrators of sexual assault were themselves victims at another point in their lives.

A regulated and peaceful Heart depends on interoceptive awareness of safety in our Kidneys. Similarly, coherence in our Heart communicates whole-body regulation that mitigates a sense of threat in our Kidneys. Understanding the dynamic relationship between the Kidneys and Heart can help providers understand the impact of their work in a "world-work" context.

The Kidneys signal threat, and the Heart gives the command to the body to respond. The Kidneys govern the primal, largely unconscious, instinctive and impulsive brain stem, while Heart governs the more thoughtful, relational, and executive frontal cortex of the brain. If fear floods the structures and functions of the brain stem, the dorsal vagus nerve must activate to put the brakes on potentially dangerous hyperarousal in the Heart. This all-consuming brake can compromise the executive functions of the frontal cortex.

Under these circumstances, the frontal cortex will no longer be available to help us manage fear, anger, or connection with ourselves or others. Our ability to digest experiences, take in a new reality, or let go of an old one will also be compromised, leaving us in a state of chaos in which the Supreme Controller has no peaceful center. We feel a sense of disconnection from ourselves and from our sense of shared humanity. We lose our capacity to trust others or connect heart-to-heart. Uncertain futures and unknown people may feel particularly threatening. Making decisions based on what is good for the whole community and our children's children feels impossible when we perceive immediate life threat.

The work of healers to restore balance and regulation in the critical dynamic between the Heart and the Kidneys can have a profound impact on healthy executive function and can improve the kinds of choices survivors make about how to live together and share our world.

One explanation for the social implications of this dynamic lies in the impact of early developmental trauma. A young child does not possess an adult's capacity to mitigate arousal using the parasympathetic function of her ventral vagus nerve when she feels threatened. A child who repeatedly experiences a sense of threat will use the dorsal vagus's brake to manage hyperarousal in her Heart. This overwhelms both the Heart and the executive functions of the frontal cortex. If this happens repeatedly, there is a risk of habituation, which limits the capacity of the young survivor's frontal cortex to inhibit antisocial behaviors as an adult. Later in life, she is more likely to act out the mobilization response that remains in her tissues, underneath the collapse engineered by her dorsal vagus nerve many years ago.

Research on adverse childhood experiences links an increase in adverse experiences in childhood to higher rates of domestic and community violence and other criminal behaviors in adulthood.[14] In one study, boys who had been sexually abused were up to forty-five times more likely to engage in dating violence in adolescence.[15]

In a study of adult males convicted of offenses including domestic violence, stalking, physical abuse of children, general violence, and sexual deviance, researchers discovered four times more adverse childhood experiences in childhood than in a paired sample. The authors concluded that neurobiologic dysregulation and attachment pathology (from adverse childhood experiences) explain the stark rates of criminal behavior. The researchers concluded that treatment interventions focusing on the crime with no attempt to heal these neurobiologic wounds are "destined to fail."[16]

When the Kidneys and the Heart and the brain stem and the frontal cortex are in healthy and dynamic relationship, better, more positive, and longer-lasting outcomes arise, enabling more peaceful and productive living. These healthy interactions between people ripple out to whole families, neighborhoods, and workplaces—as well as to our nation as a whole. An individual, community, or nation whose signaling center for threat is stuck in the on position will have a different response to perceived threat than an individual, community, or nation that feels safe, valued, and respected.

CONCLUSION

Working with the Fire Element has broad implications for whole-body regulation, cognitive function, interpersonal relationships, and social intelligence, as well as pain patterns, pleasure in sexual expression, and joy in life. Providers can help their clients heal from past heartaches, enjoy a playful life, and keep themselves and their communities safer by helping them stay in relationship and make use of the healthy executive and inhibiting functions of their prefrontal cortex. This work can help restore a regulated, coherent rhythm in the heart of individuals and in the heart of our communities.

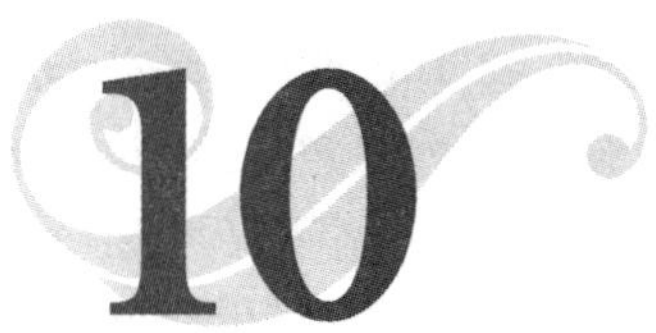

10 Earth and Late Summer: Digest the Gristle

THE FIVE STEPS OF THE SELF-PROTECTIVE RESPONSE

1. Arrest/Startle—Arousal Awakens Us Out of Exploratory Orienting. Metal.
2. Defensive Orienting—Fear Signals Threat. Water.
3. Specific Self-Protective Response—Mobilization Response Initiates. Wood.
4. Completion—Successful Defense or No Threat. Restore Coherence. Fire.
5. **Integration—Digest the Gristle. Harvest the Lessons. Earth.**

   Cycle Returns to the Metal and Restored Capacity for Exploratory Orienting.

THE EARTH ELEMENT is associated with the season of late summer. Fire creates Earth, just as heat in a compost pile creates rich humus. Summer creates late summer, a fifth season in the Chinese agricultural cycle. The Spleen and Stomach are the organ systems of the Earth Element. They serve to break down food into digestible matter, transform it into qi/energy and blood, and transport this life-giving nourishment to our body. The Spleen and Stomach also break down our experiences into digestible bits, and help us harvest and assimilate life lessons that help us navigate future threats.

The mobilize-a-response phase of the 5-SPR, organized by the Wood Element precipitates a shutdown of peristalsis in our guts. Our capacity to receive, transform, transport, and integrate nourishment is compromised while our blood and qi is directed to our muscles and joints to support fighting or fleeing. If this state becomes chronic, we may have trouble assimilating nourishment from both our food and our challenges. We may embrace lessons that contract rather than expand our worldview or find ourselves unable to trust, forever feeling like a victim. We may feel utterly lacking in confidence to move forward with life. Our trauma story may go around and around, always seeking, but not finding, adequate comfort and understanding

As you are with your client, observe her with the following questions in mind. Use them to assess the ongoing impact of an incomplete response in the integration or digest-the-gristle phase of the 5-SPR.

- *Does your client digest food easily, without excess bloating, gas, or belching?*
- *Is it challenging for her to digest her traumatic experiences, and prepare them for elimination or transformation into helpful life lessons?*
- *Are the lessons she extracts from traumatic experiences expanding or contracting to her worldview?*
- *Are her resentments, hurt feelings or trauma memories indigestible? Is her inner experience one of always being a victim?*
- *Can she receive and integrate your comfort or sympathy—and make use of it to transform her inner reality?*
- *Does she carry extra weight around her middle, suffer from an irritable bowel, or have trouble assimilating nutrients?*

CORRESPONDENCES RELATING TO THE EARTH ELEMENT'S ROLE IN THE SELF-PROTECTIVE RESPONSE

Element	*Earth*
Season	*Late summer*
Organ Systems	*Spleen, Stomach*
Emotion	*Sympathy, indifference*
Role in Self-Protective Response	*Digests the gristle, harvests the lessons*
Unsuccessful or Incomplete Self-Protective Response	*Hyperarousal: High tone in the digestive system and muscles—wiry, tight body. Dry, hard stools. Hard to receive support or nurturance.* *Hypoarousal: Low tone in the digestive system and muscles—soft, flabby body. Difficulty absorbing nutrients or transforming food into energy. Hard to harvest lessons or integrate experiences.*
Engenders	*Sensate curiosity*
Controls	*Signal for threat*
Tissue	*Flesh, muscles*
Virtue	*Selflessness*
Stores	*Nourishment*
Spirit	*Purpose, intent*
Archetypal Questions	*How do I turn life's lessons into fruit?* *How do I digest the gristle and integrate it into my flesh?*
Exercises to Enhance Regulation	*Restoring peristalsis in the viscera* *Supporting completion responses stored in the muscles and flesh* *Restoring regulation in body fluids*

ORIENTATION: THE NATURE OF THE EARTH ELEMENT

The Earth Element is associated with the time of the harvest in late summer. Fruits and vegetables hang heavy, gardens are bursting, and insects flourish in a last call for life. No more fruit or vegetables will set—but those on the vine will ripen, sweeten, and grow heavy, and if not harvested, they will fall and rot. The air feels heavy, dense, and thick. This season calls us to harvest the fruits of our year's labor, as well as the fruits of our year's experiences, and integrate all of it into our body, as well as our mind and spirit.

The functions of the Spleen and Stomach are intimately connected. The Stomach receives nourishment and "rottens and ripens it," and the Spleen transforms this nourishment into *qi*/energy and blood and transports it to the community of our body. Its primary function is to "transform and transport." Together the Spleen and Stomach create a dynamic balance between giving and receiving.[1]

Healthy, nourishing food impacts the quality of the *qi* and blood the Spleen is able to create. So too do healthy, nourishing experiences and relationships impact the lifeblood of our existence. If we are fed fear, anger, or hatred, especially as a young child, we will not enjoy healthy *qi* and blood as adults.

The key qualities of the Earth Element are nourishment and stability. When our Earth is in its most balanced and healthy state, we easily transform food and experiences into *qi*/energy and blood. We are well nourished by the food we eat and the caring actions of people in our lives. We feel grounded and embodied in our flesh. We attend well to the needs of those around us, giving nurturance and support freely. There is a healthy balance between giving and receiving in our relationships; we fully digest and embody life's experiences and eliminate what is indigestible in our meals and in our lives.

The rest-and-digest function of the digestive organs is supported by our dorsal vagus nerve when it's operating at a healthy low tone. In AAM, these organs function as an organizational unit to "process and move impure substances."[2] The gut turns last night's gristle into this morning's waste. This function is governed by our autonomic nervous system. It is completely unconscious and can't be willed.

When our Earth is out of balance, we are unable to transform or assimilate food or experiences. We may find ourselves overeating or feeling overly needy; we collect excess baggage in the form of developing obesity, fostering resentments, or perhaps even by hoarding. Our minds go around and around, thinking and thinking about an experience without fully breaking it down, digesting it, and moving on. We may find ourselves stingy in our attention for others, or we may be able to give nurturance and support but unable to receive it. We lack gratitude for life's sweetness. We feel unstable and ungrounded.

The Earth Element also has a special relationship with our muscles and flesh. The Spleen's function to create *qi* is visible in the tone and capacity of our muscles. Muscles communicate sensations that arise from our inner experience. Thwarted mobilization responses, failures of self-protection, and untransformed traumatic experiences may be stored in our muscles. What we believe and how we feel about these failures will also be found in our muscle memory and may be reflected in our posture, as well as our stance toward life. The Spleen's job in the 5-SPR is to digest the "gristle" in the stew of life, support transformation of these experiences, and build our muscular strength and resiliency.

The Stomach is said to be the "origin of fluids" in AAM classical literature's description of the entire digestive track, including the Small Intestine and Colon, as well as the Stomach. We adhere to Daniel Keown's interpretation of AAM classical literature, which embraces the entire digestive tract as the "origin of fluids."[3] Fluids enter our Stomach in the liquids we drink and the juicy foods we eat. They are absorbed into our tissues from our Small Intestine and Colon. The entire digestive system works to receive food and drink, rotten and ripen it, provide nourishment and fluids to the body, and ultimately produce "compost," or waste.

Adult bodies average between 45 and 65 percent water, with men's more muscular bodies holding the higher number, and women's higher percentage of fat resulting in the lower percentage.[4] Fluids play a role in virtually every body function. They are contained throughout our flesh, in the layers between our connective tissue, in our vessels, and in and around every cell.

Experiences that create a global response in our physiology, like exposure to toxic substances or high-voltage electricity, can dramatically impact this essential fluid matrix. The ubiquitous nature of fluids results in a global, whole-body experience of hyperarousal when we are exposed to such pervasive life threats. Neither a fight nor a flight response can successfully respond to toxic poisons or electrical shocks, and so our system, after attempting to mount such a response, may then descend into collapse. Our global fluid matrix may then express a sense of high sympathetic activation, or perhaps even the complex dynamic of high sympathetic arousal together with parasympathetic collapse. This massive dysregulation in our fluids impacts every cell, tissue, and body function that relies on fluids—essentially everything.

This global sense of an immediate threat everywhere inside our body can produce reactivity to anything that feels threatening from outside our body. This consuming sense of threat on the inside can be so strong that environmental invaders—things we can't even see, like strong smells or allergens—can trigger hypersensitivity reactions and system-wide arousal. Survivors experiencing this type of disruption often can't tolerate the detergent aisle in the grocery store, perfume on a stranger in the elevator, or the smell of new carpet, a new car, or fresh paint. They may be allergic to certain foods or preservatives, as well as things like dust, molds, grasses, and animal fur.

As you've seen in the previous four chapters, each Element stores an aspect of spirit. The Spleen stores the *yi,* translated as "thought." The *yi* influences our capacity for thinking, studying, concentration, and memorization. It helps us think through our life experiences. If the *yi* is injured, we will not be able to assimilate or learn the lessons from life's traumas; undigested, they will come around and around, again and again. We will make the same or similar mistakes over and over. We are at risk of forever feeling like a victim.

The Earth Element is most often depicted between summer's Fire and autumn's Metal circles in Five Element depictions of the seasonal cycle. In terms of the 5-SPR, this image of the Five Elements describes the Earth's role in helping us harvest the lessons for life that also hang heavy in every traumatic experience. The Earth helps us to digest the gristle in the stew of life, harvest the nourishment in that stew, and put that nourishment into long-term storage to help us manage future challenges.

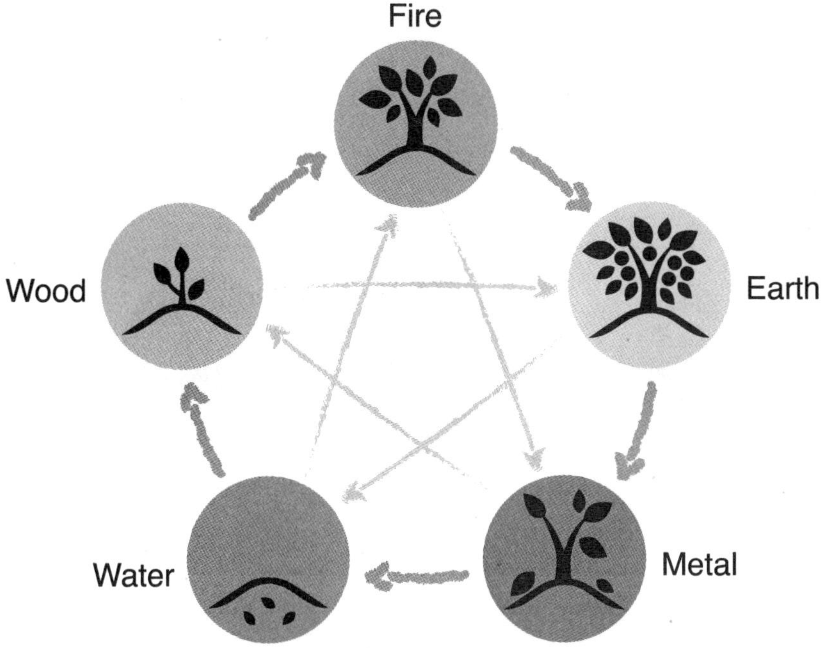

FIGURE 10.1. Five Element Cycle

The Earth is also sometimes depicted as a circle in the center of the four other circles in Five Element charts. This image speaks to the Earth's special place at the center of our existence. The history of China is replete with famines and starvation. AAM places central importance on nutrition, digestion, and nourishment as the foundation for life. Life is impossible without the Earth Element's function to receive food, transform it into *qi* and blood, and transport it to every organ, tissue, and function of the body.[5] Its importance cannot be overemphasized. It is central to the creation of the *qi*/energy and blood that gives us flesh and fuel to carry out every body function.

This depiction of the Five Element cycle metaphorically expresses the Earth's dynamic relationship with every other element.

- **Metal.** Earth creates Metal. The Earth helps us integrate life lessons. We have gained new strengths, skills, and resiliency and an expanded sense of self-confidence at the conclusion of the 5-SPR. This open, curious, and nonreactive state that we now embody is the foundation for initiating a new cycle of self-protection when we need it.

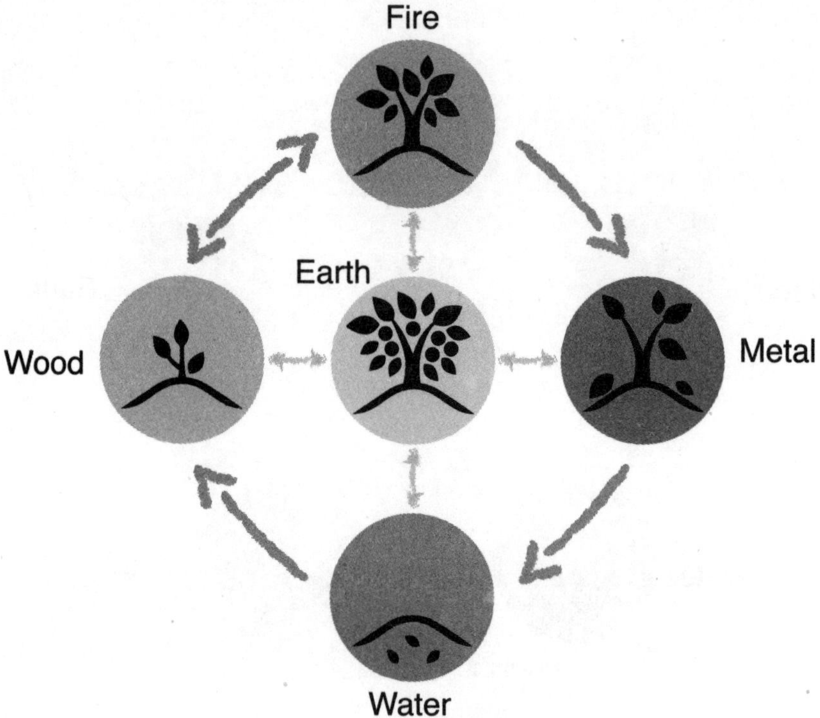

FIGURE 10.2. Five Element Cycle, Earth in Center

- **Water.** Like the banks of a stream, the Earth provides a container for the Water's fear via the control cycle. A steady, grounded, and centered Earth helps us recognize safety and contain unnecessary fear.
- **Wood.** In the context of mobilizing a response to life threat, the Wood reaches across the control cycle to shut down digestion in the Earth so that all our vital energy can be focused on mobilization in our musculoskeletal system to help ensure our immediate survival. This shutdown is a massive burden for the Earth to carry for the sake of our body's protection.
- **Fire.** The Earth plays a key role in the production of blood, which gives the spirit of the Heart a place to rest. The Heart also uses blood to transmit messages of both arousal and equanimity to the body.

Supporting the function of the Earth Element is central to the healthy functioning of every organ system and to each step in the self-protective response.

CONTEXT: THE ROLE OF THE EARTH ELEMENT IN THE SELF-PROTECTIVE RESPONSE

In response to a new stimulus in our environment—such as that twig snapping—our inner squirrel comes to rapt attention. Sensate arousal in our Metal Element wakes up our Kidneys and their close companions, the adrenal glands, to investigate the potential threat. Fear in our Kidney/adrenal system creates the impulse for us to reach across the control cycle to our Heart Protector and seek help from our tribe. But if our Heart Protector is unable to manage this threat, our Heart will be penetrated by this overwhelming experience of fear. Our Heart then sends a desperate command via the pulse to every organ system and function to respond to this message of life threat.

Part of carrying out the now necessary actions of fight or flight includes a message delivered across the control cycle from our Wood to our Earth to shut down peristalsis in our guts. The body is commanded to temporarily shut down digestion so all of our *qi*/energy can be directed to our muscles and joints to mobilize a response to this immediate threat. Like many animals experiencing a threat, we may also dump the contents of our Colon to lighten our weight and enhance our physical performance.

If we are successful in our response to this threat, our Heart will signal our return to regulation with a coherent, regular heartbeat. Peristalsis will return to our gut. We become able to digest and assimilate our food again. We are similarly able to digest this experience and learn important lessons for our future. *Don't touch a hot stove* and *Look both ways before crossing the street* are such early lessons, designed to help keep us safe.

If we are thwarted in our response to threat, this shutdown of our digestion, which AAM names the "Liver invading the Spleen," will remain in our viscera.[6] As described earlier, Western science names this phenomenon the freeze, or immobility, response. It is mediated by the parasympathetic nervous system's dorsal vagus nerve, which moves into high tone to accomplish this shutdown. In a last ditch attempt to stop overwhelming arousal and protect the Heart, our body-mind engages a massive emergency brake. This shutdown includes the functions below the diaphragm—in particular, the organs of digestion.

A freeze in the viscera has a profound impact on the enteric, or belly, brain. This brain specializes in letting us know what is safe, life sustaining, or threatening—even if we can't explain exactly why. It communicates using sensations rather than cognition to tell us who is creepy and who may become a helpful mentor or good friend—as well as just what is delightful about a ripe peach. We are referring to this belly brain when we say, "I knew it in my gut." When we lapse into a freeze state, the resulting numbing and inhibiting effect removes our awareness from the important information our gut can provide about safety, threat, comfort, self-connection, and how we feel in relation to others.

COMMON SYMPTOMS FOR THE EARTH TYPE: THE SPLEEN AND STOMACH

The impact of long-standing freeze in our viscera gives rise to diverse symptoms and often has a profound impact on our morbidity and mortality in the long term. It can manifest with digestive disturbances like irritable bowel syndrome or problems metabolizing certain nutrients. The Spleen's inability to transform food into blood and *qi* can result in an accumulation of excess weight around the middle of our body. These survivors may develop a characteristic apple-shaped body, which is associated with a greater risk for heart disease as well as the development of metabolic syndrome, in which hypertension, high cholesterol, obesity, and high blood sugar converge. It is often associated with a long-term visceral freeze.

This freeze in our viscera can cause changes in the composition of the bacteria in our gut and the integrity of our gut lining. Our gut microbiome helps metabolize food and medicine. It also produces neurotransmitters, such as serotonin and dopamine, which impact mood and mental health. It has a strong influence on the regulation of our immune system.

Often referred to as our "second brain," the visceral or enteric brain contains more neurotransmitters than the brain between our ears. More than 90 percent of our serotonin is produced in and distributed by our enteric brain, as well as 50 percent of our dopamine.[7] Five hundred million neurons—five times as many as there are in our spinal cord and brain—are embedded in our gut lining.[8]

The inflammation caused by a loss of integrity in the gut lining, often called a "leaky gut," has been shown to play a role in depression,[9] anxiety,[10] autism spectrum disorders, and schizophrenia. An increased level of inflammation in the gut and altered immune regulation has also been linked to individuals diagnosed with PTSD.[11] Access to the low-tone dorsal state, which is dominant during sleep, rest, and relaxation, supports barrier maintenance in the gut, as well as healthy immune response, particularly the calming of inflammation.[12]

The gut plays a significant role in our somatic interoception. It gives us the capacity to perceive our internal state and to use these perceptions to inform our choices. These gut messages are largely afferent—80 percent of the ANS nerves in our enteric brain send information to our central nervous system.

The disruptions in gut-brain signaling caused by a visceral freeze state can give rise to unreliable interoceptive messaging. In plain terms—we may not always be able to discern what is safe and what is not safe. Disruptions can also lead to abnormal brain function and changes in behavior, thoughts, emotions, and perceptions of pain. We may feel a gnawing inner discomfort and a lack of safety in our body. We may develop a survival strategy of ignoring warnings that show up in our visceral system, though this is not an effective long-term strategy. If we are uncomfortable attending a family reunion, for example, we may feel better in the immediate moment if we, and our guts, don't remember that a family member was once a perpetrator of a terrible crime.

The more we learn to ignore gut clues, the more bewilderment, confusion, and shame we are likely to experience. We become unable to discern what is dangerous or harmful from what is safe or nourishing, and we therefore lose trust in our ability to navigate the world safely. We struggle to identify what physical sensations mean and find it challenging to locate the words that describe our feelings. We may easily misinterpret our sensations, resulting in shutdown or panic. We become unable to trust our body and what it can tell us about the situations arising in our environment. This inability to identify our body's signals for hunger, fatigue, or safe companions contracts our life and can leave us filled with shame.[13]

In order to cope with these unwelcome feelings, we may turn to external regulation through drugs, alcohol, or medications. We may require constant reassurance or become overly submissive to authority figures. Compulsively complying with the orders or behavior of someone we perceive as more powerful than us leaves us highly vulnerable to *moral injury,* which is commonly defined as "**damage done to one's conscience or moral compass** when that person perpetrates, witnesses, or fails to prevent acts that transgress their own moral and ethical values or codes of conduct."[14] We may not even have the awareness that their behavior or actions are abuses of power until, in the dark of night, we reflect and realize that we have betrayed our values in not reporting or stopping their abusive actions. The concept of moral injury is gaining traction in the consideration of the wide-ranging impact of military service in a time of war.

Infants are particularly vulnerable to the impact of traumatic stress on this gut-brain dynamic, largely because their ventral vagus nerve is developmentally unable to help them mitigate even low-level stress. Infants rely on the ventral vagal capacity of their caregivers to soothe and comfort them and to help them manage the impact of stressful experiences. If an "external" ventral vagus nerve (via the presence of a loving caregiver) is unavailable, an infant will be left with no means of managing his arousal. His physiology will be forced into a freeze state in order to protect his Heart. If an infant continually and repeatedly lacks access to soothing, he is more likely to fall into the physiological strategy of freeze with little provocation. After prolonged or repeated exposure to such experiences, these infants and young children are at high risk of becoming habituated to a visceral freeze response—one that can extend into their adulthood.

Our capacity to perceive safety—or an embodied sense of knowing we are safe—is cultivated in childhood. Our guts learn to digest food and experiences in the context of safety in relationship. Safety and co-regulation support the development of low-tone dorsal vagus functions like sleep, peristalsis in the digestive system, assimilation of nutrients, and immune-system support.

We posit that the profound impact of developmental trauma on the enteric nervous system is a critical element in the alarming rates of adult morbidity and mortality reflected in the adverse childhood experiences (ACE) research (also explored in Chapters One, Seven, and Nine). Developmental trauma has been traced to virtually every public health concern of modern society: obesity; cardiac, pulmonary, and immune function; cigarette smoking; and drug and alcohol addiction, as well as more obvious conditions, like depression, anxiety, suicidality, and major mental illness. The ACE research demonstrates the impact of early trauma on the body as well as the mind.

The Spleen's primary function—transforming food into *qi* and blood and transporting it to every dimension of our body—is profoundly impacted by visceral freeze. Such a freeze can leave us feeling profoundly fatigued and weak and can cause us to develop blood disorders or become anemic. Disruption in the Spleen can also cause muscle wasting; we can gauge its health through the tone and vitality in the muscles.

While the physiology of our fluid system is shaped by multiple body systems, we have included the impact of poisoning and high-voltage electricity on the fluid system here in the Earth chapter because of the Earth's central role in the movement and production of fluids: The Spleen's job of transporting blood and *qi* includes the transportation of fluids, and the Stomach/gut's role to provide fluids to the flesh is central to the metabolism of fluids in AAM.

Now, we will describe healing approaches for survivors whose experience was disrupted in the Earth stage of the 5-SPR. These methods can help: restore peristalsis in the guts and interoceptive function in the visceral brain; transform messages of failed self-protection stored in our muscles; and bring stability to dysregulation in the fluids of survivors impacted by poisoning or high-voltage electricity.

REMEDIES FOR RESTORING REGULATION IN THE EARTH

Restoring function in the Spleen and Stomach supports their effort to produce *qi* and blood, thereby impacting the functioning in every body system. This restoration also helps survivors to make the best use of their experiences, helping them navigate stressful circumstances effectively in the future.

The dynamics of brace and collapse will be important for Earth survivor types and will leave a particular imprint on this Element's associated tissues—the viscera or guts, the muscles or flesh, and the fluid system.

Restoring Peristalsis in the Guts

We require a great deal of information from our gut in order to make assessments of our circumstances that can inform good judgment, reflect our needs, and steer our lives in a healthy direction. We put our survival at risk if we aren't receiving our gut's life-giving clues. We may not know when we are hungry, when we are safe, and when we need to get in out of the cold or rain. Our guts inform us about our internal state. They tell us how we are, what we need, and how we feel about our internal and external circumstances. Restoring their capacity to provide this critical information can be lifesaving for trauma survivors.

As we've seen with other survivor types, problems can arise with high tone in either the sympathetic nervous system or in the dorsal vagus nerve. Survivors with high tone in the SNS will tend to have a lean and sinewy body type. Their guts are likely to be constricted, tight, and clamped down. This leaves them challenged to make good use of the wisdom that comes from body awareness. They may not be able to pick up interoceptive insights or make sense of these insights for the rest of their body's benefit. These survivor types may not register sensations of hunger, recognize helpful companions, or know they need a hat when it's cold outside.

Survivors with high dorsal vagal tone may experience a collapse or shutdown in multiple body systems—their muscles will be more flaccid, their heart rate, blood pressure, breathing, and gut function will all be suppressed. This type of survivor will tend to have a soft and flabby body type. Their viscera lack the tone necessary to function well—or to carry messages of sensate awareness, and so their interoception is compromised. The long-term risks of such high tone in the dorsal vagus can leave these survivors even more compromised in their ability to assimilate nourishment than those with high tone in their SNS. They can be severely malnourished, in spite of the excess weight they often carry, because they often lack the capacity to assimilate essential nutritional elements. For both types, the capacity to digest food and life experiences, to learn lessons and memorize facts, and to receive interoceptive information about safety will be compromised.

Our primary goal when working with the gut is to help our client restore regulated tone in her viscera. We want to support her guts to transform food and fluids into *qi* and blood, produce neurotransmitters and support healthy immune regulation. Fundamentally, we want to support her gut's capacity to communicate interoceptive messages of safety to help her better navigate stressful situations. We are helping recalibrate her system so it can again discern what her guts have to say and can come to trust that information.

It is important for providers to model congruence between their inner state and their outer expression of affect. If, for example, your client detects that you don't feel well, and you deny that you have a mild headache, you have inadvertently compromised her increasing capacity to rely on her interoceptive awareness to inform her understanding of another person's state. Demonstrating the congruence between inner and outer states is critically important to help survivors retune their enteric brain. The bottom line: don't lie. It is much better for her if you acknowledge your headache, state your willingness to reschedule if she would prefer, and affirm that you think you are still able to offer her a good and helpful session (if that's true)—rather than deny her experience.

As always, if you are unfamiliar with the use of touch, refer to the general guidance in Chapter Five. You will be touching your client on her abdomen, which for many people feels quite vulnerable, intimate, and personal. Even though she will be fully clothed, she may feel more comfortable with a sheet over her. It is important to check in with her in advance to be sure she is comfortable with this contact. You should also have a pillow or cushion handy to support your arm so you are not resting the weight of your arm on her abdomen.

If your client has consented to your touching this part of her body, gently place your hand on her abdomen. You may choose a location over a particular organ that's playing a key role in her visceral freeze—perhaps her Stomach, Small Intestine, or Colon. If you don't know where each of these organs is located specifically, use an anatomy book to orient yourself. Absolute precision is not required in order for treatment to be effective.

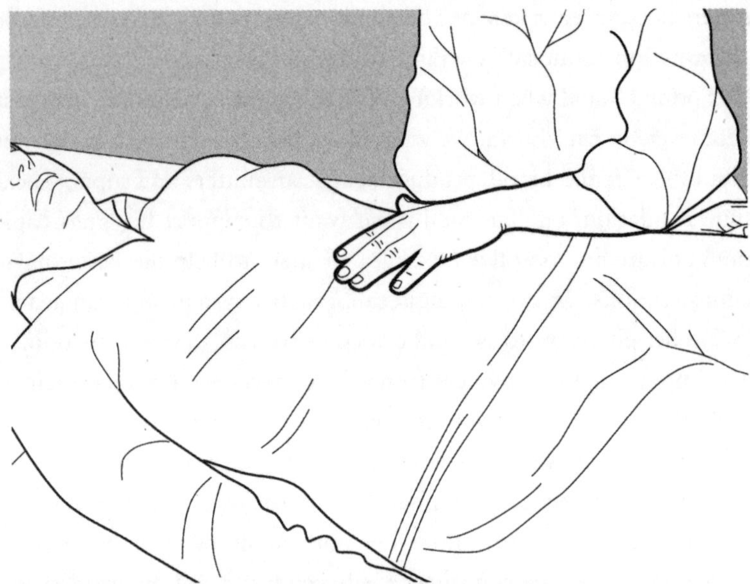

FIGURE 10.3. Touching the Viscera

If you think of the Earth Element as the primary driver of disruption for your client, choose the Stomach or Spleen as a starting place. If you think there are important dynamics between the Earth and Fire Elements, you may choose to work over the Small Intestine, a Fire organ system. If you think there are important dynamics between the Earth and her Metal Element, you may choose to work over the Colon. Similarly for her Earth and Wood Elements, leading you to work over her Gall Bladder or Liver.

The principle of titration leads us to recommend beginning in the middle of her abdomen or an area slightly higher, as the pelvis can hold complex patterns of activation related to sexual trauma and expression, as well as visceral freeze. Extreme arousal related to sexual trauma risks stimulating an even greater freeze response.

Begin slowly, simply allowing your client to notice her experience of your hand. You may want to gently "rock" her belly to bring slight movement into her viscera. Help her to tick-tock between states of arousal and comfort.

Signs of restoration of PNS function include the return of peristalsis in the guts with the gurgle of borborygmus, the rumbling of intestinal gas.

This signals the beginning of a perception of safety in the gut and should always be welcomed. We don't digest our food unless we feel safe enough to do so, which is why this is a deeply somatic indicator of a restored sense of safety. Telling your client that flatulence or belching is expected and welcomed may help her transcend cultural norms that would otherwise cause her to brace against these movements. We don't want even the slightest bracing to inhibit a return to movement in her guts.

As you perceive movement in her viscera, use your inquiry to help build her somatic interoception with questions like, "As you hear your belly gurgle, I wonder—what are you noticing in the rest of you?" or, "From the outside, I'm feeling your belly soften under my hand. What you are noticing on the inside?" You can use her experience of greater regulation in one or two dimensions of her experience to inform and facilitate system-wide regulation with questions such as, "As you hear your belly gurgle, and as your back rests more fully on the table, what do you notice in your whole body?"

Touch in the abdominal area can also give rise to nausea or even vomiting. While vomiting is rare, it is wise to have a sturdy trashcan available so you can easily reassure your client that a strong visceral response is okay and that you are prepared for it. Although vomiting is usually uncomfortable, in this context, it can be a good sign. It may indicate an attempt at reorganization within the vagus system. The Stomach *qi* is going in the wrong direction, but it is at least beginning to move, which is exactly what we want to see happen. If your client has previously experienced food toxicity or poisoning, vomiting is actually a functional, reparative response. Our body protects us in circumstances like these by expelling the contents of our Stomach.

Client Example

Sally was born septic, and she has always felt a sense of life threat from within. It is possible that her early experience of high fever initiated this imprint. She also experienced significant abuse and neglect during her childhood, as well as a long string of violent and alcoholic partners. She struggles to manage her life and is often easily preyed upon by internet schemes that promise "get rich quick" outcomes but leave her feeling, yet again, like a victim.

As an adult, she exhibits the characteristic "around the middle" obesity that survivors of developmental visceral freeze often demonstrate, as well as chronic aches and pains made worse by damp weather. Sally's Spleen doesn't manage her blood sugar well, and she has experienced chronic constipation for most of her life. She has relied on opioids to manage her pain for more than ten years, which has exacerbated her constipation.

We began Sally's treatment with the Kidney/adrenal hold to help restore her overall regulation. Sally had clamped down her guts in infancy as the only way to experience an illusion of safety. Her system required basic stability before we could invite her viscera to move. Movement in her viscera would otherwise risk a return to that primal experience of overwhelming life threat, compounding her visceral freeze. We needed to establish an embodied experience of safety to use as an anchor for any arousal that emerged alongside movement in her viscera. We would often return to the Kidney/adrenal system as a way of tick-tocking between arousal and regulation as sessions began to focus more directly on her viscera.

At first, Sally's viscera felt hard and immovable. She was barely aware of my hand on her body. I began to gently and almost imperceptibly rock her Stomach with my hand to invite movement. Over time, her Stomach began to gurgle. She became aware of the movement in her Stomach, and was able to notice that her body felt heavier and more connected to the table. Over time, she was able to associate the softening in her belly with feeling more settled and less agitated in her mind as well.

Over the course of several months, she began to report that her body felt less dense. She was able to walk increasingly greater distances, which started to shift her muscle-to-fat ratio and helped her manage her pain. She incrementally reduced her use of narcotics and within a year was completely off all narcotic medication.

These changes did not remake her apple-shaped body, and Sally's blood sugar continued to fluctuate, but she was now free of narcotics and proud of herself for finding new ways to manage the pain she experienced.

Supporting Completion Responses Stored in the Muscles/Flesh

Survivors use different tissues to help them manage, contain, or control an overwhelming experience. The tissue they "choose" depends on the nature of their trauma, their constitutional type, and the management strategy they utilized.

The muscles, or flesh, are the tissues associated with the Earth Element. Our muscles carry body memories of our inner experiences. They hold the record of our history of failed self-protection. What we believe and how we feel about failures of self-protection will be found in our muscles.

When we are upright, our muscle system is engaged in struggle against gravity. If this were not the case, we would simply fall down, as happens when we faint. So we expect a certain level of tension within the muscle system, even when someone is seated. What we are looking for in assessing the muscle system for unresolved self-protective impulses is a sense that the anti-gravity effort is out of place—it's either more than what is required under the current circumstances, or the muscle system is not sufficiently engaged to hold the body fully upright.

While it would be an oversimplification to divide our muscle system into only two categories—postural and movement-oriented muscles—this division can help us understand how our clients retain unresolved patterns of self-protection.

Our mobilizing muscles are typically large and oriented around movement. They are attached to our long bones and have a thick belly in their middle, with thin ends. Mobilizing muscles assist with repetitive movement for a specific amount of time and will fatigue if used for extended periods. They enable us to reach, push, grab, and move ourselves through space. They directly support our self-protective impulse and so will often more clearly indicate experiences of thwarted self-protection than will our postural muscles.

In contrast, our postural muscles are primarily small, flat, and situated close to our bones—such as the paravertebral muscles found all along the spine. Postural muscles provide low-grade sustained contraction. Their role in the mobilization response is to help hold us stable and upright. They typically won't fatigue over time, unless they are called on to sustain weight or movement, as if they were movement-oriented muscles. For example, carrying a heavy load on our back for an extended period of time will exceed the functional capacity of the small postural muscles found along the spine—and will give rise to back pain.

There are other categories of muscles that may be important to account for in trauma responses, including internal muscles, such as the heart and those in the walls of the digestive tract. These internal muscles can also contain and express hyperarousal and hypoarousal responses. We have already demonstrated the importance of reengaging tone in the digestive system, which includes the muscles contained there. The Heart, in AAM, resides in its chamber and should not be touched directly. The Pericardium and the mediastinum serve as its protectors. We help restore regulation to the Heart through its relationship with other organs—notably the other organ systems of the Fire Element and the critical dynamics in the Kidney/Heart axis.

Our muscle system, particularly our mobilizing muscles, tends to be loud and distracting in terms of our interoceptive awareness. Muscles contain and convey strong sensations we are meant to feel—their tension or relaxation, their pain when we strain them, and their experience of weight and movement are meant to inform how we use them. They can be braced and uncomfortable, or they can be weak, collapsed, and lacking in tone. Because they easily capture our attention with their clear and available sensations, they can cloud the more subtle information from other systems that may also need help.

As practitioners, we must be aware that some of our clients will report only the muscle-oriented information that is readily available to them: "I have pain in my back and tension in my neck, and I feel stiff all over." While we should attend to this information appropriately, we should also remember that there are quieter and less easily accessible interoceptive indicators within other systems that can also inform our choice of interventions. As noted previously, we want to support our clients in developing their capacity to notice all aspects of their internal experience, not just the most vocal systems.

We are meant to feel our muscles. They carry important information about our history of self-protection and the direction and strength of the effort necessary to perform the task at hand. Their loud voice can also mean their information can override other aspects of awareness. We are not meant to directly feel more subtle body information, such as digestion or heartbeat, and so we are easily distracted by the louder signals of the muscles. We may miss the more subtle information from these more diffuse sensations of interoception, which may be more important in restoring the self-protective response than are the muscles, so we need to stay attentive to the quieter signals as well.

The nature of interoception is that it tends not to be specific; it is often described by clients as "a sense of something," while the muscle information can be very specific and therefore more noticeable. We can support better interoception in our clients by helping them bring attention to these quieter forms of self-communication. A helpful practice to use with clients is the comparing of notes about what you are both noticing: "From the outside, I'm noticing this. What are you noticing from the inside?" That guides the client's attention in an invitational way toward other parts of their interoceptive experience, which they may have had little access to previously.

As providers, we need to develop our own interoceptive and observational skills in order to help guide our client's awareness: "From the outside, I just noticed a little gurgle in your stomach as your muscles relaxed. What did you notice on the inside?" It simply takes practice—and then more practice—to become well versed and seamless in using this somatic vocabulary. If this is unfamiliar to you, you can trust that over time your hesitancy will transform, and you will develop the skills to support your clients to similarly use this somatic vocabulary and attention to help ensure that "louder" systems, like the muscles, aren't always commanding your attention.

When working with the muscles, we want to support our clients in their transition from a braced or locked posture to a more regulated state—or if survivors are primarily more collapsed, we want to support them in restoring their tone and capacity to be upright in an effortless way. This can manifest in different ways. Some people will move from brace into collapse and then rebound into a more balanced tone. Others may move from collapse to tension and then toward balance.

Some people will be more tolerant (and others less tolerant) of letting go in order to transition out of a braced state. A survivor who has coupled his sense of safety with holding his muscles tightly will have a relatively more rigid body system. He will be more prone to injury, and the transition out of brace will be more challenging for him. Help this type of survivor cultivate body awareness in an area where he feels more resilient and malleable. He may find it easier to cultivate flexibility in certain locations, which can then inform other regions of his body that feel more rigid. Help him notice and harvest how experiences of greater muscle flexibility mirror expanded flexibility in his interpersonal relationships—all as a result of cultivating regulated tone in his muscle system.

While each mobilizing muscle has the potential to carry experiences of thwarted defense, we will use as an example the psoas muscle—the only muscle that connects our spine to our legs. This muscle supports both a twist in our torso when our legs are anchored, and will support flexion and external rotation of our legs when our torso is stable and not moving. The psoas is the primary muscle engaged in the opposing impulses of standing our ground and fighting or twisting away and fleeing. Thus, it tends to hold the history of any dilemmas we've faced about our choice to fight or to flee. If we have been indecisive in a moment of mobilization, the psoas will be vulnerable to spasm. This may contribute to the common experience of lower back pain reported by many trauma survivors.

While the psoas is best known for its powerful role in our core's stability, flexibility, and balance, it is also an intelligent structure that communicates our life experiences of safety and threat and embodies our impulse for survival. Traumatic stress can leave the psoas shortened, dry, tight, and exhausted, resulting in lower back or groin pain, sciatica and hip tension, as well as poor bladder function, menstrual pain, or digestive upset.[15]

The location of its origin, at the twelfth thoracic vertebra, is particularly potent. The twelfth thoracic vertebra has anatomical features of both a thoracic and a lumbar vertebra. Its upper half is shaped like our thoracic vertebrae, which are designed to support the twisting of our torso—and our flight response. Its lower half is shaped like our lumbar vertebrae, which are designed to allow flexion and extension, to support stability, standing our ground, and our fight response. Thus, this vertebra carries the dilemma between fight and flight in its essential structure, as well as its function. The burden of carrying these opposing impulses is great—it is the vertebra most likely to be broken in the spine.

The twelfth thoracic vertebra is also the site in the body where the respiratory diaphragm attaches to the spine, and so it may contain experiences held in the diaphragm system, as described in Chapter Six. The Spleen lies between the ninth and twelfth ribs, and will bring its influence to this vertebra's region as well.

When working with a client's psoas, the client should lie on his back, fully clothed. A pillow or bolster under the knees will help relax the psoas, making it more available to your touch and better positioned to release any brace it may be holding. Refer to Chapter Five for general guidance on touch.

You may want to begin with your hand under the nearby Kidney/adrenal system to establish a sense of safety and regulation before moving to the psoas. Then, when you and your client are ready, slide your hand over to the origin of the psoas, where the lower end of the rib cage meets the spine at the twelfth thoracic vertebra in the middle of the back. Invite your client to simply notice your hand and any movement or stillness, images, or sensations that may emerge.

Your client may notice movement going down his legs, which may be an expression of a thwarted fight-or-flight response. Give him plenty of time to allow this response to complete—trauma is often experienced as "too much, too fast," and so the gift of time can be extraordinarily helpful for a survivor to organize his body's experience of completion.

Help your client tick-tock between any states of arousal that emerge and his experience of safety. If he becomes hyperaroused—anxious, afraid, or jumpy—you may direct his attention to his experience of the table as grounded and stable; or you may choose to move your hand back to the Kidney/adrenal system. Let your pace be slow. Allow time for states of greater regulation to settle in.

As the tension in his psoas is released, he may notice that his back is flatter on the table, his back pain has reduced, and his sense of anxiety is calmed. After he gets off the table, if he takes some time to walk slowly and mindfully, it may help him integrate the greater function in his psoas.

This example of working with the psoas muscle can be used with any mobilizing muscle carrying a thwarted response. Bring your hand and your attention to any mobilizing muscle—perhaps one carrying pain or lacking function—and observe any subtle or gross movements that emerge. Use the same principles of titration, tick-tock, and cultivation of somatic interoception.

Look for subtle movement within the muscle, enhanced range of motion, and more integrated functional expression in the musculoskeletal system. Help your client notice changes in the tone or flexibility of his emotional experience, as well as the meaning he carries about his trauma experience.

Client Example

> *Brian came to see me with chronic lower back pain, which he attributed to a long-ago back injury from lifting a heavy toolbox. As he settled onto the table, I noticed that his lower back was so arched it wasn't even touching the table. At the same time, he kept his arms somewhat flexed, with his hands floating above his abdomen, rather than resting there. Even when I placed a bolster under his knees and invited him to relax, this posture persisted.*
>
> *His body position gave the impression of someone accelerating forward, not someone relaxing while lying down. I gently asked about other injuries, accidents, or experiences in which he had felt threatened. After pausing for a long time, he slowly looked over at me, and said, "I haven't thought about this in such a long time. I'd forgotten it even happened."*
>
> *He then related an experience from college, when he was walking home drunk one night. He noticed two men on the other side of the street who seemed to be taking too much interest in him. It was late, and the street was deserted. He decided to turn around and go back to the house he'd just left, but as he started to turn, he noticed the men running across the street toward him. He was just drunk enough that he couldn't coordinate his movements sufficiently to defend himself, and the two men pummeled him until he was on the ground. They took his wallet and ran off. He managed to get back to his friends' house, and they took him to the emergency room. He remembered being both frightened and embarrassed by the experience, but he hadn't thought about it in years.*
>
> *I asked Brian if he would be okay with me putting my hands under his low back, and he agreed that would feel somehow reassuring. When I touched his low back, the entire area of the psoas attachments, and his entire lower back felt rigid and contracted. I gently*

invited him to bring his attention to his low back, and to feel my contact and support. As he did so, his legs began to tremble. He reported feeling a sense of confusion about what he should do. I invited him to simply notice what his body wanted to do, and slowly he became aware of a sense of wanting to move his legs. He did that slowly and gently, which decreased the trembling.

Together, we then noticed that his hands were clenched tightly into fists. As he brought his attention to that area of brace, he also noticed that the muscles in his arms were clenched. I continued to support his lower back but also encouraged him to slowly let his arms complete whatever movements they wanted to make. In slow motion, his arms came up to protect his head, his fists opened, and he used his hands to cover his face and the top of his head. At the same time, he rolled onto his side and curled into a ball on the table. I kept my hand on his lower back as he did this, helping him to move in a controlled and titrated way.

He lay in that position for about ten minutes, then slowly, slowly uncurled and returned to lying on his back. As he did so, we both noticed that his lower back had relaxed and was resting fully on the table. His arms came down by his sides and his hands rested comfortably on his abdomen.

We both felt he had finally been able to revisit the dilemma he had experienced during the assault: Should he run away? Try to fight off his attackers? Or simply submit and wait until the attack was over? He felt a deep sense of the "rightness" of not fighting back, of just letting the attackers have what they came for and protecting himself from injury by covering his head. After this one session, his back pain was reduced by about 50 percent.

Impact of Poisoning and Electrocution on the Fluid System

As stated earlier, our body composition is 45 to 65 percent water. Fluids play a crucial role in virtually every body function, forming a global system within our body. If we have been exposed to toxic substances, a drug overdose, or high-voltage electricity—or possibly even if we have had a strong allergic reaction—we may experience a state of elevated and global arousal. This global arousal may "transmit" through our global fluid system, in which every drop of body fluid carries the complex dynamic of either high-tone sympathetic arousal or high-tone parasympathetic collapse—or perhaps both together.

The nature of fluids—the fact that they are everywhere—means that when our fluids are carrying the imprint of this type of stress response, they propagate stress everywhere. This type of dysregulation may be found in people with hypersensitivity reactions. These survivors can't tolerate anything that may provoke a sense of toxicity, such as strong odors or exposure to cleaning products or chemicals. They may be highly allergic to a whole host of substances. The functional orbit of their lives is often highly contracted as a result.

You can most easily access the fluid system in soft, squishy areas. Using a touch location like the calf muscle or the back of the upper arm is often the easiest place to begin. The squishy areas of the abdomen also hold the complexity of underlying organs, and so we do not recommend you use the abdomen. You will likely want to start by establishing core regulation with the Kidney/adrenal work.

In most cases, you will work over your client's clothing. Before you begin, give yourself a few moments to quiet your mind and bring presence to your hand. Then place your hand gently on the fleshy, soft area at the back of the client's calf or upper arm. Take a few moments to arrive with your quiet and full attention. Once you have settled in with your contact, let your attention sink into his flesh. Begin "looking" with your hand for subtle movement, almost like a tidal rhythm.

If trauma has affected the fluids, it can be difficult to contain the high level of activation you will encounter, simply because the fluids inherently tend to propagate such a reaction. Providers will need to titrate their work carefully. You may make use of the Kidney/adrenal hold as a resource to return to if hyperarousal emerges. Go slow and remain steady.

Interestingly, if there is no trauma related to the fluids, accessing the fluid system can often be highly restorative, nourishing, and relaxing. Clients may find an experience akin to the tide moving through their body.

Client Example

Miguel suffered from a host of health issues, mostly related to sensitivities. His diet was severely restricted because many foods upset his digestion. He had trouble gaining weight, was sensitive to extreme temperatures, and spent a lot of time managing his exposure to things he felt would provoke reactions, such as scented products, especially laundry soaps, which gave him rashes. He also reported feeling something like a high-pitched vibration or buzzing in his body a lot of the time, especially when trying to sleep.

We worked first with Miguel's Kidney/adrenal system, which helped somewhat with the buzzing sensations and seemed to help him sleep a little better. In our third session, I suggested we do some fluid work, and Miguel agreed. My intention was to simply imagine the fluid system as something like kelp responding to the tides—and to join that rhythm as I found it, while contacting his calf muscle. However, as I put my hand on Miguel's calf—holding the kelp image in my mind—Miguel exploded into something resembling a seizure. I quickly took my hand away and spent a few minutes helping Miguel track his breathing and settle again. I was able to return to Kidney/adrenal contact with no further reactions. We decided to delay the work with fluids for another few sessions and take the time to develop a more settled state in Miguel's system.

The second time we worked with fluids, we agreed that I wouldn't use touch at the beginning, that Miguel would simply imagine a fluid breath moving in his legs. He again felt a strong sense of contraction and energy running through his whole body. We took a break and then conducted the exercise again, this time with me touching his arm as he again imagined a fluid breath moving through him. As we again felt the surge of energy in his system, Miguel remembered an accident he experienced when he was working on a construction site—he had nearly died from being electrocuted when a piece of machinery malfunctioned. He realized that what he was feeling was a mild version of that electrocution experience, when the electricity was running through his system, causing his muscles to spasm. A coworker who had managed to unplug the equipment saved his life.

We spent the next few months not only working with Miguel's fluids but also trying to complete the self-protective responses in his muscles and harvest his gratitude for the coworker who saved his life. During the months we worked together, Miguel noticed that the buzzing reduced to almost nothing. He still experienced sensitivity, but he was more able to manage his anxiety in relation to these experiences.

THE SOCIAL IMPLICATIONS FOR RESTORING REGULATION IN THE EARTH ELEMENT

As reflected in the CDC's adverse childhood experiences research, adult survivors of developmental trauma fill our social welfare system, flood our public health clinics, and are disproportionately represented in our criminal justice system.[16] While there is a paucity of research on the specific and long-term impact of the freeze response on the viscera early in life, one possible explanation comes from AAM.

The Earth Element can be shut down even with low-level sympathetic arousal in infancy, when the mitigating influence of the ventral vagus nerve is less available. The Earth plays a central role in the creation of *qi* and blood—and in supporting the function of all other Elements. A disruption early in life in this critically nourishing and supportive center will play a role in disruption everywhere.

The cost of developmental trauma is surely found in survivors' diminished quality of life, but it also has a profound impact on our community life. The financial costs in our social safety net are staggering. Developmental trauma robs children of academic success in school, steals opportunities for healthy relationships in adulthood, is a foundation for criminal behavior and addiction, and profoundly affects the health and welfare of individuals, families, and communities. Our growing understanding of the impact of developmental trauma on adult morbidity and mortality has given rise to valuable programs that teach parenting skills, address early trauma, and transform early childhood education.[17]

In the Earth Element, the Spleen's job to harvest the nourishment in our food and in our life experiences is central to the meaning we take away from traumatic experiences. What do we assimilate from our experience of a purse snatching? What lessons are harvested? Did we learn never to go to that part of town? To never carry a purse? Not to go out at night? That we are old and vulnerable and unsafe even in our own neighborhood? That we shouldn't trust people of the same gender or ethnicity as the person who stole our purse? Such questions and suspicions contract our life and our world.

There are other lessons in such experiences that are also available to be harvested—lessons that instead expand our world and create a better place for all of us to cohabitate. Providers can help survivors restore their sense of safety, digest their experiences, and transform these experiences of contraction.

Different conclusions can emerge from a traumatic experience: Our community would benefit from inter-generational activities. Young people need jobs. Young people need mentors. Who is this young person? What's his experience like at school or at home? What's happening in his life that lets him think that it's okay to snatch my purse? Can he be saved from committing other criminal acts, which are so destructive to him and to our community? What can I do to prevent such things from happening again—to me or to others?

With proper treatment and attention, expansion can replace contraction. Instead of growing suspicion and mistrust, we grow service, sincere understanding, compassion, and the fabric of community. Our world becomes a better, more supportive place.

CONCLUSION

We have successfully explored and completed each step of the self-protective response. We have integrated our experience of balance and regulation along the way. We harvested insights about how to respond to similar experiences in the future. We appreciate the skills we have learned and the person we have become. We never thought we could be grateful for the traumatic experience we endured, but we are a bigger person now because of it.

We can enjoy the sweetness of life. Our Heart returns to its regulated state. It signals our successful completion via the blood to every crevice of our body, mind, emotions, and spirit. The easy rise and fall between sympathetic arousal and parasympathetic restoration is restored. Peristalsis returns to our digestive organs. All of our sense organs are relaxed, curious, and available—but they are not activated.

The self-protective response flows into the Metal Element, where it began. Our felt sense, or animal soul, is again available to us. We feel safe enough to explore broadly without focusing our energies on scanning the environment for perceived threat. We have returned to a state of curiosity and capacity for connection that allows interaction with others and our environment. We are living in the open, sensate curiosity of the Metal. From this state, if circumstances require it, we can awaken our arousal response and initiate a new cycle of self-protection.

APPENDIX 1

Chart of Correspondences of the Five Elements

Element	*Metal*	*Water*	*Wood*	*Fire*	*Earth*
Season	*Autumn*	*Winter*	*Spring*	*Summer*	*Late Summer*
Organ Systems	*Lung* *Colon*	*Kidney, Bladder*	*Liver and Gall Bladder*	*Heart, Small Intestine;* *Heart Protector, Triple Heater*	*Spleen* *Stomach*
Emotion	*Inspiration/ Grief*	*Wisdom/* *Fear*	*Hope/* *Anger*	*Joy/* *Panic*	*Sympathy/* *Indifference*
Role in Successful Self-Protective Response	*Restores curiosity. Awakens arousal.* *Foundation for interoceptive awareness.*	*Signaling center; Power to fuel the mobilization response*	*Mobilizing a Response. Orient to threat. Strategize, implement plan for fight or flight.*	*Restore Coherence*	*Digests the gristle. Harvests the lessons*
Unsuccessful or Incomplete Self-Protective Response	*Hyperarousal: Anxious, jumpy, rapid breathing* *Hypoarousal: shallow breathing, empty or "hollow" presentation, fatigued*	*Hyperarousal: Panic, agitation, hypervigilance* *Hypoarousal: collapse, phobias*	*Hyperarousal: rigid impulses, thoughts, emotions and tissues; constantly mobilizing for threat with chronic and unreasonable anger and volatility, tight, painful tissues.* *Hypoarousal: flaccid or passive impulses, thoughts, emotions, and tissues; little initiative to respond to threats; a sense of not taking up space.*	*Hyperarousal – panic attacks, mania, "dark" humor, insomnia, racing thoughts.* *Hypoarousal - Dissociation, flat eyes and emotions, hard to connect, poor memory and focus.*	*Hyperarousal – high tone in the digestive system and muscles – wiry, tight body. Dry, hard stools. Hard to receive support or nurturance.* *Hypoarousal – low tone in the digestive system and muscles - soft, flabby body. Difficulty absorbing nutrients or transforming food into energy. Hard to harvest lessons or integrate experiences.*
Engenders	*Signal for threat*	*Power for mobilization*	*Cardiac coherence*	*Digestion and Harvesting*	*Sensate curiosity*

Controls	*Mobilization, orientation to threat*	*Cardiac coherence*	*Integration and digestion*	*Sensate Curiosity*	*Signal for Threat*
Tissue	*Skin and Body Hair*	*Bones, Brain, Spinal chord*	*Ligaments, tendons, sinews*	*Vessels*	*Flesh/Muscles*
Virtue	*Justice*	*Wisdom*	*Benevolence*	*Propriety*	*Selflessness*
Stores	*Qi/energy,* *Breath*	*Genetic potential or jing*	*Blood*	*Spirit of Mind*	*Nourishment*
Spirit	*Po, or Animal Soul*	*Willpower, or zhi*	*Etheric Soul, or the hun*	*Consciousness* *Presence*	*Purpose, Intent*
Archetypal Question	*Can I let go, allow breath to penetrate?* *Can I tolerate imperfection?*	*Do I have enough crops stored away? Do I have enough fuel? Can I survive this cold winter?*	*How do I navigate obstacles as I sprout and grow?* *Is there hope for my growing season?*	*How do I find the one great heart that beats in all hearts?* *Can I find love and joy with other beings?*	*How do I turn life's lessons into fruit?* *How do I digest the gristle and integrate it into my flesh?*
Exercises to Enhance Regulation	*Awakening interoception* *Creating embodied awareness of the skin as a protective container* *Restoring regulation in the diaphragm system after traumatic stress*	*Building a felt sense of safety* *Repairing boundary ruptures* *Building capacity in the Kidney/adrenal system* *Restoring regulation in the fear/terror centers in the brain stem* *Supporting bone flexibility and resilience*	*Restoring protective/ defensive responses in the secondary diaphragms* *Integrating motor and sensory function in the orientation system* *Restoring vitality in the blood*	*Restoring interoception in the gates of the Heart Protector* *Using co-regulation to restore auto-regulation* *Restoring the infrastructure for connection* *Restoring the spirit of the Heart*	*Restoring peristalsis in the viscera* *Supporting completion responses stored in the muscles/flesh* *Restoring regulation in body fluids*

APPENDIX 2

The Twelve Organ Systems or "Officials" in AAM

AAM views the organization of the body and its organs as a kingdom. Each organ system is described poetically as an official in charge of one of twelve different functions or departments critical to the smooth and coherent operation of this kingdom. They are described as follows:[1]

The **Heart** holds the office of lord and sovereign. The radiance of the spirit stems from it.

The **Lung** holds the office of minister and chancellor. The regulation of the life-giving network stems from it.

The **Liver** holds the office of general of the armed forces. Assessment of circumstances and conception of plans stem from it.

The **Gall Bladder** is responsible for what is just and exact. Determination and decision stem from it.

The **Pericardium** has the charge of resident as well as envoy. Elation and joy stem from it.

The **Spleen** and **Stomach** are responsible for the storehouses and granaries. The five tastes stem from them.

The **Colon,** or **Large Intestine,** is responsible for transit. The residue from transformation stems from it.

The **Small Intestine** is responsible for receiving and making things thrive. Transformed substances stem from it.

The **Kidneys** are responsible for the creation of power. Skill and ability stem from them.

The **Triple Burner** is responsible for opening up passages and irrigation. The regulation of fluids stems from it.

The **Bladder** is responsible for regions and cities. It stores the body fluids. The transformations of the *qi* then give out their power.

Each of these organ systems is paired with another in a *yin/yang* relationship. Together, each pair of organ systems belongs to an Element, and shares a set of resonant correspondences. The organ systems work together to both support and contain each other.

APPENDIX 3

Helpful Phrases To Enhance Interoception

- Where do you notice that in your body?
- From the outside, I'm noticing *this* (e.g., the muscles in your face softening, a rhythmic pulsing in your Kidney, your belly softening under my hands, your Liver expanding and becoming more juicy). I wonder—what are you noticing from the inside?
- As you notice *this* (e.g., the muscles in your back softening, your Kidney sinking, your deeper breath), what do you notice in the rest of you?
- As you took that deeper breath, I wondered: what you noticed in the rest of your body?
- That was a nice gurgle in your belly—and from the outside, your body appears softer. I wonder—what does that feel like on the inside?
- As you experience *this* and *this* (e.g., hear your belly gurgle, feel your back resting on the table, your belly soften, your Kidney sink, your muscle let go), what do you notice in your whole body?
- From the outside, it appears your jaw is getting tight. I wonder—if you brought your attention to wherever this chair feels the most comfortable or supportive, what would happen in your jaw?

- I'm noticing a faraway look in your eyes. I wonder—if you brought your attention back to this room and the color blue, how many things you would find that are blue?
- Can you find another place in your body that feels the same as this place we're contacting (or focusing) on?
- Can you find another place in your body that feels different than this place we're contacting (or focusing) on?
- If I bring my attention to your *this* (e.g., bone, skin, muscle), does that feel different than when I bring my attention to your *this* (e.g., bone, skin, muscle)? (Or this question can be about the client's own attention: "If you bring your attention to…")
- Is there anything about noticing your *this* (e.g., bone, skin, muscle) that feels the same as noticing your *this* (e.g., bone, skin, muscle)?
- If you take your attention to your *this* (e.g., bone, skin, muscle), then bring your attention to your *this* (e.g., bone, skin, muscle)—is there one you prefer to the other? Is there one whose sensations you like—or dislike?
- We are not at a formal event. I celebrate any movement in your guts as a sign of restoration of your system's vitality. I don't want you to brace against any movements in your guts. I welcome—even celebrate—your burps or farts.

NOTES

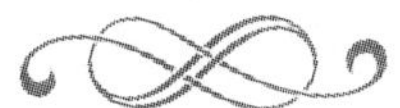

1 Margaret Reed MacDonald, *Three Minute Tales: Stories from around the World to Tell or Read When Time Is Short* (Little Rock, AR: August House, 2004), 145.

PREFACE

1 "How to Listen for a Leading," QuakerSpeak, http://quakerspeak.com/how-to-listen-for-a-leading.
2 Somatic Experiencing Trauma Institute, https://traumahealing.org.
3 Somatic Practice: Trainings with Kathy L. Kain, www.somaticpractice.net.

INTRODUCTION

1 Bessel van der Kolk, *The Body Keeps the Score: Brain, Mind, and Body in the Healing of Trauma* (New York: Viking. 2014), 47.
2 Van der Kolk, *Body Keeps the Score.*
3 Hippocrates, *On Ancient Medicine,* trans. Francis Adams (Whitefish, MT: Kessinger, 2010).
4 Peter Levine and Ann Frederick, *Waking the Tiger: Healing Trauma* (Berkeley, CA: North Atlantic Books, 1997).
5 Ted J. Kaptchuk, *The Web That Has No Weaver,* 2nd ed. (New York: McGraw-Hill, 2000), xix.

CHAPTER 1

1 Jonathan Shay, *Achilles in Vietnam: Combat Trauma and the Undoing of Character* (New York: Scribner, 1994); Jonathan Shay, *Odysseus in America: Combat Trauma and the Trials of Homecoming* (New York: Scribner, 2002). For a later example of a poet's interest in trauma, see Jessica Toomer, *This Veteran Is Using Shakespeare to Heal: Who Knew Shakespeare Could Help Veterans with PTSD?* www.guideposts.org/inspiration/people-helping-people/this-veteran-is-using-shakespeare-to-heal.

2 Cecilia Tasca, Mariangela Rapetti, Mauro Giovanni Carta, and Bianca Fadda. "Women and Hysteria in the History of Mental Health," *Clinical Practice and Epidemiology in Mental Health* 8, 110–19. http://doi.org/10.2174/1745017901208010110.

3 "History of PTSD in Veterans: Civil War to DSM-5," PTSD: National Center for PTSD, U.S. Department of Veterans Affairs, www.ptsd.va.gov/public/PTSD-overview/basics/history-of-ptsd-vets.asp.

4 "How Common Is PTSD?" PTSD: National Center for PTSD, U.S. Department of Veterans Affairs, www.ptsd.va.gov/public/PTSD-overview/basics/how-common-is-ptsd.asp.

5 "What Is Posttaumatic Stress Disorder?" American Psychiatric Association www.psychiatry.org/patients-families/ptsd/what-is-ptsd.

6 A. A. Stone "Post Traumatic Stress Disorder and the Law: Critical Review of the New Frontier," *Bulletin of the American Academy of Psychiatry and the Law* 21, no. 1 (1993).

7 Peter Levine, *In an Unspoken Voice: How the Body Releases Trauma and Restores Goodness* (Berkeley, CA: North Atlantic Books, 2010).

8 Stephen W. Porges, *The Polyvagal Theory: Neurophysiological Foundations of Emotions, Attachment, Communication, and Self-Regulation* (New York: W. W. Norton. 2011).

9 Levine and Frederick, *Waking the Tiger.*

10 Wayne B. Jonas, Joan A. G. Walter, Matt Fritts, Richard C. Niemtzow, "Acupuncture for the Trauma Spectrum Response: Scientific Foundations, Challenges to Implementation," *Medical Acupuncture* 23, no. 4 (2011): 249–62.

11 Rachel Karr-Morse and Meredith Wiley, *Scared Sick: The Role of Childhood Trauma in Adult Disease* (New York: Basic Books, 2012), 20–21.

12 Bruce S. McEwen, Jason D. Gray, and Carla Nasca, "*Recognizing Resilience: Learning from the Effects of Stress on the Brain*," *Neurobiology of Stress* 1 (2015): 2.

13 Robert M. Sapolsky, *Why Zebras Don't Get Ulcers: The Acclaimed Guide to Stress, Stress-Related Diseases, and Coping*, 3rd ed. (New York: Henry Holt 2004), 11.

14 Bruce S. McEwen and J. C. Wingfield, "The Concept of Allostasis in Biology and Biomedicine," *Hormones and Behavior* 43, no. 1 (2003): 2–15.

15 Bruce S. McEwen,"Allostasis and the Epigenetics of Brain and Body Health Over the Life Course: The Brain On Stress," *JAMA Psychiatry* 74, no. 6 (2017).

16 Bruce S. Ewen and Eliot Stellar, "Stress and the Individual: Mechanisms Leading to Disease" *Archives of Internal Medicine* 153, no. 18 (1993): 2093–101, doi:10.1001/archinte.1993.00410180039004.

17 Robert-Paul Juster, "From Stressed Neurons to Resilient Neighborhoods: Discussion with Drs. Lia N. Karatsoreos and Bruce S. McEwen," *Mammoth Magazine* 13, Summer 2013.

18 Daniel J. Siegel, *Mindsight: The New Science of Personal Transformation* (New York: Bantam, 2011).

19 David W. Brown, Robert Anda, Henning Tiemeier, Vincent J. Felitti, Valerie J. Edwards, Janet B. Croft, and Wayne H. Giles, "Adverse Childhood Experiences and the Risk of Premature Mortality," *American Journal of Preventative Medicine* 37, no. 5 (2009): 389–96.

20 Kathy L. Kain and Stephen J. Terrell, *Nurturing Resilience: Helping Clients Move Forward From Developmental Trauma—An Integrative Somatic Approach* (Berkeley, CA: North Atlantic Books, 2018).

21 Peter Levine, *In an Unspoken Voice: How the Body Releases Trauma and Restores Goodness* (Berkeley, CA: North Atlantic Books, 2010).

22 Nityamo Sinclair-Lian, Michael Hollifield, Margaret Menache, Teddy Warner, Jenna Viscaya, Richard Hammerschlag, "Developing a Traditional Chinese Medicine Diagnostic Structure for Post-Traumatic Stress Disorder," *Journal of Alternative and Complementary Medicine* 12, no.

1 (2006): 45–57; and Michael Hollifield, Nityamo Sinclair-Lian, Teddy Warner, Richard Hammerschlag, "Acupuncture for Posttraumatic Stress Disorder: A Randomized Controlled Pilot Trial," *Journal of Nervous and Mental Disease* 195, no. 6 (2007): 504–13.

23 See Hollifield 2011; Charles Engel, Elizabeth H. Cordova, David M. Benedek, Xian Liu, Kristie Gore, Christine Goertz, Michael C. Freed, Cindy C. Crawford, Wayne B. Jonas, Robert J. Ursano, "Randomized Effectiveness Trial of a Brief Course of Acupuncture for Post Traumatic Stress Disorder, *Medical Care* 52, no. 12 (2014), Suppl. 5; and Wayne Jonas, Dawn Bellanti, Charmagne Paat, Alaine Duncan, Ashley Price, Weimin Zhang, Louis M. French, Heechin Chae, "A Randomized Exploratory Study to Evaluate Two Acupuncture Methods for the Treatment of Headaches Associated with Traumatic Brain Injury," *Medical Acupuncture* 28, no. 3 (2016).

24 Courtney Lee, Cindy Crawford, Dawn Wallerstedt, Alexandra York, Alaine Duncan, Jennifer Smith, Meredith Sprengel, Richard Welton, and Wayne B. Jonas, "The Effectiveness of Acupuncture Research Across Components of the Trauma Spectrum Response (TSR): A Systematic Review of Reviews, *Systematic Reviews* 1 (2012): 46.

25 Courtney Lee, Dawn Wallerstedt, Alaine Duncan, Alexandra York, Michael Hollifield, Richard Niemtzow, Stephen Burns and Wayne B. Jonas, "Design and Rationale of a Comparative Effectiveness Study to Evaluate Two Acupuncture Methods for the Treatment of Headaches Associated with Traumatic Brain Injury," *Medical Acupuncture* 23 no, 4 (2011).

26 Laura Krejci, Kennita Carter, and Tracy Gaudet, "Whole Health: The Vision and Implementation of Personalized, Proactive Patient-Driven Health Care for Veterans," *Medical Care* 52, no. 12 (2014): Supplement 5; and Tracy Gaudet, "Turning the Promise of Truly Integrative Medicine into Reality," *Alternative Therapies in Health and Medicine* 14, no. 4 (2008): 66–75.

27 Josephine P. Briggs, "Perspectives on Complementary and Alternative Medicine Research," *Journal of the American Medical Association* 310, no. 7 (2013): 691–92.

28 Wayne B. Jonas, Richard Welton, Roxana Delgado, Sandra Gordon, Weimin Zhang, "CAM in the United States Military: Too Little of a Good Thing?" *Medical Care* 52 (2014): S9–S12.

29 Amanda Hull, Matthew Reinhard, Kelly McCarron, Nathaniel Allen, Michael Corey Jecman, Alaine Duncan, and Karen Soltes, "Acupuncture and Meditation for Military Veterans: First Steps of Quality Management and Future Program Development, *Global Advances in Health and Medicine* 3, no. 4 (2014): 27–31.

30 Bessel van der Kolk, Laura Stone, Jennifer West, Alison Rhodes, David Emerson, Michael Suvak, and Joseph Spinazzolla, "Yoga as an Adjunctive Treatment for Posttraumatic Stress Disorder: A Randomized Controlled Trial," *Clinical Psychiatry* 75, no. 6 (2014): e559–65; and Daniel J. Libby, Felice Reddy, Corey Pilver, and Rani Desi, "The Use of Yoga in Specialized VA PTSD Treatment Programs," *International Journal of Yoga Therapy* 22 (2012): 79–87.

31 Anthony J. Lisi and Cynthia A. Brandt, "Trends in the Use and Characteristics of Chiropractic Services in the Department of Veterans Affairs," *Journal of Manipulative Physiolical Therapeutics* 39, no. 5 (2016): 381–86.

32 F. Zangrando, G. Piccinini, C. Tagliolini, G. Marsilli, M. Iosa, and T. Paolucci, "The Efficacy of a Preparatory Phase of a Touch-Based Approach in Treating Chronic Low Back Pain: A Randomized Controlled Trial," *Journal of Pain Research* 10 (2017): 941–49.

33 Kathryn M. Magruder, Nancy Kassam-Adams, Siri Thoresen, and Miranda Olff, "Prevention and Public Health Approaches to Trauma and Traumatic Stress: A Rationale and a Call to Action," *European Journal of Psychotraumatology* 7 (2016).

34 Vincent J. Felitti, Robert Anda, Dale Nordenberg, David F. Williamson, Alison M. Spitz, Valerie Edwards, Mary P. Koss, and James S. Marks, "Relationship of Childhood Abuse and Household Dysfunction to Many of the Leading Causes of Death in Adults," *American Journal of Preventative Medicine* 14, no. 4 (1998).

35 "Adverse Childhood Experience (ACE) Questionaire," National Council of Juvenile and Family Court Judges, www.ncjfcj.org/sites/default/files/Finding%20Your%20ACE%20Score.pdf.

36 Bruce S. McEwen, Jason Gray, and Carla Nasca, "Recognizing Resilience: Learning from the Effects of Stress on the Brain," *Neurobiology of Stress* 1 (2015), 1–11.

37 Jamie L. Hanson, Amitabh Chandra, Barbara L. Wolfe, and Seth D. Pollak, "Association Between Income and the Hippocampus," *PLoS One* 6 (2011), https://doi.org/10.1371/journal.pone.0018712.

38 Peter J. Gianaros, Jeffrey A. Horenstein, Sheldon Cohen, Karen A. Matthews, Sarah M. Brown, Janine D. Flory, Hugo D. Critchley, Stephen B. Manuck, and Ahmad R. Hariri, "Perigenual Anterior Cingulate Morphology Covaries with Perceived Social Standing," *Social Cognitive and Affective Neuroscience* 2 (2007), 161–73.

39 Peter J. Gianaros, Ahmad Hariri, Lei K. Sheu, Matthew Muldoon, Kim Sutton-Tyrrell, and Stephen B. Manuck, "Preclinical Atherosclerosis Covaries With Individual Differences in Reactivity and Functional Connectivity of the Amygdala," *Biological Psychiatry* 65 (2009): 943–50.

40 Shanta R. Dube, Vincent J. Felitti, Maxia Dong, Daniel P. Chapman, Wayne H. Giles, and Robert F. Anda, "Childhood Abuse, Neglect and Household Dysfunction and the Risk of Illicit Drug Use: The Adverse Childhood Experience Study," *Pediatrics* 111, no. 3 (2003): 564–72.

41 Susan D. Hillis, Robert F. Anda, Vincent J. Felitti, and P. A. Marchbanks. "Adverse Childhood Experiences and Sexual Risk Behaviors in Women: A Retrospective Cohort Study," *Family Planning Perspectives* 33 (2001): 206–11.

42 Charles L. Whitfield, Robert F. Anda, Shanta R. Dube, and Vincent J. Felitti, "Violent Childhood Experiences and the Risk of Intimate Partner Violence in Adults: Assessment in a Large Health Maintenance Organization," *Journal of Interpersonal Violence* 18, no. 2 (2003): 166–85.

43 David F. Williamson, T. J. Thompson, Robert F. Anda, W. H. Dietz, and Vincent J. Felitti. "Body Weight, Obesity, and Self-Reported Abuse in Childhood," *International Journal of Obesity* 26 (2002): 1075–82.

44 Maxia Dong, Wayne H. Giles, Vincent J. Felitti, Shanta R. Dube, J. E. Williams, Daniel P. Chapman, Robert F. Anda, "Insights Into Causal Pathways for Ischemic Heart Disease: Adverse Childhood Experiences Study," *Circulation* 110 (2004): 1761–66.

45 Robert F. Anda, David W. Brown, Shanta R. Dube, J. Douglas Bremner, Vincent J. Felitti, and Wayne H. Giles, "Adverse Childhood Experiences and Chronic Obstructive Pulmonary Disease in Adults," *American Journal of Preventative Medicine* 34, no. 5 (2008): 396–403.

46 Maxia Dong, Robert F. Anda, Shanta R. Dube, Vincent J. Felitti, and Wayne H. Giles, "Adverse Childhood Experiences and Self-Reported Liver Disease: New Insights into a Causal Pathway," *Archives of Internal Medicine* 163 (2003): 1949–56.

47 Shanta R. Dube, DeLisa Fairweather, William S. Pearson, Vincent J. Felitti, Robert F. Anda, and Janet B. Croft, "Cumulative Childhood Stress and Autoimmune Disease," *Psychomatic Medicine* 71 (2009): 243–50.

48 Daniel P. Chapman, Anne G. Wheaton, Robert F. Anda, Janet B. Croft, Valerie J. Edwards, Yong Liu, Stephanie L. Sturgis, and Geraldine S. Perry, "Adverse Childhood Experiences and Sleep Disturbances in Adults," *Sleep Medicine* 12 (2011): 773–79.

49 Daniel P. Chapman, Robert F. Anda, Vincent J. Felitti, Shanta R. Dube, Valerie J. Edwards, and Charles L. Whitfield. "Adverse Childhood Experiences and the Risk of Depressive Disorders in Adulthood, *Journal of Affective Disorders* 82 (2004): 217–25.

50 Shanta R. Dube, Robert F. Anda, Vincent J. Felitti, Daniel P. Chapman, David F. Williamson, and Wayne H. Giles, "Childhood Abuse, Household Dysfunction and the Risk of Attempted Suicide Throughout the Life Span: Findings from Adverse Childhood Experiences Study," *Journal of the American Medical Association* 286 (2001): 3089–96.

51 Heather Larkin, Joseph J. Shields, and Robert F. Anda, "The Health and Social Consequences of Adverse Childhood Experiences (ACE) Across the Lifespan: An Introduction to Prevention and Intervention in the Community," *Journal of Prevention and Intervention in the Community* 40, no. 4 (2012): 263–70.

52 Katie A. Ports, Derek C. Ford, and Melissa T. Merrick, "Adverse Childhood Experiences and Adult Sexual Victimization," *Child Abuse and Neglect* 51 (2016): 313–22.

53 Robert F. Anda, Vincent J. Felitti, Vladimir I. Fleisher, Valerie J. Edwards, Charles L. Whitfield, Shanta R. Dube, and David F. Williamson.

"Childhood Abuse, Household Dysfunction, and Indicators of Impaired Worker Performance," *Permanente Journal* 2004;8(1): 30–38.

54 Kain and Terrell, *Nurturing Resilience.*

55 Laurie Leitch, "Action Steps Using ACEs and Trauma InforMedical Care: A Resilience Model," *Health Justice* 5 (2017): 5; and Carmela DeCandia and Kathleen Guarino, "Trauma-Informed Care: An Ecological Response," *Journal of Child and Youth Care Work* (2015): 7–32.

56 Robert F. Anda, Vincent J. Felitti, J. D. Walker, Charles Whitfield, J. Douglas Bremner, Bruce D. Perry, Shanta R. Dube, and Wayne H. Giles, "The Enduring Effects of Abuse and Related Adverse Experiences in Childhood: A Convergence of Evidence from Neurobiology and Epidemiology," *European Archives of Psychiatry and Clinical Neuroscience* 56, no. 3 (2006): 174–86.

CHAPTER 2

1 Porges, *Polyvagal Theory.*

2 Stephen W. Porges and Senta A. Furman, "The Early Development of the Autonomic Nervous System Provides a Neural Platform for Social Behavior: A Polyvagal Perspective," *Infant and Child Development* 20, no. 1 (2011): 106–18, http://doi.org/10.1002/icd.688.

3 Porges and Furman, 2011.

4 Elizabeth R. Sowell, Bradley Peterson, Paul M. Thompson, and Arthur W. Toga, "Mapping Cortical Change Across the Human Life Span," *Nature Neuroscience* 6, no. 3 (2003): 309–15.

5 Stephen W. Porges, "Love: An Emergent Property of the Mammalian Autonomic Nervous System," *Psychoneuroendochrinology* 23, no. 8 (1998): 837–61.

6 Sebastian Junger, *Tribe: On Homecoming and Belonging* (New York: Hachette Book Group, 2016).

7 Stephen Porges, personal communication, July 23, 2018.

8 Junger, *Tribe.*

9 Karin Roelofs, "Freeze for Action: Neurobiological Mechanisms in Animal and Human Freezing," *Philosophical Transactions of the Royal Society B: Biological Sciences* 372, no. 1718 (2017), http://doi.org/10.1098/rstb.2016.0206.

CHAPTER 3

1 Lao Tzu and Sam Torode, *The Tao te Ching: The Book of the Way,* based on translation by Dwight Goddard. (Nashville, TN: Ancient Renewal, 2013).

2 Angela Hicks, John Hicks, and Peter Mole, *Five Element Constitutional Acupuncture,* 2nd ed. (London: Churchill Livingstone, 2011).

3 Claude Larre and Elisabeth Rochat de la Vallée, *Survey of Traditional Chinese Medicine* (Paris: Institut Ricci and Columbia, MD: Traditional Acupuncture Institute, 1986).

4 Harriet Beinfeld and Efrem Korngold, *Between Heaven and Hearth* (New York: Ballantine Books, 1991), 30.

5 Levine, *An Unspoken Voice,* 2010.

6 Kaptchuk, *Web That Has No Weaver,* 43–46.

7 Giovanni Maciocia, *The Foundations of Chinese Medicine* (London: Churchill Livingston, 1989), 35–38.

8 Maciocia, *Foundations of Chinese Medicine,* 46–47.

9 Wayne B. Jonas, Joan A. G. Walter, Matt Fritts, and Richard C. Niemtzow, "Acupuncture for the Trauma Spectrum Response," *Medical Acupuncture* 23, no. 4 (2011): 249–62.

10 Jonas, Walter, Fritts, and Niemtzow, "Acupuncture for the Trauma Spectrum Response."

11 Michael Hollifield, "Acupuncture for Posttraumatic Stress Disorder: Conceptual, Clinical, and Biological Data Support Further Research," *CNS Neuroscience and Therapeutics* 17 (2011): 769–79.

12 Manfred Porkert, *Theoretical Foundations of Chinese Medicine: Systems of Correspondence,* East Asian Science Series (Boston: MIT Press, 1974).

13 Levine and Frederick, *Waking the Tiger.*

14 John R. Worsley, *Traditional Acupuncture: Vol II Traditional Diagnosis* (London: The College of Traditional Acupuncture, 1990).

15 Hicks, Hicks, and Mole, *Five Element Constitutional Acupuncture.*

16 See appendix two for a list of the organ systems described in the *Huang Di Neijing (Yellow Emperor's Classic of Internal Medicine).* This textbook of internal medicine is 2,500 years old and is oldest known medical text in the world.

17 Hicks, Hicks, and Mole, *Five Element Constitutional Acupuncture.*

18 John Hicks and Angela Hicks, *Healing Your Emotions: Discover Your Element Type and Change Your Life* (London: Thorsons, 1999).

19 Claude Larre and Elisabeth Rochat de la Vallée, The Secret Treatise of the Spiritual Orchid: Neijing Suwen Chapter 8, 2nd ed. (Cambridge: Monkey Press. 1992), 49–57.

20 Ibid, 115–18.

CHAPTER 4

1 Deanne Juhan, *Job's Body: A Handbook for Bodywork,* 2nd ed. (New York: Barrytown/Station Hill Press, 2003).

2 Ruth Feldman, *Maternal Touch and the Developing Infant: The Handbook of Touch,* ed. M. J. Hertenstein and S. J. Weiss (New York: Springer, 2011), 373–407.

3 Allan N. Schore, "Early Interpersonal Neurobiological Assessment of Attachment and Autistic Spectrum Disorders," *Frontiers in Psychology* 5 (2014): 1049, doi:10.3389/fpsyg.2014.01049.

4 Bruce Perry and Maia Szalavitz, *Born for Love: Why Empathy is Essential—and Endangered* (New York, Harper Collins, 2010).

5 K. M. Penza, C. Heim, and C. Nemeroff, "Neurobiological Effects of Childhood Abuse: Implications for the Pathophysiology of Depression and Anxiety" *Archives of Womens Mental Health* 6 (2003): 15–22.

6 Allan N. Schore, "Early Organization of the Nonlinear Right Brain and Development of a Predisposition to Psychiatric Disorders," *Development and Psychopathology* 9, no. 4 (1997): 595–631.

7 Allan N. Schore and Ruth P. Newton, "Using Modern Attachment Theory to Guide Clinical Assessments of Early Attachment Relationships," in *Attachment-Based Clinical Work with Children and Adolescents, Essential Clinical Social Work Series,* ed. J. E. Bettmann and D. Demetri Friedman (New York Springer, 2013).

8 John Bowlby, *Separation, Anxiety and Anger* (New York. Basic Books, 1976).

9 Victoria Latifses, Debra Bendell Estroff, Tiffany Field, and Joseph P. Bush, "Fathers Massaging and Relaxing Their Pregnant Wives Lowered Anxiety and Facilitated Marital Adjustment," *Journal of Bodywork and Movement Therapies* 9, no. 4 (2005): 277–82.

10 Tiffany Field, Nancy Grizzle, Frank Scafidi, Sonya Abrams, Sarah Richardson, Cynthia Kuhn, and Saul Schanberg, "Massage Therapy for Infants of Depressed Mothers," *Infant Behavior and Development* 19 (1996): 107–12.

11 Kate White, ed. *Touch: Attachment and the Body* (London: Karnac Books, 2004).

12 Erik Ceunen, Johan W. S. Vlaeyen, and Ilse Van Diest, "On the Origin of Interoception," *Frontiers in Psychology* 7 (2016): https://doi.org/10.3389/fpsyg.2016.00743.

13 Rollin McCraty and Maria A. Zayas, "Cardiac Coherence, Self-Regulation, Autonomic Stability, and Psychosocial Well-Being," *Frontiers in Psychology* 5 (2014): 1090, http://doi.org/10.3389/fpsyg.2014.01090.

14 Robert Whitehouse and Diane Poole-Heller, "Heart Rate in Trauma: Patterns Found in Somatic Experiencing and Trauma Resolution," *Biofeedback* 36, no. 1 (2008): 24–29.

15 McCraty and Zayas, "Cardiac Coherence."

16 "Resonance," HowStuffWorks, August 25, 2009, https://science.howstuffworks.com/resonance-info.htm.

17 Encyclopaedia Britannica Online, s.v. "Resonance," accessed September 24, 2018, https://www.britannica.com/science/resonance-vibration

18 McCraty and Zayas, "Cardiac Coherence."

19 Richard Lannon, Fari Amini, and Thomas Lewis, *A General Theory of Love* (New York: Random House, 2000).

20 Jack Kornfield, *The Wise Heart: A Guide to the Universal Teachings of Buddhist Psychology* (New York: Bantam Books. 2008), 17.

21 Junger, *Tribe.*

22 Joselyn A. Sze, Anett Gyurak, Joyce W. Yuan, and Robert W. Levenson, "Coherence Between Emotional Experience and Physiology: Does Body Awareness Training Have An Impact?" *Emotion* 10, no. 6 (2010): 803–14. Doi:10.1037/a0020146.

23 Antonio R. Damasio, "Subcortical and Cortial Brain Activity During the Feeling of Self-Generated Emotions," *Nature Neuroscience* 3, no. 10 (2000): 1049–56.

24 Graham Scarr, *Biotensegrity: The Structural Basis of Life* (East Lothian, Scotland, Handspring, 2014).

CHAPTER 5

1 Kain and Terrell, 2018.

2 Jonas, Walter, Fritts, and Niemtzow, "Acupuncture for the Trauma Spectrum Response."

3 James Giordano and Joan A. G. Walter, "Pain and Psychopathology in Military Wounded: How Etiology Epidemiology Sustain an Ethics of Treatment," *Practical Pain Management* 7, no. 6 (2007): 34–42.

4 Ron *Kurtz,* Body-Centered Psychotherapy: The Hakomi Method *(Mendocino, CA: LifeRhythm, 2007).*

5 Eugene T. Gendlin, *Focusing,* 2nd ed. (New York: Bantam Books, 1982).

6 Oliver G. Cameron, "Interoception: The Inside Story—A Model for Psychosomatic Processes," *Psychosomatic Medicine* 63, no. 5 (2001): 697–710.

7 Kathrin Malejko, Birgit Abler, Paul L. Plener, and Joana Straub, "Neural Correlates of Psychotherapeutic Treatment of Post-Traumatic Stress Disorder: A Systematic Literature Review," *Frontiers in Psychiatry* 8 (2017): 85. DOI=10.3389/fpsyt.2017.00085.

8 Martin P. Paulus and Murray B. Stein, "Interoception in Anxiety and Depression," *Brain Structure and Function* 214 (5–6) (2010): 451–63. doi:10.1007/s00429-010-0258-9.

9 Porges, *Polyvagal Theory,* 79.

10 "Direction of Cure," The School of Homeopathy, www.homeopathyschool.com/why-study-with-us/what-is-homeopathy/direction-of-cure.

11 "Hering's Laws of Cure Help Us Understand How Homeopathy Works," Joette Calabrese, Practical Homeopathy, https://joettecalabrese.com/blog/homeopathy/herings-laws-of-cure-help-us-understand-how-homeopathy-works.

12 J. A. Horton, P. R. Clance, C. Sterk-Elifson, and J. Emshoff. "Touch in Psychotherapy: A Survey of Patient's Experiences," *Psychotherapy* 32, no. 3 (1995): 443–57. Doi:10.1037/0033-3204.32.3.443.

13 For a deeper exploration of scope of practice, we suggest you consult Ben E. Benjamin and Cherie Sohnen-Moe, *The Ethics of Touch* (Tucson, AZ: Sohnen-Moe Associates, 2013).

14 Eugene Gendlin, *Focusing* (New York: Bantam Dell, 2007).

15 Ron Kurz, *Body Centered Psychotherapy* (Mendocino, CA: Life Rhythm Books, 1990).

16 Levine, *In an Unspoken Voice.*

17 Pat Ogden, Kekuni Minton, and Clare Pain, *Trauma and the Body: A Sensorimotor Approach to Psychotherapy*, 1st ed. (New York: W. W. Norton, 2006).

18 Francine Shapiro. *Eye Movement Desensitization and Reprocessing (EMDR) Therapy,* 3rd ed. (New York: Guilford Press. 2018).

19 Jonathan E. Sherin and Charles B. Nemeroff, "Post-Traumatic Stress Disorder: The Neurobiological Impact of Psychological Trauma," *Dialogues in Clinical Neuroscience*, 13, no. 3 (2011): 263–78.

20 Shira Segev, Maayan Shorer, Yuri Rassovsky, Tammy Pilowsky Peleg, Alan Apter, and Silvana Fennig, "The Contribution of Posttraumatic Stress Disorder and Mild Traumatic Brain Injury to Persistent Post Concussive Symptoms Following Motor Vehicle Accidents," *Neuropsychology* 7 (2016): 800–810, http://dx.doi.org/10.1037/neu0000299.

CHAPTER 6

1 Descriptions of the nature and function of the Metal Element are drawn from Hicks, Hicks, and Mole, *Five Element Constitutional Acupuncture,* 130–51.

2 Larre and Rochat de la Vallée, *Secret Treatise of the Spiritual Orchid,* 49–57.

3 Hicks and Hicks, *Healing Your Emotions,* 11.

4 Larre and Rochat de la Vallée, *Secret Treatise of the Spiritual Orchid,* 115–18.

5 Karen McCune, personal correspondence and class notes from her study with Nikki Bilton.

6 A. D. Craig, "How Do You Feel? Interoception: The Sense of the Physiological Condition of the Body," *Nature Reviews Neuroscience* 3, no. 8 (2002): 655–66. doi:10.1038/nrn894.

7 Martin P. Paulus and Murray B. Stein, "Interoception in Anxiety and Depression," *Brain Structure and Function* 214, nos. 5–6 (2010): 451–63. doi:10.1007/s00429-010-0258-9.

8 Kathrin Malejko, Birgit Abler, Paul L. Plener, and Joana Straube, "Neural Correlates of Psychotherapeutic Treatment of Post-Traumatic Stress Disorder: A Systematic Literature Review" *Frontiers in Psychiatry* 8 (2017): 85.

9 Porges, *Polyvagal Theory.*

10 Lisa Feldman Barrett and W. Kyle Simmons, "Interoceptive Predictions in the Brain." *Nature Reviews Neuroscience* 16, no. 7 (2015): 419–429. doi:10.1038/nrn3950.

11 A. D. (Bud) Craig, "How Do You Feel—Now? The Anterior Insula and Human Awareness," *Nature Reviews Neuroscience* 10, no. 1 (2009): 59–70.

12 Our acknowledgment and thanks to Peter Levine, the founder of Somatic Experiencing model for trauma resolution for the basis of this exercise. It is routinely taught in his Somatic Experiencing training program.

13 Ofer Zur, "Touch in Therapy and the Standard of Care in Psychotherapy and Counseling: Bringing Clarity to Illusive Relationships," *United States Association of Body Psychotherapists Journal (USABPJ)* 6, no. 2 (2007): 61–93, 84.

14 Susan Standring, *Gray's Anatomy: The Anatomical Basis of Clinical Practice,* 41st ed., (London: Elsevier, 2015).

15 Kain and Terrell, *Nurturing Resilience.*

CHAPTER 7

1 Descriptions of the nature and function of the Water Element are drawn from Hicks, Hicks, and Mole, *Five Element Constitutional Acupuncture,* 152–77.

2 Daniel Keown, *The Spark in the Machine: How the Science of Acupuncture Explains the Mysteries of Western Science*, (London: Singing Dragon, 2014).

3 Maciocia, *Foundations of Chinese Medicine,* 95.

4 Sapolsky, *Why Zebras Don't Get Ulcers.*

5 Van der Kolk, *Body Keeps the Score*, 30.

6 Stan Tatkin. *Wired for Love: How Understanding Your Partner's Brain and Attachment Style Can Help You Defuse Conflict and Build a Secure Relationship* (Oakland, CA: New Harbinger Publications, 2011).

7 Waldemar Iwańczuk, Piotr Guźniczak, "Neurophysiological Foundations of Sleep, Arousal, Awareness and Consciousness Phenomena. Part 1." *Anaesthesiology Intensive Therapy* 47, no. 2 (2015): 162–67. doi:10.5603/AIT.2015.0015.

8 Van der Kolk, *Body Keeps the Score.*

9 National Death Index, CDC, www.cdc.gov/nchs/ndi/index.htm.

10 Adverse Childhood Experiences (ACEs), CDC, www.cdc.gov/violenceprevention/acestudy/index.html.

11 Karr-Morse and Wiley, *Scared Sick.*

12 C. Brudey, J. Park, J. Wiaderkiewicz et al. "Autonomic and Inflammatory Consequences of Posttraumatic Stress Disorder and the Link to Cardiovascular Disease," *American Journal of Physiology: Regulatory, Integrative, and Comparative Physiology* 309, no. 4 (2015): R315–R321; A. O'Donovan, B. Cohen, K. Seal et al. "Elevated Risk for Autoimmune Disorders in Iraq and Afghanistan Veterans with Posttraumatic Stress Disorder," *Biological Psychiatry* 77 (2015): 365–74; and Karr-Morse and Wiley, *Scared Sick.*

13 Ted Kaptchuk. *The Web That Has No Weaver.*

14 Rachel Yehuda, Nikolaos P. Daskalakis, Linda M. Bierer, Heather N. Bader, Torsten Klengel, Florian Holsboer, and Elisabeth B. Binder, "Holocaust Exposure Induced Intergenerational Effects on FKBP5 Methylation," *Biological Psychiatry* 80 (2016): 372–80.

15 Rachel Yehuda, and L. M. Bierer, "Transgenerational Transmission of Coritsol and PTSD Risk," *Progress in Brain Research* 167 (2007): 121–35.

16 Laura C. Schulz, "The Dutch Hunger Winter and the Developmental Origins of Health and Disease," *Proceedings of the National Academy of Science* 107, no. 39 (2010): 16757–58.

17 Natan P. F. Kellerman, "Epigenetic Transmission of Holocaust Trauma: Can Nightmares Be Inherited?" *The Israel Journal of Psychiatry and Related Sciences* 50, no. 1 (2013). AMCHA, the National Israeli Center for Psychosocial Support of Survivors of the Holocaust and the Second Generation, Jerusalem, Israel; and Bruce Perry, "Childhood Experience and the Expression of Genetic Potential: What Childhood Neglect Tells Us about Nature and Nurture," *Brain and Mind* 3 (2002): 79–100.

18 Carey B. Maslow, Kimberly Caramanica, Jie Hui Li, Steven D. Stellman, and Robert M. Brackbill, "Reproductive Outcomes Following Maternal

Exposure to the Events of September 11, 2001, at the World Trade Center, in New York City," *American Journal of Public Health* 106, no. 10 (2016): 1796–803, doi: 10.2105/AJPH.2016.303303.

19 Christopher Kuzawa and Elizabeth Sweet, "Epigenetics and the Embodiment of Race: Developmental Origins of US Racial Disparities in Cardiovascular Health," *American Journal of Human Biology* 21, no. 1 (2009): 2–15.

20 Teresa Brockie, Morgan Heinzelmann, and Jessica Gill, "A Framework to Examine the Role of Epigenetics in Health Disparities among Native Americans," *Nursing Research and Practice* 2013 (2013), Article ID 410395.

21 Yehuda, Daskalakis, Bierer, Bader, Klengel, Holsboer, and Binder, "Holocaust Exposure."

22 Kellerman, "Epigenetic Transmission of Holocaust Trauma."

CHAPTER 8

1 Heather Dorst, personal correspondence and class notes from her study with Julia Measures.

2 Claude Larre and Elizabeth Rochat de la Vallee, *The Liver,* 2nd ed. (Cambridge: Monkey Press, 1999).

3 Descriptions of the nature and function of the Wood Element are drawn from Hicks, Hicks, and Mole, *Five Element Constitutional Acupuncture,* 53–77.

4 Larre and Rochat de la Vallée, Secret Treatise of the Spiritual Orchid, 53.

5 Larre and Rochat de la Vallée, *The Liver,* 8.

6 Claude Larre and Elisabeth Rochat de la Vallée, *Essence, Spirit, Blood and Qi,* (Cambridge: Monkey Press, 1999).

7 "How to "Read" a Skull: Eye Placement and Size," Skeleton Museum, www.museumofosteology.org/museum-education/3/How-to-quotReadquot-a-Skull-Eye-Placement-and-Size.htm.

CHAPTER 9

1 Descriptions of the nature and function of the Fire Element are drawn from Hicks, Hicks, and Mole, *Five Element Constitutional Acupuncture,* 78–104.

2 Larre and Rochat de la Vallée, *Secret Treatise of the Spiritual Orchid,* 33.
3 Rollin McCraty, Mike Atkinson, Dana Tomasino, and Raymond Trevor Bradley, *The Coherent Heart*, HeartMath Institute. 2006.
4 McCraty and Zayas, "Cardiac Coherence."
5 Larre and Rochat de la Vallée, *Secret Treatise of the Spiritual Orchid,* 34.
6 Larre and Rochat de la Vallée, *Secret Treatise of the Spiritual Orchid,* 90–108.
7 Keown, *Spark in the Machine.*
8 Larre and Rochat de la Vallée, *Secret Treatise of the Spiritual Orchid,* 142–45.
9 Larre and Rochat de la Vallée, *Survey of Traditional Chinese Medicine,* 209.
10 Hicks, Hicks, and Mole, *Five Element Constitutional Acupuncture.*
11 Junger, *Tribe.*
12 Descriptions of the symptoms of dysregulation in the Fire Element are drawn from Hicks, Hicks, and Mole, *Five Element Constitutional Acupuncture*, 78–104.
13 Porges, *Polyvagal Theory.*
14 Bryanna Hahn Fox, Nicholas Perez, Elizabeth Cass, Michael T. Baglivio, and Nathan Epps, "Trauma Changes Everything: Examining the Relationship between Adverse Childhood Experiences and Serious, Violent and Chronic Juvenile Offenders," *Child Abuse and Neglect* 46 (2015): 163–73.
15 Naomi N. Duke, Sandra L. Pettingell, Barbara J. McMorris, and Iris W. Borowsky, "Adolescent Violence Perpetration: Associations with Multiple Types of Adverse Childhood Experiences," *Pediatrics* 125, no. 4 (2010): e778–86.
16 James A. Reavis, Jan Looman, Kristina Franco, and Briana Rojas, "Adverse Childhood Experiences and Adult Criminality: How Long Must We Live Before We Possess Our Own Lives?" *The Permanente Journal* 17, no. 2 (Spring 2013).

CHAPTER 10

1 Descriptions of the nature and function of the Earth Element are drawn from Hicks, Hicks, and Mole, *Five Element Constitutional Acupuncture,* 105–28.

2 Maciocia, *Foundations of Chinese Medicine,* 69.

3 Keown, *Spark in the Machine,* 247.

4 P. E. Watson, I. D. Watson, and R. D. Batt, "Total Body Water Volumes for Adult Males and Females Estimated from Simple Anthropometric Measurements," *The American Journal of Clinical Nutrition* 33, no. 1 (1980): 27–39, https://doi.org/10.1093/ajcn/33.1.27.

5 Maciocia, *Foundations of Chinese Medicine.*

6 Maciocia, *Foundations of Chinese Medicine,* 227–28.

7 Alper Evrensel and Mehmet Emin Ceylan, "The Gut-Brain Axis: The Missing Link in Depression," *Clinical Psychopharmacology and Neuroscience* 13, no. 3 (2015): 239–44.

8 Emeran A. Mayer, Rob Knight, Sarkis K. Mazmanian, John F. Cryan, Kirsten Tillisch, "Gut Microbes and the Brain: Paradigm Shift in Neuroscience," *Jounal of Neuroscience* 34, no. 46 (2014): 15490–96.

9 A. Naseribafrouei, K. Hestad K, E. Avershina, M. Sekelja, A. Linløkken R. Wilson, K. Rudi, "Correlation Between the Human Fecal Microbiota and Depression," *Neurogastroenterology and Motility* 26 (2014): 1155–62.

10 Jane A. Foster and Karen Anne McVey Neufeld, "Gut-Brain Axis: How the Microbiome Influences Anxiety and Depression," *Trends in Neurosciences* 36 (2013): 305–12.

11 Stellenbosch University, "Role of Gut Microbiome in Posttraumatic Stress Disorder: More Than a Gut Feeling," *Science Daily,* www.sciencedaily.com/releases/2017/10/171025103140.htm.

12 M. Maes, M. Kubera, J. C. Leunis, "The Gut-Brain Barrier in Major Depression: Intestinal Mucosal Dysfunction with an Increased Translocation of LPS from Gram Negative Enterobacteria (Leaky Gut) Plays a Role in the Inflammatory Pathophysiology of Depression," *Neuroendocrinology Letters* 29, no. 1 (2008).

13 Marilia Carabotti, Annunziata Scirocco, Maria Antonietta Maselli, Carola Severi, "The Gut-Brain Axis: Interactions Between Enteric Microbiota, Central and Enteric Nervous Systems," *Annals of Gastroenterology : Quarterly Publication of the Hellenic Society of Gastroenterology* 28, no. 2 (2015): 203–9.

14 "What Is Moral Injury," The Moral Injury Project, Syracuse University, http://moralinjuryproject.syr.edu/about-moral-injury.

15 Liz Koch, *The Psoas Book: A Comprehensive Guide to the Iliopsoas Muscle and Its Profound Influence on the Body, Mind and Emotions*, 30th anniversary edition (Lawrence, KS: Guinea Pig Publications, 2012).

16 Adverse Childhood Experiences (ACEs), CDC, www.cdc.gov/violenceprevention/acestudy/index.html.

17 Trauma Center at Justice Resource Institute, www.traumacenter.org/clients/clients_landing.php.

APPENDIX 2

1 Larre and Rochat de la Vallée, Secret Treatise of the Spiritual Orchid, 151–52. This list of officials is a translation of the *Huang Di Neijing (Yellow Emperor's Classic of Internal Medicine)*. It is approximately 2,500 years old and is the oldest known textbook of internal medicine.

INDEX

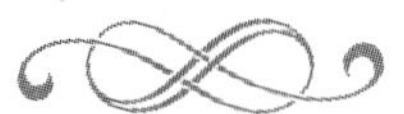

B

C

D

E

F

G

H

I

J

K

L

P

Q

R

S

T

V

W

Y

Z

ABOUT THE AUTHORS

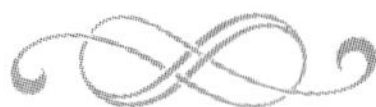

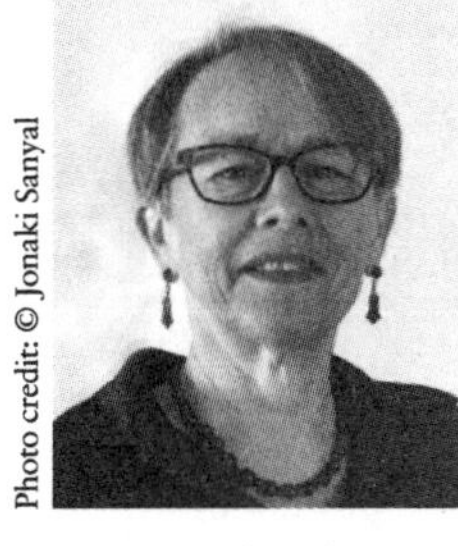

Photo credit: © Jonaki Sanyal

ALAINE DUNCAN, MAC, LAC, integrates the wisdom of Acupuncture and Asian Medicine with the study of neurobiology and traumatic stress in the classroom and her treatment room. She served as founding director of Crossings Healing and Wellness and is a charter member of the Integrative Health and Wellness program at the DC Veterans Administration, an adjunct faculty member at Maryland University of Integrative Health, and founder of the National Capitol Area Chapter of Acupuncturists Without Borders. Her research background includes studies assessing integrative medicine for compassion fatigue in military caregivers and the use of acupuncture for treating Gulf War Veterans Illness as well as combat-related traumatic stress, chronic pain, and chronic headaches. Duncan lives in Hyattsville, Maryland.

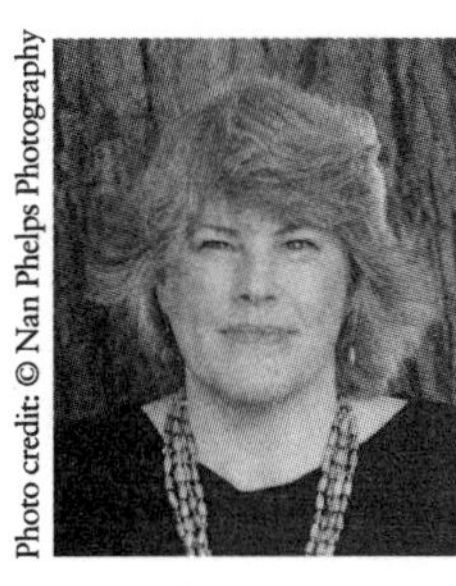

Photo credit: © Nan Phelps Photography

KATHY L. KAIN, PHD, has been practicing and teaching bodywork and trauma recovery for thirty-seven years. A senior trainer in the Somatic Experiencing trauma resolution model, she is an expert in integrating touch into the practice of psychotherapy and trauma recovery, as well as in somatic approaches to working with developmental and complex trauma. Kain teaches therapists how to incorporate touch into their practices through her popular program "Touch Skills Training for Trauma Therapists," as well as in the "Somatic Resilience and Regulation" program she co-teaches with Stephen Terrell. She is the coauthor of *Nurturing Resilience: Helping Clients Move Forward from Developmental Trauma* and the principal author of *Ortho-Bionomy: A Practical Manual.* She lives in Portland, Oregon.

About North Atlantic Books

North Atlantic Books (NAB) is a 501(c)(3) nonprofit publisher committed to a bold exploration of the relationships between mind, body, spirit, culture, and nature. Founded in 1974, NAB aims to nurture a holistic view of the arts, sciences, humanities, and healing. To make a donation or to learn more about our books, authors, events, and newsletter, please visit www.northatlanticbooks.com.